Early Modern Literature in History

Within the period 1520–1740, this large, very well-established series with notable international representation discusses many kinds of writing, both within and outside the established canon. The volumes may employ different theoretical perspectives, but they share an historical awareness and an interest in seeing their texts in lively negotiation with their own and successive cultures. This series is approaching a hundred titles on a variety of subjects including early modern women's writing; domestic politics; drama, performance and playhouses; rhetoric; religious conversion; translation; travel and colonial writing; popular culture; the law; authorship; diplomacy; the court; material culture; childhood; piracy; and the environment.

More information about this series at
http://www.palgrave.com/gp/series/14199

Sophie Chiari · Samuel Cuisinier-Delorme
Editors

Spa Culture and Literature in England, 1500–1800

palgrave
macmillan

Editors
Sophie Chiari
Clermont-Ferrand, France

Samuel Cuisinier-Delorme
Vichy, France

ISSN 2634-5919 ISSN 2634-5927 (electronic)
Early Modern Literature in History
ISBN 978-3-030-66567-8 ISBN 978-3-030-66568-5 (eBook)
https://doi.org/10.1007/978-3-030-66568-5

Cover credit: Gibon Art/Alamy Stock Photo

This Palgrave Macmillan imprint is published by the registered company Springer Nature Switzerland AG
The registered company address is: Gewerbestrasse 11, 6330 Cham, Switzerland

Acknowledgements

This book finds its origins in an international conference on the 'Great Spas of Europe', a group of eleven spa towns nominated to UNESCO for inscription on the World Heritage List. This event took place in Vichy, one of the eleven towns concerned, in October 2019.

We are both grateful to our research team, IHRIM ('Institut d'Histoire des Représentations et des Idées dans les Modernités'), for its generous support without which our symposium could not have taken place. We would also like to thank the mayor and municipal staff of the city of Vichy—we acknowledge, in particular, our indebtedness to Yves-Jean Bignon—as well as the staff of 'Vichy Communauté' and the 'Pôle Universitaire de Vichy' for their help and wonderful hospitality.

This edited collection is also the product of several helpful conversations with the authors who contributed a piece to this volume. We would like to thank them for their patience, insights and encouragements. Needless to say, we are also grateful to the anonymous readers whose expertise and invaluable feedback have allowed us to improve the contents of the present book.

Our most sincere thanks go to Eileen Srebernik, our editor at Palgrave Macmillan, whose precious guidance and personal commitment have been crucial to the completion of this volume, as well as to Shreenidhi Natarajan and Jack Heeney, who also took care of the project coordination.

Finally, and above all, we would like to extend our gratitude to those among our families and friends whose love and confidence have helped to sustain us.

Introduction

[...] [T]he bath for my help lies
Where Cupid got new fire: my mistress's eyes.

(Shakespeare, Sonnet 153, l. 13–14)

Hoping to restore his health in a bubbling bath presumably healing 'strange maladies' (l. 8), the poet of Shakespeare's *Sonnets* soon realizes that the only cure for his diseased self turns out to be his mistress's eyes: love's fire is not easily quenched.[1] Capturing the rich ambivalence of spring waters, our collection examines the emerging and complex relationship between English spa culture and literature and its societal, spiritual, humoral, medicinal, as well as deep historical contexts, since it is articulated in a range of literary texts, movements, and expressions all over the sixteenth, seventeenth, and eighteenth centuries.

'Spa' is thus the key notion examined in the following pages. If the definition of the word is relatively simple—the *OED* defines it, in its general usage, as '[a] medicinal or mineral spring or well' (2.a)'—its origins seem to be more uncertain. The term possibly 'derives from the Walloon French *espa*, 'waterfountain', of which the most famous example was the thermal well at Spa (Belgium)' (Kelly 2008–2009, 99). Yet, as James Kelly acknowledges, 'the word has also been given a Latin etymology, which points to the fact that the therapeutic benefits of mineral water

[1] On sonnet 153, see also Richard Kerridge's Coda in this volume.

were recognized long before the identification of Spa in the fourteenth century'.

For all its apparent simplicity, the definition given above is somewhat perplexing when applied to early modern resorts. Indeed, the *OED* assumes that spas, or 'spaws', were not seen as medicinal springs or wells before 1626.[2] Yet, sixteenth-century literature already mentions them and several treatises of the period duly insist on the manifold functions of these English resorts, which were both spiritual and therapeutic places.

Balneology: A Very Brief History

As stated above, *Spa Culture and Literature in England, 1500–1800* aims at highlighting the various uses of water in sixteenth-, seventeenth- and eighteenth-century England, while exploring the tensions between those people who praised the curative virtues of waters and those who rejected them for their supposedly harmful effects.

These tensions cannot be correctly grasped without a basic knowledge of the history of curative waters, which is in fact a complex one. If bathing was considered as hygienic and, therefore, necessary in the Greek and Roman cultures, James Kelly reminds us that 'balneotherapy fell into disfavour following the Christianisation of Europe and the decline of the Roman Empire because of the association of bathing with bodily indulgence and immorality, and the identification of prayer and personal self-denial as the true sources of wellbeing' (Kelly 2008–2009, 99). Then, during the Middle Ages, steam baths, whose purpose was more recreational than regenerative, flourished in many Christian cities. Yet the bad reputation of 'stews', i.e. dry or moist heated baths, was rapidly re-established: over time they were increasingly regarded as places that facilitated prostitution and promiscuity. After his ascension to the throne, King Henry VIII came to regard public baths as places of debauchery in which infections and contaminations easily spread. When he himself developed syphilis, he ordered the closing down of baths. As a result, in the Tudor era, they became synonymous with forbidden practices. No wonder that, in Shakespeare's *Measure for Measure*, Duke Vincentio describes

[2] The first example given is taken from Deane's *Spadacrene Anglica. Or, The English spaw-fovntaine*: '1626 E. Deane *Spadacrene Anglica* 9: Doctor Timothy Bright [...] first gave the name of the *English Spaw* vnto this Fountaine about thirty yeares since, or more' (*OED*, 2.a).

how corruption will 'boil and bubble / Till it o'errun the stew' (Shakespeare 2016, 2264; 5.1.307), 'stew' being synonymous with 'brothel' in such a context. Turkish baths, famed for their exoticism, were also seen as privileged places for 'illicit sexuality' (Stanivukovic 2007, 68) and, in particular, for female eroticism and, as is suggested in Thomas Washington's translation of *The nauigations, peregrinations and voyages, made into Turkie by Nicholas Nicholay Daulphinois, Lord of Arfeuile, chamberlaine and geographer ordinarie to the King of Fraunce* (1585).

The early modern period marked a decisive shift in spa activities. So far, healing waters had been regarded differently according to faith: Catholics understood them ritualistically and superstitiously, Protestants pragmatically. Towards the end of the sixteenth century, however, the various treatises published on the issue of spas no longer systematically described water as a sacred or sacramental element, examining instead its curative properties. Dr William Turner, a pioneer of spamedicine in England, drafted the first English-language treatise on hot springs, namely *A Book of the natures and properties of the baths in England and other baths in Germany and Italy*. Published in 1562, the volume recorded the healing properties of spawaters for nearly a hundred diseases, compared Bath with spa towns on the continent, and pleaded for improvements to be undertaken in the English city. As part of the 'generall rules to be obserued of all them that will entre into anye bath or drinke the water of anye bath', Turner made clear that 'no man' should 'enter into any bath before his bodye be purged [...] [f]or if any man go on prepared and unpurged to the bath, he maye fortune neuer come home agayne or if he come home, he commeth home most commonly with a worse disease then he brought to the bath with him' (Turner 1562, 15).

A few decades later, in 1626, Elizabeth Farrow discovered a spring in Scarborough. The publication in 1660 of *Scarbrough Spaw, or, A description of the nature and vertues of the spaw at Scarbrough in Yorkshire*, by Dr Robert Wittie, made Scarborough one of the most important spa resorts of the time. Wittie's observations were extended in the second edition of the book (*Scarbrough–Spaw: or a description of the nature and vertues of the spaw at Scarbrough Yorkshire*, 1667)[3] in which he provided a description of the benefits of water on nerves and lungs as well as on mental

[3] The book was then translated into Latin under the title *Fons scarburgensis*, published in 1678.

health. According to him, water restores the balance of the humours and can even cure 'Hypochondriack Melancholy, suppressing the vapours which fly up to the head, and cheering the heart' (Wittie 1667, 182). While Bath, Bristol, and Harrogate were recognized as established spa towns, Scarborough's reputation soared when spa treatments developed there and when seawaterbaths were introduced in addition to springwater ones.

Illustrious physicians, in the meantime, kept publishing treatises promoting the therapeutic dimension of spas. Robert Pierce was one of them. He settled in Bath in 1653, and 44 years later, in 1697, he published his *Bath Memoirs,* in which he asserted the exceptional properties of mineral waters and foregrounded their curative quality. Bathing and drinking the waters proved especially beneficial to infertile women desiring to bear children, he explained. He mentioned, for example, the case of 'My Lord *Blessington*'s Lady, Daughter to the Countess of *Montwroth*, from the Kingdom of *Ireland*, a very weakly and sickly Person, having been some Years marry'd, and never had a Child' came to Bath 'for Health, as well as for Children'. As a result, Pierce noticed, 'she not only recover'd a better State of Health, but afterwads [sic] became a Mother of Children' (Pierce 1697, 197). Towards the very end of the century, in 1699, Benjamin Allen wrote a medical treatise dedicated to the health benefits of spas called *The natural history of the chalybeat and purging waters of England with their particular essays and uses*. He notably insisted on the necessity of drinking the waters, and not just of bathing in them, to recover from physical troubles: 'The Repetition of drinkingPurgingWaters three or four times, sufficiently answers the general Design of washing the Body, though the more stubborn disorders of some Bodies, make a longer use of them necessary' (Allen 1699, 176).

In the seventeenth century, spa activities kept pace with changes in social mores. Many people began to fear that hot water could infuse their bodies with dangerous humours. As a result, they turned, domestically, to waterless grooming achieved by rubbing or wiping the skin. The habit of bathing only became general relatively late, when public baths reopened in London at the end of the century, and bathing came back into fashion as a medical resource only in the mid-1750s. Coldwater was then favoured since it was believed to be invigorating and to regulate blood circulation.

Actually, the many attractions of spa resorts, including relaxation, music, and congenial company, soon became even more important than the curative properties of the waters. As a result, beyond its medical dimension, the social and cultural life of spa towns, frequently described in the literary productions of the early modern period, needs examination. At the beginning of the eighteenth century, Bath had become a fashionable holiday destination for the English aristocracy and the upper middle classes. Queen Anne's visit in 1702 and the arrival there of Richard 'Beau' Nash in 1704 turned Bath into the most elegant resort in Georgian England. Not only did people go to Bath for spa treatments, but also for entertainment: concerts, dances, card games and gambling thrived in this curative city. The eighteenth century marked both the absolute climax and the slow decline of spa waters. Indeed, as observed by Alain Corbin, 'cure takers began rushing toward the seashore around 1750' (Corbin 1994, 57): new places of wellness and entertainment emerged in the second half of the century, and more and more seasonal resorts were now to be found near the coasts. Ronald W. Cooley thus rightly comments on 'a shift in fashion from inland to coastal spas, and from drinkingmineral water to sea bathing as a form of hydropathy' (Cooley 2015, 111). Spa towns had to reinvent themselves and some of them, such as Tunbridge Wells, became permanent places of residence rather than occasional locations for times of leisure.

The State of the Art

We have just seen that water has been used for recreational or therapeutic purposes, shaping landscapes, cleansing bodies and spirits alike throughout the centuries. While balneology has frequently been studied in connection with classical Antiquity or with more recent times (in particular the nineteenth century, often seen as the Golden Age of spa activities), much work remains to be done regarding its significance in the early modern period.

It is true that, capitalizing on the renewed interest in watering places all over Europe,[4] a number of books have recently been published on early

[4] 'Great Spas of Europe', for example, 'is a group of eleven spa towns across seven countries that has been nominated to UNESCO for inscription on the World Heritage List as a transnational serial 'property''. URL: https://greatspasofeurope.org (accessed September 12, 2020).

modern spa literature and on the changing attitudes to mineral water.[5] Most of them, however, highlight the fashion of watering places in the eighteenth century, and they are often related to the history of medicine. By contrast, we intend to reconsider spa culture and literature over a broader period which encompasses three centuries, from the sixteenth to the eighteenth century, and we aim at emphasizing a variety of overlapping aspects (literary analysis, anthropology, social history) too often neglected in spa literature. We thus intend to lay the groundwork for filling the gaps in the existing criticism related to early modern spa culture and to arouse new interest in the field. Taking stock of current research on the various existing interconnections between literature, culture, baths, and hydrotherapy in early modern England, this collection of essays sheds fresh light on the activities and daily life in spa towns at the time.

As a result, it delineates new approaches and takes baths and spa culture as vectors of aesthetic, sociological and scientific concerns that articulate new kinds of connections between leisure, arts and science from Edmund Spenser to Jane Austen. Doing so, it proposes nuanced answers to a number of questions. Were English curative venues elite locations only? Were these locations gendered? Was bathing considered more as a medical or as a leisure activity? Can we truly say that taking the waters in towns like Bath, Tunbridge Wells, Harrogate, as well as Hampstead and Islington in London, only became fashionable in the eighteenth century and mainly corresponded to an emerging travel industry?

It seems that the ideals of the hierarchy of fashion so often foregrounded by scholars specializing in eighteenth-century studies had not always been so deeply inscribed in spa culture. In sixteenth-century England for example, water cures chiefly became the object of medical interest. So far, they had mainly been regarded as religious sites and were frequently endowed with papist connotations, which should come as no surprise. Indeed, as noted by Barbara M. Benedict, '[s]pas have always offered a mixture of religious and physical cure: Roman, Medieval, and Renaissancesprings attracted pilgrims for both practical and spiritual reasons' (Benedict 1995, 203). Nevertheless, in Shakespeare's time, a growing number of medical guides started to focus especially on the English baths whose virtues were extolled. One primarily came there to

[5] See for example Borsay (Anne) 1999; Borsay (Peter) 2000; Cossic-Péricarpin and Galliou 2006; Eglin 2005; Hembry 1990; Jennings 2006; Large 2015.

improve one's health. Gradually, the scientific aspect of these watering-places became compatible with religious thinking. This is corroborated, for example, by Dr Walter Baily's *Brief Discours of certaine Bathes or Mineral Waters in […] Newenam Regis*, published in 1582, and republished five years later under a slightly different title, in which 'mineral' was aptly replaced by 'medicinal'.[6] Baily writes in his Introduction that

> […] it is not altogither a vaine coniecture, to thinke that God in these daies miraculously reuealed wels and springs of medicinall waers neuer knowen before, to worke effects strange and maruellous in our sights, thereby to induce all men to forsake such puddle pits which mans deuise hath digged, and drinke onely of the cleere fountains of his word, thence onely to fetch remedy for our diseased soules. The bathes of Bathe and Buckstan for their antiquitie and long proofe in times past, are of great fame, and no doubt as of more efficacie than others, may iustly most be accounted of […]. (Baily 1587, n.p.)

Phyllis Hembry makes clear that '[t]he particular interest of the *Discours* lies in the argument of the introduction, linking the new role of medicinal waters with Anglican theology, and it places Baily foremost among those employed to promote the English baths' (Hembry 1990, 16). By the end of the seventeenth century, '[o]wing to the poor health of his wife', the clergyman Anthony Walker 'became a regular visitor to Tunbridge Wells, where he appears to have occasionally preached' (Smith 2008, n.p.). In his sermons at the spa resort, he hoped 'that [the waters] may occasion neither Sin nor Sickness, nor any Inconvenience to us: but prove useful and beneficial to us, for the continuance, restauration, and confirmation of Health to our frail Bodies' (Walker 1685, 142).

At that time, springspas had already become sites of high sociability in Britain. These sites did not only appeal to men in quest of fresh air and new professional networks, but also to women—and, in particular, elite women. Peter Borsay observes that 'one of the most striking characteristics of resorts was the female profile of their population' and mentions, as a result, a 'social system […] more than usually geared to [women's] needs and aspirations' (Borsay 2000, 795–96). As shown by Amanda

[6] See Walter Baily, *A briefe discours of certain bathes or medicinall waters in the Countie of Warwicke neere vnto a village called Newnam Regis*, London, 1587, STC (2nd ed.) / 1191.

E. Herbert, 'while vacationing at health towns, women used their elite educations to help facilitate female sociability; they exercised their feminine knowledge of medical care, cookery and artistic expression discursively, joining with other women in these activities to create or deepen female social alliances' (Herbert 2009, 362). It must be said, however, that '[c]ure remained the moral justification for the pursuit of pleasure' (Benedict 1995, 209) and that spa literature, in the eighteenth century, generally 'present[ed] spas as a social environment that would cure their visitors' urban ills' (Benedict 1995, 209). Be that as it may, individuals could thus (re)fashion their identities while sojourning in spa towns, and this volume interrogates the multiple processes of self-fashioning which were then made possible by the British watering places.

A Survey of the Volume

The present collection of essays is divided into three different parts which explore, in turn, baths from an aesthetic, recreational, and medical perspective—three dimensions which are ultimately shown to overlap. Therefore, throughout the volume as a whole, we have tried to promote a coherent, yet varied approach, as the thirteen chapters all discuss plays, poems and novels condemning or deriding baths, or essays and treatises that either praise or criticize the curative use of water.

In a first part entitled 'Generic Explorations: Baths and Waters in Poetry, Drama and Prose', Alix Desnain addresses the issues of baths in Spenser's *The Faerie Queene* (1590), where images of water, and particularly of baths, are recurrent. Desnain shows that baths, in *The Faerie Queene*, often simultaneously weaken and strengthen the individual. Interestingly, to these baths are sometimes added flowers and herbs, some associated with lust and syphilis, while others suggest love and virginity. Desnain then turns to another type of contrast present in the poem, since Spenser'sbaths both conceal and reveal, as the account of Duessa bathing in Book I makes clear. This finally leads the author to study bathing in correlation with metamorphosis and, in particular, with the female body. The poem's bathing scenes are indeed often tinged with eroticism, and the combination of concealing and revealing tropes is reminiscent of the allure and threat of Spenser's female creatures. It is significant that, while the voyeuristic tropes used by the poet make the reader and the male protagonist part of the scene he describes, they are nonetheless kept on the margins, as outsiders looking in.

The second chapter, by François Laroque, is devoted to waters and baths in one of Spenser's most eminent literary heirs, namely John Webster. *The Duchess of Malfi* (1614), he explains, is a play fraught with allusions to ponds and fountains and which culminate in a general blood-bath at the end. In an intriguing historical parallel, Laroque reminds us that Countess Elizabeth Bathory of Hungary was arrested in her castle in 1610 owing to the bloodbaths she took after a series of mass killings of servants and young girls in the hope of rejuvenating her skin. Through its recurrent imagery, Webster's tragedy also evokes some hospital riddled with infectious diseases. In the play, Laroque contends, the many water images suggest the idea of purgation and purification while ultimately showing that, in a world where evil and irrational passion run so deep, such a cure is impossible to achieve. Indeed, the tragedy sadly exposes the insidious work of poisoned words and polluted waters that reverse the beneficent action of holy, or simply purgative, waters. Cariola's idea of 'a progress to the baths / At Lucca' or of a visit to 'the Spa / In Germany' (3.2.301–303) temporarily creates the fantasy of female companionship and evokes the tradition of women's bath in Turkey as described by Nicolas de Nicolay's *Peregrinations and voyages...into Turquie* (1585).

The next chapter discusses a highly self-conscious prose romance first published in 1621. Tiffany Jo Werth dwells on Lady Mary Wroth's *The Countess of Montgomery's Urania*, whose characters engage in a variety of hydrotherapeutic cures to erase or enflame love's afflictions. Even the 'sage' Melissa, the story's enchantress and revered source of counsel, operates what appears to be a kind of spa on the island of Delos. Werth's chapter examines three specific episodes in which water cures recur as a motif with various forms of hydrotherapy administered throughout *Urania*. It explores how the newly revived interest in the healing properties of mineral waters in late sixteenth-century England infiltrates the imaginative landscape of romance. What do these episodes reveal—and foretell—about changing social attitudes towards the wonder of the natural world? How might these imagined cures facilitate later theories that ministered healing water for both physical and mental health?

In Chapter 4, Anne Rouhette pays special attention to the third and last volume of *Evelina* (published in three volumes in 1778), in which Frances Burney has her heroine go to Bristol Hotwells 'for the recovery of [her] health' and visit briefly '[t]he charming city of Bath'. This plan is so successful that, in the process, Evelina also recovers her name and her father and acquires a husband, a brother and a sister of sorts in the most lavish happy ending of all of Burney's novels. However, while short vignettes of fashionable places or touristic spots abound in the novel, Rouhette observes that neither the Hotwells nor the city of Bristol receive any kind of description, and Evelina never actually leaves what was supposed to be a temporary place of residence. After examining the 'permanent transience' of Evelina's stay at Bristol, she focuses on the surprising vagueness of the setting to bring out its literary dimension, highlighting parallels with and differences from Smollett's *Humphry Clinker* (1772) and Anstey's *The New Bath Guide*, discussed in the eighth chapter.

Marie-Laure Massei-Chamayou follows up on Rouhette's chapter with an analysis of Bath in Jane Austen's *Northanger Abbey* and *Persuasion*, both published in 1817. While the choice of Bath in *Northanger Abbey* is linked to Austen's literary project to parody generic conventions and experiment with fiction, *Persuasion* is a novel that conveys a more complex decor: even though Bath appears as a site of ironic dislocation, synonymous with alienation and social competition, its urban space nonetheless enables the blissful reunion of Anne Elliot and Captain Wentworth. The two texts, however, explore the interdependent economies of health, sickness, marriage and gossip to uncover what actually lies beneath the genteel surface of harmonious architecture, polite manners and civilized conventions.

The second part of the volume, 'Taking the Waters: Myth, Recreation and Satire', promotes a slightly different approach to springs and baths by questioning the history and practice of balneology. Tiffany Stern starts with a two-part reassessment of an omnipresent, yet rarely studied myth, that of King Bladud in connection with the city of Bath. Part one tells the intriguing tale of Bladud, as first related by Monmouth in the eleventh century, up until now, showing the changes and permutations it underwent over time. Part two tells the story of Bath over the same period, revealing how Bladud's founding myth was reconceived whenever beliefs about the hot water changed. Both parts consider what unfixed foundation mythology reveals about its spa city. To what extent has Bladud's story shaped Bath and its baths, and to what extent has Bath and its baths shaped what is, in more than one sense, the fluid tale of Bladud?

Amanda E. Herbert then supplies a detailed exploration of the seventeenth-century transformations of the British spa. Drawing upon travel guides, government documents, private correspondence and medical case-books from spa cities, she examines the various ways in which early modern Britons used bodies of water—specifically, the supposedly miraculous waters of medical springs in cities such as Bath, Tunbridge Wells, and Epsom—to refigure and reimagine themselves. Early modern Europeans firmly believed in the curative powers of mineral waters, and at these sites, Herbert shows that many different kinds of people sought relief from disease and injury: women, men, and children; poor as well as rich; people from Britain and abroad. By drinking British springwater, pumping it over their bodies, and plunging into mineral pools to swim, these health-seekers attempted to change themselves for the better.

The next chapter by Shaun Regan examines Christopher Anstey's *The New Bath Guide* and the resort satires that it inspired. The literary sensation of 1766, Anstey's poem was praised by contemporary readers and frequently imitated during the decades that followed. Over the course of 15 verse epistles, the *Guide* details the attempts made by the unfortunate Blunderhead family to adapt to the culture and behavioural codes of Bath's society. Through narrating the family's mishaps, the poem offers a lively satiric exposé of the social rituals going on at Britain's leading resort for bathing and medicinal waters. Yet for all its fun at the expense of the Blunderhead clan and of Bath itself, Regan argues that the poem also conveys the resort's many attractions—the contemporary allure of the 'Fine Balls, and fine Concerts, fine Buildings, and Springs, / Fine Walks, and fine Views, and a Thousand fine Things' on offer to the city's seasonal visitors (Anstey 2010, 115).

Then, in a ninth chapter bridging the gap between the second and the third sections of the volume, Pierre Degott deals with music in connection with spa culture. Just as baths and spawaters were praised for their curative virtues or discarded for their supposedly harmful effects on the body and morals, Degott reminds us that music, in spa towns, could often be regarded as a noisy and omnipresent nuisance in the same way that it could be extolled for its charm, elegance and recreational power. Denounced by some bathers for the disruptive tumult brought about by unwelcome band-players, music could rank as one of the many attractions afforded by notable English spas. Not only the cultural but also the social life of most bathers was organized around activities involving the presence of musicians or band-players. In a context in which ailment and entertainment would inevitably go hand in hand, Degott suggests that music could be seen as a curative and restorative element, able not only to please the senses but also to bring spiritual and physical comfort.

Logically enough, then, the last section of this collection examines spa culture from a therapeutic perspective. Mickaël Popelard offers a stimulating chapter on the role of balneology in Bacon's *New Atlantis* (1626) and *Historia vitae et mortis* (1623). Taking the last-named opus as a starting point for his discussion of balneology, he makes it clear that, in *New Atlantis*, baths fulfil both a medical and a social (or political) function. On closer inspection, Bacon's medical works are also suffused with sensuous undertones that transcend the ambit of sheer medical thinking. What looks like a purely medical line of reasoning at first sight is finally revealed to be a twofold meditation on how to increase longevity while also enhancing the quality and sensuousness of life.

In Chapter 11, Lowell Duckert notices that many medical manuals of the mid- to late-seventeenth century advised against the ingestion of coldwater, as it was believed that an excessive amount of cold essentially plugged the body's pores, trapping its unhealthy elements inside the skin. This chapter draws from a range of literary and natural-philosophical texts invested in the un/healthy effects of cold contact, chiefly the *Scarbrough Spaw* (1660) by Robert Wittie, an English physician who successfully managed to turn his country's exposed eastern coast into a thriving therapeutic resort. While he is persuasive in his defence of a salubrious north and of the physiological benefits that come from its coldness, Wittie's most notable accomplishment, Duckert argues, is in situating the spa-going human subject in wider global-local waters, collapsing hydro-spatial distance by eliminating the separation between embodiment and environment. Returning to Wittie'sspa-derived macro-microcosmic model, Duckert believes, can reinsert us in the precarious water cycles of today's cryosphere, calling our attention to its porous bodies most at risk.

Sophie Vasset, as to her, proposes to take an interest in the treatment of infertility by mineral waters in order to examine, on the basis of this specific object, the social diversity of water users, as well as the diversity of medical theories that justify the internal and external prescription of water for women who were considered infertile. She thus turns to the representation of the treatment for barrenness in eighteenth-century popular literature (miscellanies) and examines the recurrent trope of the adulterous woman who pretends that she was cured by the waters.

To conclude this third and last part, Vaughn Scribner studies the perceptions of mineral water and alcohol in eighteenth-century medical literature. He notices that while modern science generally equates consuming water with health and alcohol with illness, eighteenth-century

Britons hardly relied upon such dyads. As this chapter demonstrates, alcohol, mineral water, taverns, and spas were to be understood as homogenous rather than heterogenous. Labelled as 'intoxicants' by eighteenth-century physicians, mineral water and alcohol could do as much harm as good if not consumed correctly. Mineral spas and taverns, finally, necessarily entered the larger conversation over the supposed social health of the British Empire: might they be civilizing schools or dens of debauchery? Who should attend them and why? Who shouldn't?

In fine, the Coda to the volume offers the reader new ecocritical perspectives and branches out into deep waters. Richard Kerridge asks what inflection an environmental concern with ecological processes has given to the tropes explored in our edited collection and he goes through the three waves of ecocriticism that have been widely identified in the ecocritical community. He examines the first wave's assertion of the value of literal approaches to nature alongside metaphorical and symbolic uses; the second wave's emphasis on environmental justice and cultural diversity; and the third wave's New Materialist re-conceptualizing of non-human agency, trans-corporeality and systemic life. After looking especially at the concern of hydro-feminists Stacy Alaimo and Astrida Neimanis with deep water and deep origin, he finally discusses some practical examples of these ecocritically inflected tropes in contemporary environmental writing. The need for ecological familiarity with depth and origin stands in difficult but energetic dialectical relation to the traditional need for mystery, Kerridge concludes.

Kerridge's Coda thus explains why the spa-related issues examined in our edited collection still resonate in today's society. Over the last few years, ecocriticism has steadily gained footing within the larger arena of early modern scholarship, and this volume testifies to this new trend: the ecocritical concern made obvious in this very last section actually runs throughout our collection. Ecocritical thinking has sensitized us more than ever before to the tremendous importance of water for human life and, in its own peculiar way, the present book intends to be part of the current reflection on the cultural use and representation(s) of water. There is no denying that spa resorts, with their growing number of visitors over the centuries, have enduringly modelled the English land/mindscapes. By simultaneously addressing the varied early modern attitudes to resort tourism, approaches to health issues, and literary expressions of spa culture, we aim at providing our readers with new interpretive tracks in the rapidly emerging and intersecting fields of literary ecology and water studies.

Sophie Chiari
Samuel Cuisinier-Delorme

Works Cited

Primary sources

Allen, Benjamin. 1699. *The natural history of the chalybeat and purging waters of England with their particular essays and uses*. A1018. London: Printed and sold by S. Smith and B. Walford, Wing.

Baily, Walter. 1587. *A briefe discours of certain bathes or medicinall waters in the Countie of Warwicke neere vnto a village called Newnam Regis*. 2nd ed. 1191. London: STC.

Nicolay, Nicolas de. 1585. *The nauigations, peregrinations and voyages, made into Turkie by Nicholas Nicholay Daulphinois, Lord of Arfeuile, chamberlaine and geographer ordinarie to the King of Fraunce*. trans. Thomas Washington. 2nd ed., 18574. London: Printed by Thomas Dawson, STC.

Pierce, Robert. 1697. *Bath memoirs: Or, observations in three and forty years practice, at the bath what cures have been there wrought*. 2nd ed., P2163. Bristol: Printed for H. Hammond, Wing.

Shakespeare, William. 2016. *The Complete Works. Modern Critical Edition*. [eds.]. Gary Taylor, John Jowett, Terri Bourus and Gabriel Egan. Oxford: Oxford University Press.

Turner, William. 1562. *The seconde part of Vuilliam Turners herball wherein are conteyned the names of herbes in Greke, Latin, Duche, Frenche, and in the apothecaries Latin, and somtyme in Italiane, wyth the vertues of the same herbes wyth diuerse confutationes of no small errours, that men of no small learning haue committed in the intreatinge of herbes of late yeares. Here vnto is ioyned also a booke of the bath of Baeth in Englande, and of the vertues of the same wyth diuerse other bathes moste holsum and effectuall, both in Almany and Englande*. 2nd ed., 24366. Cologne: Printed by Arnold Birckman, STC.

Walker, Anthony. 1685. *Fax fonte accensa, fire out of water: or, An endeavour to kindle devotion, from the consideration of the fountains God hath made Designed for the benefit of those who use the waters of Tunbridg-Wells, the Bath, Epsom, Scarborough, Chigwell, Astrop, Northall, & c. Two sermons preached at New Chappel by Tunbridg-Wells*. London: Printed for Nathaniel Ranew, Wing.CD-ROM, 1996, W302A.

Wittie, Robert. 1660. *Scarbrough Spaw, or, A description of the nature and vertues of the spaw at Scarbrough in Yorkshire*. 2nd ed., W3231. London: Printed by Charles Tyus, Thomason/E.1830[2]; Wing.

Wittie, Robert. 1667. *Scarbrough–Spaw: or a description of the nature and vertues of the spaw at Scarbrough Yorkshire*. 2nd ed., W3232. York: Printed by A. Broad for Tho. Passenger, Wing.

Secondary sources

Benedict, Barbara M. 1995. Consumptive Communities: Commodifying Nature in Spa Society, *The Eighteenth Century*, Vol. 36 (Autumn), No. 3: 203–219.

Borsay, Anne. 1999. *Medicine and Charity in Georgian Bath: A Social History of the General Infirmary, c. 1739–1830*. History of Medicine in Context. Aldershot: Ashgate.

Borsay, Peter. 2000. Health and Leisure Resorts 1700–1840. In *The Cambridge Urban History of Britain*. Cambridge: Cambridge University Press, 2: 775–804.

Borsay, Peter. 2000. *The Image of Georgian Bath, 1700–2000: Towns, Heritage, and History*. Oxford: Oxford University Press.

Cooley, Ronald W. 2015. 'Sexy in a 'Tunbridge Wells' Sort of Way': A Study in the Literary Iconography of Place, *Journal for Early Modern Cultural Studies*, Vol. 15, No. 1 (Winter): 90–118.

Corbin, Alain. 1994. *The Lure of the Sea: The Discovery of the Seaside in the Western World, 1750–1840*. Cambridge: Polity.

Cossic-Péricarpin, Annick, and Galliou, Patrick (eds.). 2006. *Spas in Britain and in France in the Eighteenth and Nineteenth Centuries*. Newcastle: Cambridge Scholars Press.

Eglin, John. 2005. *The Imaginary Autocrat: Beau Nash and the Invention of Bath*. London: Profile.

Hembry, Phyllis. 1990. *The English Spa, 1560–1815: A Social History*. London: Athlone Press.

Herbert, Amanda E. 2009. Gender and the Spa: Space, Sociability and Self at British Health Spas, 1640–1714, *Journal of Social History*, Vol. 43, No. 2 (Winter): 361–83.

Jennings, Eric Thomas. 2006. *Curing the Colonizers: Hydrotherapy, Climatology, and French Colonial Spas*. Durham, NC: Duke University Press.

Kelly, James. 2008–2009. Drinking the Waters: Balneotherapeutic Medicine in Ireland, 1660–1850, *Studia Hibernica*, No. 35: 99–146.

Large, David Clay. 2015. *The Grand Spas of Central Europe: A History of Intrigue, Politics, Art, and Healing*. Lanham, MD: Rowman & Littlefield.

Smith, Hannah. 2008. Walker, Antony (bap. 1622, d. 1692), Clergyman, *Oxford Dictionary of National Biography*. Oxford: Oxford University Press.

Stanivukovic, Goran V. 2007. Cruising the Mediterranean: Narratives of Sexuality and Geographies of the Eastern Mediterranean in Early Modern English Prose Romance. In *Remapping the Mediterranean World in Early Modern English Writings*, [ed.] Goran V. Stanivukovic. New York: Palgrave Macmillan: 59–74.

Contents

Editors and Contributors

About the Editors

Sophie Chiari is Professor of early modern studies at Université Clermont Auvergne and a member of the IHRIM research unit ('Institut d'Histoire des Représentations et des Idées dans les Modernités'). She has published several books on Shakespeare and his contemporaries, including Love's Labour's Lost*: Shakespeare's Anatomy of Wit*, and As You Like It: *Shakespeare's Comedy of Liberty* (Presses Universitaires de France, 2014 and 2016). She has edited several collections of essays such as *The Circulation of Ideas in Early Modern English Literature* (Ashgate, 2015; Routledge, 2016), *Spectacular Science, Technology and Superstition in the Age of Shakespeare* coedited with Mickaël Popelard (Edinburgh University Press, 2017), *Freedom and Censorship in Early Modern English Literature* (Routledge, 2019), and *Performances at Court in the Age of Shakespeare* co-edited with John Mucciolo (Cambridge University Press, 2019). Her latest monograph is entitled *Shakespeare's Representation of Weather, Climate and Environment* (Edinburgh University Press, 2019). She is currently working on an Arden Dictionary entitled *Shakespeare's Environment: A Dictionary* (Bloomsbury).

Samuel Cuisinier-Delorme is a Senior Lecturer in English literature at Université Clermont Auvergne and a member of the IHRIM research unit. In 2013, he completed a Ph.D. dissertation on dancing in Shakespeare's works. His research interests include connections between Renaissance drama and dance, as well as dance history. He is currently working on an edited collection entitled *Écrire la danse dans l'Europe de la Renaissance aux Lumières.* He is also interested in British contemporary drama. He has published several articles on Sarah Kane's works and in 2015, he co-edited with Susan Blattès *Le Théâtre In-Yer-Face aujourd'hui : bilans et perspectives* (*Coup de Théâtre*, #29).

Contributors

Pierre Degott is Professor of English studies at Université de Lorraine, Metz, where he mainly teaches eighteenth-century literature. Published at Éditions L'Harmattan, his Ph.D. was a study on the themes and poetics of Handel's oratorio libretti. His current research is on the following subjects: 1. librettology and the reflexivity of the sung text; 2. the representation of musical and operatic performances in Anglo-Saxon fiction; 3. opera and oratorio in translation. Even though his research covers all eras concerned by operatic practise, he mainly concentrates on eighteenth-century musical forms (opera, semi-opera, oratorio, odes, ballad-opera, musical plays). He has published about a hundred academic articles and organized several conferences, mainly on musico-literary subjects. He is currently Dean of the UFR Arts, Lettres et Langues in Metz.

Alix Desnain is a Doctoral Fellow at Université Clermont Auvergne, where she also teaches. A specialist of English literature and a member of the IHRIM research unit, she wrote a master's thesis on the transformation of the Arthurian legend throughout the Middle Ages. Her dissertation, under the supervision of Prof. Sophie Chiari, focuses on its resurgence in the literature and the culture of Early Modern England.

Lowell Duckert is Associate Professor of English at the University of Delaware, where he specializes in early modern literature, environmental criticism, and the various 'new materialisms'. He has recently written articles on lagoons, premodern weather, the north wind, and Shakespeare's 'humming water'. With Jeffrey Jerome Cohen, he is the editor of 'Eco-materialism' (*postmedieval: a journal of medieval cultural studies* 4.1); *Elemental Ecocriticism: Thinking with Earth, Air, Water, and Fire*; and *Veer Ecology: A Companion for Environmental Thinking* (nominated for the Association for the Study of Literature and Environment's Ecocriticism Book Award). His book *For All Waters: Finding Ourselves in Early Modern Wetscapes* was published by the University of Minnesota Press in 2017 and was short-listed for the SLSA's Michelle Kendrick Memorial Book Prize for the best academic book on literature, science, and the arts. He is currently working on a book project about the early modern cryosphere and its potential intersections with contemporary climate change activism.

Amanda E. Herbert is Associate Director at the Folger Institute of the Folger Shakespeare Library, where she runs the Fellowships Program. She holds a Ph.D. in History from the Johns Hopkins University, and is the author of *Female Alliances: Gender, Identity, and Friendship in Early Modern Britain* (Yale, 2014) winner of the Best Book Award from the Society for the Study of Early Modern Women. She edits *The Recipes Project* and co-directors *Before 'Farm to Table': Early Modern Foodways and Cultures*, a $1.5 million Mellon initiative in collaborative research; as part of this project she co-curated an exhibit at the Folger in 2019, 'First Chefs: Fame and Foodways from Britain to the Americas'. She is at work on two book projects, *Water Works: Faith, Public Health, and Politics in the British Atlantic*, and *Leftovers: The Afterlives of Early Modern Food.*

Richard Kerridge is a nature writer and ecocritic. At Bath Spa University, he leads the MA in Creative Writing and co-ordinates research and postgraduate studies in Literature and Creative Writing. He has published essays on ecocritical topics ranging from Shakespeare and Thomas Hardy to present-day fiction, poetry, nature writing and film. In 1998, he co-edited *Writing the Environment*, the first collection of ecocritical essays to be published in the UK. Other work has been published in *BBC Wildlife*, *Poetry Review* and *Granta*. Richard was awarded the 2012 Roger Deakin Prize by the Society of Authors, and he has twice received the BBC Wildlife Award for Nature Writing. *Cold Blood: Adventures with Reptiles and Amphibians* (2014) is a mixture of memoir and nature writing. Richard's most recent publication is a new annotated edition of J.H. Prynne's place-based poem-sequence *The Oval Window*, using previously unavailable archive material. He also reviews nature writing for *The Guardian.*

François Laroque, Professor Emeritus at Université Sorbonne Nouvelle-Paris 3, is the author of *Shakespeare's Festive World* (Cambridge University

Press, 1991) and several books and articles on Shakespeare and the Elizabethan and Jacobean drama. His last two publications are *Dictionnaire amoureux de Shakespeare* (Plon, 2016) and *John Webster.* The Duchess of Malfi (Ellipses, 2018).

Marie-Laure Massei-Chamayou is a Senior Lecturer in English studies at the University of Paris 1-Panthéon Sorbonne and a member of the 'Centre d'Histoire du XIXe Siècle'. She is the author of two books on Jane Austen's novels: *La Représentation de l'argent dans les romans de Jane Austen: L'Être et l'avoir* (L'Harmattan, 2012) and *Between Secrets and Screens.* Sense and Sensibility*: Jane Austen, Ang Lee* (CNED/PUF, 2015). She has also published articles on Jane Austen's fictional responses to the economic and social transformations of her time. Her current research explores how novels written by women during the Georgian and Victorian eras address female concerns about property, inheritance, consumption, or the domestic economy, and engage with increasingly complex financial realities.

Mickaël Popelard is Professor of early modern literature at Université de Caen Normandie. He has written several books and articles on early modern literature and philosophy, with a special interest in William Shakespeare and Francis Bacon. His current research interests focus on the two-way relationship between science and literature in early modern England. With Sophie Chiari, he has recently co-edited *Spectacular Science, Technology and Superstition in the Age of Shakespeare* (Edinburg University Press, 2017) and he is currently working on a French translation of some of Bacon's literary works, to be published by Classiques Garnier.

Shaun Regan lectures on eighteenth-century and romantic literature at Queen's University Belfast. He has published extensively on satire, prose fiction, mid-eighteenth-century literature and the early Black Atlantic. He is the author of *Making the Novel: Fiction and Society in Britain, 1660–1789* (Palgrave 2006, with Brean Hammond), and editor of *Reading 1759: Literary Culture in Mid-Eighteenth-Century Britain and France* (Bucknell 2013) as well as *The Culture of the Seven Years' War: Empire, Identity, and the Arts in the Eighteenth-Century Atlantic World* (Toronto 2014, with Frans De Bruyn). His most recent articles have appeared in the journals *Textual Practice*, *Forum for Modern Language Studies*, *Irish University Review* and *The Eighteenth Century: Theory and Interpretation.*

Anne Rouhette is a Senior Lecturer in eighteenth- and nineteenth-century British literature at Université Clermont Auvergne. Her main field of interest is women's fiction from the late eighteenth and the early nineteenth centuries and she has published in particular on Mary Shelley, Frances Burney and Jane Austen. She is currently working on a critical edition of an eighteenth-century translation of *Evelina* and on a volume on dreams and literary creation in women's fiction (in the eighteenth and nineteenth centuries), co-edited with Isabelle Hervouet.

Vaughn Scribner is an Assistant Professor of History at the University of Central Arkansas. He has published numerous articles which investigate eighteenth-century British leisure spaces such as spas, taverns, and pleasure gardens through the lens of science, urbanity, and the environment. He also recently published *Inn Civility: Urban Taverns and Early American Civil Society* (New York University Press, 2019), which utilizes the colonial American urban tavern to understand colonists' efforts (and failures) at realizing a monarchical 'civil society'. His last book is entitled *Merpeople: A Human History* (Reaktion Books, 2020).

Tiffany Stern is Professor of early modern drama at The Shakespeare Institute, University of Birmingham. She specializes in literary criticism, theatre, book history and editing from the sixteenth to the eighteenth century. She is the author of *Rehearsal from Shakespeare to Sheridan* (2000), *Making Shakespeare* (2004), *Shakespeare in Parts* (with Simon Palfrey, 2007) and *Documents of Performance in Early Modern England* (2009). She co-edited a collection of essays with Farah Karim-Cooper, *Shakespeare's Theatres and the Effects of Performance* (2013), and edited the anonymous *King Leir* (2001), Richard Brinsley Sheridan's *The Rivals* (2004), George Farquhar's *Recruiting Officer* (2010), and Richard Brome's *Jovial Crew* (2014). She has recently edited a collection of essays entitled *Rethinking Shakespeare's Theatrical Documents* (2019). She is also a General Editor of the New Mermaids play series and Arden Shakespeare 4. Her current projects are a book on early modern theatre and popular entertainment, *Playing Fair*, exploring the cultural exchanges between playhouses and fairgrounds, and a book on *Shakespeare Beyond Performance*, looking at the theatrical documents produced in the light of a play's performance—ballads, chapbooks, commonplace books, 'noted' texts.

Sophie Vasset is a Senior Lecturer at Université de Paris. She has published extensively on eighteenth-century British literature (*The Physics of Language*, PUF, 2010), eighteenth-century history of medicine (*Décrire, Prescrire, Guérir*, Hermann, 2011; *Bellies Bowels and Entrails in the Eighteenth Century* with S. Kleiman-Lafon and R. Barr) and she is currently working on mineral waters in eighteenth-century Britain and Europe. She is part of the steering committee of 'The Person in Medicine Institute' at the Université de Paris, and she obtained a CNRS research grant at the IHRIM research unit, Université Clermont Auvergne, in 2019–21. She is also the Director of the 'Fondation des États-Unis', Cité Internationale Universitaire de Paris.

Tiffany Jo Werth is an Associate Professor of English at UC Davis. Her work on the thorny relationship of romance to the long English Reformation has appeared in article form in the *Shakespearean International Yearbook* and *English Literary Renaissance* and as her first monograph *The Fabulous Dark Cloister: Romance in England after the Reformation* (Johns Hopkins University Press, 2011). Her current book project, entitled *The English Lithic Imagination from More to Milton*, argues that the mineral (clay, rocks, stones, bezoars, iron) offers an unsettling touchstone for rethinking Renaissance humanism and literary creation. She has published on the more-than-human world as editor of a special issue of *The Shakespearean International Yearbook* and in various articles. She co-edited a never-before-printed academic drama, *The Converted Robber or Stonehenge, a Pastoral*, in *English Literary Renaissance*, as well as a collection of essays with Vin Nardizzi, *Premodern Ecologies in the Modern Literary Imagination* (University of Toronto Press, 2019).

List of Figures

Chapter 6

Chapter 9

Chapter 13

PART I

Generic Explorations: Baths and Waters in Poetry, Drama and Prose

CHAPTER 1

'Bathing [...] in Origane and Thyme': Baths in Spenser's *The Faerie Queene*

Alix Desnain

Spenser's national epic is peppered with references to water, among which we can find several bathing scenes that will be the focus of this chapter. While the nudity implied in bathing would suggest a certain amount of disclosure, bathing in *The Faerie Queene*[1] quickly appears to be much more complex, and rife with symbolism as Spenser's allegorical logic demands. From the down-to-earth references to famous thermal springs and their virtues to a more poetic use of the bath, Spenser's waters seem to be imbued with a serpentine essence that wards off any singular general interpretation. Similar to Spenser's poem, water symbolism seems to divaricate and change course as the poem unfolds. The substantial intermingling of classical, biblical and folkloric sources adds to the complex and mutable character of water and bathing in Spenser's national epic. As the *OED* defines the verb 'bathe' as 'immers[ing] (the body, or any part of it) in water or other liquid, for the sake of some effect (e.g. health,

[1] All quotations from *The Faerie Queene* are from Spenser 2013.

A. Desnain (✉)
Département d'Études Anglophones, Université Clermont Auvergne, Clermont-Ferrand, France

S. Chiari and S. Cuisinier-Delorme (eds.), *Spa Culture and Literature in England, 1500–1800*, Early Modern Literature in History,
https://doi.org/10.1007/978-3-030-66568-5_1

warmth, cleansing) promoted by the action of the liquid' (I.1.a), I will deal with bathing in springs, wells and fountains alike, and I will focus on the direct and indirect effects of bathing, as they are of paramount importance in the literary landscape of the first three books of *The Faerie Queene*. I will indeed argue that water in Spenser has a transformative power and the bathing scenes in *The Faerie Queene* are interesting to analyse through this particular lens as its meanings and symbols shift but tend toward a poetics of transformation through water.

1 From Therapeutic to Erotic Waters

At the end of Book I, during the battle against the dragon, Redcrosse falls into water and this is what eventually allows him to defeat his opponent. In canto xi, he is losing the battle when he is thrown into the well of life whose virtues are described in stanza 30:

> For vnto life the dead it could restore,
> And guilt of sinfull crimes cleane wash away,
> Those that with sicknesse were infected sore,
> It could recure, and aged long decay
> Renew, as one were borne that very day.
> (I.xi.30)

The properties of this well seem astounding as the water is '[f]ull of great vertues, and for med'cine good' (I.xi.29). It can cure diseases, rejuvenate and can even bring the dead back to life. As a matter of fact, the water not only heals Redcrosse, but it also gives him the physical and mental strength to slay the dragon, as the virtues of this well are physical as well as spiritual. It can 'guilt of sinfull crimes cleane wash away' (I.xi.30) and consequently, his being immersed in water has often been seen as a symbolic baptism,[2] especially given that a few stanzas later, when he rises from the water, he is described as '[s]o *new* this *new-borne* knight to battell *new* did rise' (I.xi.34, my emphasis). The baptismal analogy is rather evident here, with the emphasis on the renewal Redcrosse has undergone, and it adds another layer to the interaction between bodies and water.

[2] See Hester Lees-Jeffries (2003, 135–176), for an example of such interpretation.

The description of the virtues of the well of life during Redcrosse's battle leads to the mention of famous waters: 'Both *Silo* this, and *Iordan* did excell, / and th'English *Bath*, And eke the german *Spau*, / Ne can *Cephise*, nor *Hebrus* match this well' (I.xi.30). While it is said that these are no match for the waters of the well of life, the very fact that this comparison is made creates a link between these waters and the sacred well presented in this episode. Their properties are famous enough to warrant their being used as a foil and while they may not raise the dead, they benefit from this mention in a trickling down effect. The waters of Bath are specifically brought up again in Book II when Arthur and Guyon read a 'chronicle of Briton kings' (II.x.Argument):

Behold the boyling Bathes at Cairbadon,
Which seeth with secret fire eternally,
And in their entrailles, full of quick Brimston,
Nourish the flames, which they are warmd vpon,
That to their people wealth they forth do well,
And health to euery forreyne nation.
(II.x.26)

These waters are given an origin story in which king Bladud,[3] versed in the 'arts', is responsible for the warm waters of the city of Bath. Once again, the fact that a stanza is devoted to Bath—here called by its Welsh name 'Cairbadon'—in this fictional chronicle is significant as it hints at the importance of the city of Bath at the time. The inclusion of its story in Spenser's chronicle, within his national epic, suggests that it is a landmark, a way to recognize Britain, in the same way as in the passage from Book I, it was 'th'*English* Bath' (I.xi.30, my emphasis). It is the coalescing of water and fire or water and heat, presented here as one of the properties of the waters of Bath, that is responsible for its restorative power. The water–heat combination is also a key element in the conception of Belphoebe and Amoret in Book III where its generative potential is exemplified:

In a fresh fountaine, far from all mens vew,
She bath'd her brest, the boyling heat t'allay;
She bath'd with roses red and violets blew,

[3] For more on Bladud and the foundation of Bath, see Tiffany Stern's chapter on the subject in this collection.

And all the sweetest flowres, that in the forest grew. [...]
The sunbeames bright vpon her body playd,
Being through former bathing mollifide,
And pierst into her womb, where they embayd
With so sweet sence and secret power vnspide,
That in her pregnant flesh they shortly fructifide.
(III.vi.6–7)

In this scene, the conception of the twins is explicitly linked to Chrysogone—their mother—bathing. This passage of sexless conception places the bath at the centre of the process as bathing essentially prepares ('mollifide') her body to accept the sun (the masculine element here) as it 'pierst into her womb'. This conjunction of water and heat as a generative phenomenon is spelt out in the following stanza: 'But reason teacheth that the fruitfull seades / Of all things liuing, through impression / Of the sunbeames in moyst complexion, / Doe life conceiue' (III.vi.8), an Aristotelian idea still at play during the Renaissance (Hamilton 2014, 'medicine' 461), and it is also a large part of the alchemical process which is already suggested in Chrysogone's name as it combines χρῡσός 'gold' and γόνος 'that which is begotten' (Liddell and Scott 1940), and alchemy is concerned with gold-making. This bathing scene could therefore be read as an alchemical process which results in Amoret and Belphoebe.

While this passage appears quite innocent at first glance, one actually detects here an underlying voyeurism characteristic of such bathing scenes (especially those which partake of the Acteon myth in the poem). Indeed, it is specified that Chrysogone is 'far from all mens vew' (III.vi.6–7) which suggests that this transgressive behaviour should be absent here, but then the lines 'Vpon her fell all naked bare *displayd*; / The sunbeames bright vpon her body playd' (my emphasis) conveys the chaste sensuality of the scene, but still suggests a certain transgression as 'to display' is 'to open up or expose to view, exhibit to the eyes, show' (*OED* 3.a).

2 Threatening Transgressions

The nudity implied in the act of bathing leads to a fair deal of voyeurism in *The Faerie Queene*. In the first bathing scene of the poem (I.ii.40–43)—when Fradubio gives Redcrosse his account of how he came to be changed into a tree—many words have to do with the male gaze and appearances. In this passage, Duessa is revealed to Fradubio and the reader for the first time, 'in her proper hew'. The transgression and the threat stem from the very act of looking: 'For danger great, if not assurd decay / I saw before mine eyes' (I.ii.41). Duessa who, so far, had been a beautiful woman, becomes in this scene 'a filthy foul old woman' (I.ii.40) when she bathes. However, water seems to both reveal and conceal in this instance. The beginning of stanza 41 ('Her neather partes misshapen, monstruous, / Were hidd in water, that I could not see, / But they did seeme more foule and hideous, / Than womans shape man would beleeue to bee') presents the reader with a description of her deformity, but it is hidden in water, and Fradubio 'see[s] her in her proper hew' (I.ii.40), but at the same time, he 'could not see' (I.ii.41).

This motif of water as both transparent and opaque is expanded upon in the scene depicting the knight Guyon's and the Palmer's arrival at the Bower of Bliss (II.xii.60–72) in which they come upon 'two naked Damzelles' (II.xii.63) bathing in a fountain, and there follows what could be called an erotic game of hide-and-seek (Chiari 2009) in which the two damsels 'wrestle wantonly' (II.xii.63). The sapphic undertones as they play together in order to attract Guyon's attention and let him spy on them heighten the eroticism of the scene. In addition to the insistence on gazing in this scene,[4] this voyeuristic interplay is punctuated by a recursive process of veiling and unveiling that is at the core of stanzas 64 to 67. Water here serves as a veil, sometimes hiding, sometimes revealing parts of the women's bodies as they tantalize Guyon so that he strays from his quest:

> The whiles their snowy limbes, as through a vele,
> So through the christall waues appeared plaine:
> Then suddeinly both would themselues vnhele,
> And th'amarous sweet spoiles to greedy eyes reuele.
> (II.xii.64)

> The wanton Maidens him espying, stood
> Gazing a while at his vnwonted guise;
> Then th'one her selfe low ducked in the flood,

[4] There are numerous words related to sight from stanzas 62 to 68: 'see', 'espyde', 'vew', 'eyd', 'greedy eyes', 'saw', 'espying', 'gazing', 'auise', 'spectacle', 'lookers', 'looking', 'spyde', etc.

Abasht, that her a straunger did auise:
But thither rather higher did arise,
And her two lilly paps aloft displayd,
And all, that might his melting hart entyse
To her delights, she vnto him bewrayd:
The rest hidd vnderneath, him more desirous made.
(II.xii.66)

This play on covering and uncovering echoes the juxtaposition—at the beginning of the scene—of chaste and erotic elements, even though eroticism overtakes any semblance of chastity by the end of the passage. In stanza 63, when the two damsels are first described, the reference to the Laurel trees brings to mind the Ovidian story of Daphne and the preservation of her virginity (Ovid 1965, 18–20). The two damsels, however, are never described as chaste, and the only moment one of them acts somewhat demurely is in stanza 66, but this is undermined right away by the other one exposing herself even more. The more demure one also ends up rising from the water in stanza 67, although she is still covered by her hair, which replaces the water as a veil, but 'a veil tantalises the spectator, piques the curiosity, by swathing what lies beneath in an aura of mystery' (Dauber 1980, 165). The insistence on this sensual, tantalizing game the two play with Guyon heightens the potential threat to his quest.

A threatening sexuality thus underscores Spenser's poetry, especially through the temptation represented by the two bathing damsels. In Fradubio's story (I.ii.40–43), the first bathing scene of *The Faerie Queene*, the threat is very explicit: a disquieting atmosphere is at play, with the use of words such as 'monstruous', 'danger', 'assurd decay', 'diuelish', etc. The reference to thyme suggests that the threat is in part sexual given that this herb, as noted by Hamilton, was used to cure syphilis (Spenser 2013, 52, footnote). The contrast with the episode of Amoret and Belphoebe's conception (III.vi.4–7) is apparent as 'roses and violets' replace 'thyme and origane' in the water. Traditionally, roses were associated with love and marriage as a symbol of Venus/Aphrodite and could also be linked to the Virgin Mary, while violets, also associated with the Virgin Mary, symbolized humility and gentleness[5] (Faircloth and Thomas

[5] The virtue at the centre of Book III is Chastity, embodied by the female knight Britomart. Amoret and Belphoebe serve as her counterparts in the representation of

2014, 292–293; 347). In Fradubio's scene, even the herbs used for bathing suggest a dangerous sexuality, and this menace is only reinforced by Fradubio's voyeurism as this is the reason for his punishment. Reminiscent of Acteon's myth, Duessa turns Fradubio into a tree for having seen her 'in her proper hew' (I.ii.40), and his only salvation is to be 'bathed in a livuing well' (I.ii.43), which implies that, in this particular case, the act of bathing is both the catalyst for the punishment as well as the hope of salvation.

Duessa has another bathing scene, in canto vii of the same book, that has a negative effect on Redcrosse and suggests a sexual threat. It takes place in what seems, at first, to be a *locus amoenus,* but Duessa and Redcrosse bathing together results in him losing his strength as seen in stanza 6: 'Eftsoones his manly forces gan to fayle, / and mightie strong was turnd to feeble frayle' (I.vii.6). The first explanation, the one we are given, is that the waters of this fountain are cursed since a nymph was punished for her idleness and was turned to water by the goddess Diana. This is explained in stanza 5 and 'Thenceforth her waters wexed dull and slow, / And all that drinke thereof, do faint and feeble grow' (I.vii.5) and it is based on the myth of Salmacis and Hermaphroditus. A more symbolic interpretation of this episode is that '[t]he knight is enfeebled as the result of his first act of venery with Duessa, the drink he takes of the fountain is the metaphor for that act' (Shroeder 1962, 145) and that the fountain 'promotes impotence through sexual overindulgence' (Silberman 1995, 55). The implied sexual intercourse between Duessa and Redcrosse[6] therefore seems to lead to Redcrosse's emasculation.

In this scene, Redcrosse's divesting himself of his armour in order to bathe is significant, not only because it leaves him vulnerable physically, but also because it symbolically strips him of his identity. Indeed, he is 'the Redcrosse knight' because his armour is adorned by a red cross (Lees-Jeffries 2003, 154–155). As a matter of fact, the first canto of the first book begins with the description of this knight, especially through his armour and shield (I.i.1–2). So when he goes 'To rest him selfe, foreby a fountaine side, disarmed all of yron-coted Plate' (I.vii.2), his nakedness

Chastity, and their immaculate conception and their being 'enwombed in the sacred throne/ Of [Chrysogone's] chaste bodie' (III.vi.5) only drives in the point.

[6] Hester Lees-Jeffries suggests that 'Duessa becomes the fountain, and that Redcrosse's drinking stands for his fornication' in her article 'From the Fountain to the Well: Redcrosse Learns to Read' (2003, 157).

is more than physical and his very identity is threatened because of his bathing.[7] As Krier writes, 'Spenser consistently elides the self-estranging violence of Petrarchan eros in the direction of gradual change or sustained transformation, acknowledging but defusing the threat of rupture in time' (Krier 1990, 117–118). If we apply this idea to the threat posed by water, and if we examine several bathing episodes in *The Faerie Queene*, transformation seems linked with water, more often than not.

3 The Shiftiness of Spenser's Waters

In the Middle Ages, fountains were often depicted as a portal to another world and Spenser resorts to fountains as an entrance into a world of change, of metamorphosis. In *The Spenser Encyclopedia,* fountains are described as 'manifestations of radical mutability' (Hamilton 2014, 'fountains', 314) and while the symbolic baptism of Redcrosse at the end of Book I is a spiritual change, I would now like to focus on the more physical ones, especially if we consider that, as Austin Denis Britton writes, 'Ovidian metamorphosis is more powerful than baptism' (2014, 77).

At the beginning of Book II, canto ii, the Palmer actually explains the virtues of waters to Guyon after the latter tries in vain to wash Ruddymane's hands of blood: 'But know that secret vertues are infusd / In euery fountaine, and in euerie lake, / Which who hath skill them rightly to have chusd /, To proofe of passing wonders hath full often vsed' (II.ii.5). The Palmer speaks of the secret virtues of waters and the popularity of some and then goes on recounting the story of this well, whose purity is explained by the story of a metamorphosis. Indeed, a chaste nymph fleeing from Faunus wept and prayed to Diana who turned her to stone so that she could remain undefiled. This purity extends to the waters as it is said that they, similarly, cannot be stained. Here the outcome is rather positive and gives an etiological myth as a basis for the properties of water:

> Lo now she is that stone, from whose two heads,
> As from *two weeping eyes*, fresh streames do flow,
> Yet colde through feare, and old conceiued dreads;
> And yet the stone her semblance seemes to show,
> *Shapt like a maide*, that such ye may her know;

[7] On masculine pleasure and vulnerability, see Campana (2009, 465–496).

> And yet her vertues in her water byde:
> For it is chaste and pure, as purest snow,
> Ne lets her waues be with any filth be dyde,
> But euer like her selfe vnstayned hath beene tryde.
> (II.ii.9, my emphasis)

Whether physically or by the properties of her waters, this well *is* the nymph. This adequation between the fountain and the nymph[8] echoes what happens in canto i of the same book when Guyon comes upon Amavia: 'Pitifull spectacle of deadly smart, / Beside a bubling fountaine low she lay, / Which shee increased with her bleeding hart, / And the cleane waues with purple gore did ray; / [...] For in her streaming blood he [a louely babe] did embay' (II.i.40). Amavia has stabbed herself after her lover's death, and the image of her blood increasing the stream of the fountain is a powerful one. Her own blood merges with the water of the fountain and her son finds himself bathed in 'her streaming blood'. The 'streaming blood', in addition to the fact that her bleeding wound is referred to as 'the floodgate' (II.i.43) three stanzas later, actually suggests that her own body has become a fountain, not unlike the nymph.

This correspondence between fountains and the female body is used slightly differently in the scene of the Bower of Bliss. The description of the fountain in which the two damsels are bathing takes up two stanzas (II.xii. 60–61). The fountain 'Was ouerwrought, and shapes of naked boyes, / Of which some seemd with liuely iollitee, / To fly about, playing their wanton toyes, / Whylest others did them selues embay in liquid ioyes' (II.xii.60). At first, the description of the boys seems to refer to real ones rather than to sculptures, as they are 'flying about, playing and bathing'. This deceit is said to be true of the ivy in the next stanza as 'That wight, who did not well auis'd it vew, / Would surely deeme it to bee yuie trew: / Low his lasciuious armes adown did creepe' (II.xii.61). The personification of the ivy with its 'lasciuious armes', in addition to its misleading verisimilitude and that of the boys, should make the reader wary of appearances. The ekphrasis presented here with the description of the fountain in all its vividness corresponds to what Grogan

[8] A parallel could also be drawn with canto 4 of the Song of Solomon: 'My sister, my spouse is as a garden enclosed, as a spring shut up, and a fountain sealed up' (Geneva Bible). In Spenser, fountains are not sealed however, which hints at the mutability always at play in *The Faerie Queene*, as water is almost always moving.

calls '*energeia*—the commitment to creating intensely vivid images in the mind's eye of the reader' (Grogan 2009, 168) but, as she shrewdly demonstrates, '[w]here allegory cautiously enwraps, ekphrasis flagrantly reveals' (Grogan 2009, 167), and Spenser's allegorical poem does not lose its didactic intent in such moments. Indeed, the enticing description of the fountain creates a very clear image in which the reader, like Guyon, might get absorbed, but in the middle of the second descriptive stanza, the line 'That wight, who did not well auis'd it vew' (II.xii.61) should alert the reader: it 'reinsert[s] a critical distance into the reader's experience' and 'separate[s] the perspective of the viewing hero from that of the reader at the very optimum moment of absorption: a destabilising of the identification between reader and hero' (Grogan 2009, 128). The sight presented in the Bower of Bliss seems to have an arresting power on Guyon who appears to be attracted to this deceitful picture. As Theresa Krier remarks, '[a]nother frequent danger to the male viewer contemplating feminine beauty in Spenser's work is the arresting power of that beauty [...] [which] is a drastic disruption, a breaking of time's continuity by a rupture that Spenser is ever anxious both to acknowledge and to overcome' (Krier 1990, 116–117). Of course, this passage takes place in the Bower of Bliss, therefore it stands to reason that appearances are made to be deceiving, but the fact that this fountain and the two damsels bathing in it are Guyon's first introduction to it make it significant. Indeed, not only does the lengthy description of the fountain and the interplay taking place in it slow down the narrative in a way that mirrors the threat to Guyon's quest, but the rampant sexuality at play here also turns this bathing scene into a dangerous one not unlike a refracted image in which things are not as they seem.

However, these deceiving appearances are somewhat counteracted by the last image of Book III in the 1590 version—*i.e.* the image on which the whole poem ended before the addition of Books IV to VI. In this version, the poem concludes on the vision of the union of Scudamour and Amoret which is described as follows[9]:

> Had ye them seene, ye would haue surely thought,
> That they had beene that faire Hermaphrodite,
> Which that rich Romane of white marble wrought,
> And in his costly Bath causd to bee site:

[9] For a detailed analysis of the 1590 ending, see Cheney (1972).

> So seemd those two, as growne together quite[.]
> (III.xii.46*)

As Lauren Silberman notes, '[i]f the statue represents the metamorphosed Hermaphroditus, the bath itself must evoke the infamous fountain of Salmacis whose waters must cause men to become effeminate' (Silberman 1987, 222). The 1590 version therefore ends on the image of a bath linked with a metamorphosis, while 'Britomart and Spenser's reader are onlookers' (Silberman 1987, 221). In itself, the fact that the lovers are compared to a work of art suggests their transformation, from two separate beings to one work of art that is fixed in time. This artefact being a statue of Hermaphroditus adds another layer to the metamorphosis of the young man. When Hermaphroditus dives into the pool of which Salmacis is the nymph, the latter becomes so enamoured with him that she asks the gods to unite them. When Hermaphroditus sees that his body has fused with the nymph's and that he has become half-man, half-woman, he asks his divine parents to curse the fountain so that any man drinking from it would become half a man (Ovid 1965, 98–99). This is what happens to Redcrosse in Book I when he bathes with Duessa, and Spenser's explanation for the effect of the fountain (I.vii.5) aligns with Ovid's story. The last image of the poem in its first version echoes a key event from Book I, but it focuses on the creative aspects of the myth of Hermaphroditus, instead of the debilitating effects. From its origins, the story is a story of disintegration, of the destruction of the individual, but it also represents the synthesizing of something new and it seems to mimic the way water, in Spenser, serves as both the medium of dissolution and of combination, always shifting and deceiving. The conjunction of Hermaphroditus and the bath can suggest an alchemical reading, as this last image of the poem seems to represent an alchemical bath and Hermaphroditus is a recurrent trope in alchemical representations. As Pinkus writes, the combination of the male and female elements 'in a chemical bath or oven (*copulatio*, chemical nuptials), to produce Gold (the philosopher's stone, wisdom, truth, resurrection, salvation, the Son)' is one of the stages of alchemy. If we take into account the fact that 'in many of the variants of alchemy, the primary stage(s) of the transformation process is depicted as a wedding' (Pinkus 2006, 102) then this image of Hermaphroditus in the bath opens up a new layer of interpretation. The union of Scudamour and Amoret is depicted as two entities dissolving into a single one. Even their names can easily be combined into Scudamoret, which Norhnberg refers to as the 'impending mutualization' (1976, 607) of Spenser's lovers' names. There is a hermaphroditic logic to Spenser's couples, and the last image of the 1590 version uses that in the representation of the wedding. Britomart is an onlooker and she is 'halfe enuying their blesse' (III.xii.46*), as they seem to represent a perfect union ('No word they spake, nor earthly thing they felt, / But like two senceles stocks in long embracement dwelt', III.xii.45*). The use of the word 'halfe' in reference to Britomart is not trivial and it suggests that Britomart is still only half of one. She is not yet a whole entity, whereas the wedded couple in the (alchemical) bath appears to be complete in their hermaphroditic union, Britomart—as well as the reader, who is put in an observational position with the line 'Had ye them seene' (III.xii.46*)—is left out, and once again, while Book III appears to end on a happy note, there are some dissonances under the surface.

4 Conclusion: Liquid Poetics

Baths, in Spenser's national epic, clearly have a symbolic meaning, but that meaning seems to fluctuate as we move from one bathing scene to another. The complex representations make it hard for the reader and the characters to see through appearances. Similarly to the damsels in the Bower of Bliss, Spenser conceals and reveals information to his reader, playing with their perception and at times tantalizing them, only to throw them off once again, misleading the reader on their quest to find meaning, to see through appearances. And while Spenser acknowledges the virtues of baths with his mention of famous ones and his putting Bath in the chronicle of England, his use of the bathing imagery reminds us of the fluidity of water. It has no fixed form, it changes as the poem goes along, from sensual and erotic to a symbol of chastity, from threat to salvation, from opaque to transparent, as if the poetic matter itself takes on the liquid form it describes. The fact that water defies any clear-cut definition allows Spenser to use this imagery to tend towards a form of liquid poetics which renders his poem deceivingly fluid. This fluidity is part of the transformative power of baths, as it softens the matter and changes its form. There is a protean logic behind the bathing scenes that culminates in the 1590 version with the image of the Hermaphrodite statue, and therefore a metamorphosis, while allowing for an underlying alchemical reading that ties into other bathing scenes in the poem.

Works Cited

Primary Sources

Spenser, Edmund. 2013. *The Faerie Queene* (1590), eds. Albert C. Hamilton, Hiroshi Yamashita and Toshiyuki Suzuki. Revised second edition. Longman Annotated English Poets. London, New York: Routledge, Taylor & Francis Group.

Secondary Sources

Britton, Dennis Austin. 2014. *Becoming Christian: Race, Reformation, and Early Modern English Romance*. New York: Fordham University Press.

Campana, Joseph. 2009. Boy Toys and Liquid Joys: Pleasure and Power in the Bower of Bliss. *Modern Philology* 106 (3): 465–496.

Cheney, Donald. 1972. Spenser's Hermaphrodite and the 1590 Faerie Queene. *PMLA* 87 (2): 192–200.

Chiari, Sophie. 2009. 'Désirs Masculins et Plaisirs Féminins à La Renaissance'. Presented at the séminaire IRIS, Paris 3-Sorbonne Nouvelle, October 26.

Dauber, Antoinette B. 1980. The Art of Veiling in the Bower of Bliss. *Spenser Studies* 1 (January): 163–175.

Faircloth, Nicki, and Vivian Thomas. 2014. *Shakespeare's Plants and Gardens: A Dictionary*. Arden Shakespeare Dictionary. London: Bloomsbury.

Grogan, Jane. 2009. "So Liuely and So Like, That Liuing Sence It Fayld": *Enargeia* and Ekphrasis in *The Faerie Queene*. *Word & Image* 25 (2): 166–177.

Hamilton, A.C., ed. 2014. *The Spenser Encyclopedia*. Longman Annotated English Poets. London, New York: Routledge, Taylor & Francis Group.

Krier, Theresa M. 1990. *Gazing on Secret Sights: Spenser, Classical Imitation, and the Decorums of Vision*. Ithaca: Cornell University Press.

Lees-Jeffries, Hester. 2003. From the Fountain to the Well: Redcrosse Learns to Read. *Studies in Philology* 100 (2): 135–176.

Liddell, Henry George, and Scott, Robert. 1940. *A Greek-English Lexicon*. Revised and Augmented throughout by Sir Henry Stuart Jones with the Assistance of Roderick McKenzie. Oxford: Clarendon Press.

Nohrnberg, James. 1976. *The Analogy of 'The Faerie Queene'*. Princeton University Press.

Ovid, and Arthur Golding. 1965. *Metamorphoses: The Arthur Golding Translation, 1567*. Ed. John Frederick Nims. New York: Macmillan.

Pinkus, Karen. 2006. Hermaphrodite Poetics. *Arcadia* 41 (1): 91–111.

Shroeder, John W. 1962. Spenser's Erotic Drama: The Orgoglio Episode. *ELH* 29 (2): 140–159.

Silberman, Lauren. 1987. The Hermaphrodite and the Metamorphosis of Spenserian Allegory. *English Literary Renaissance* 17 (2): 207–223.
Silberman, Lauren. 1995. *Transforming Desire: Erotic Knowledge in Books III and IV of The Faerie Queene*. Berkeley, CA: University of California Press.

CHAPTER 2

Fountain, Waters and Spas in John Webster's *The Duchess of Malfi*: From Blood Baths to 'Turkish Delights'

François Laroque

John Webster's *The Duchess of Malfi* (first performed in 1613–1614) is often seen as a sensationalist tragedy teeming with horrors of various sorts.[1] Maria Aberg's 2018 RSC production of the play at the Swan in Stratford exaggerated the horror of the tragedy by literally turning its second half into a shambles and smudging the whole stage platform with blood as described in the following review:

> By the end of this production of John Webster's [...] *The Duchess of Malfi*, the stage is swamped in blood. Initially seeping out of a gash in the huge, headless carcass of a beast hanging by its feet behind the action,

[1] All quotations from the play refer to Webster 2015 (Michael Neill's edition of *The Duchess of Malfi*).

F. Laroque (✉)
Département Monde Anglophone, Université
Sorbonne Nouvelle–Paris 3, Paris, France
e-mail: flaroque@orange.fr

S. Chiari and S. Cuisinier-Delorme (eds.), *Spa Culture and Literature in England, 1500–1800*, Early Modern Literature in History,
https://doi.org/10.1007/978-3-030-66568-5_2

> the blood spreads until it's tracked into every footprint. None of the characters escapes it, soaking into their clothes and smearing their skin. It's overwhelming, and it overwhelms Maria Aberg's staging. (Wicker 2018, online)

The imagery of blood which is recurrent in Webster's play visibly refers to Shakespeare's *Macbeth*, particularly when the title part affirms that 'blood will have blood' (Shakespeare 2015, 3.4.101) and, as the above critical review shows, modern directors are not afraid to take it quite literally and make it physically present onstage. Once blood is being shed it will, as it seems, initiate an unstoppable movement with the overriding impression that it is then impossible to wash it away:

> Will all great Neptune's ocean wash this blood
> Clean from my hand? No, this my hand will rather
> The multitudinous sea incarnadine,
> Making the green one red.
> (Shakespeare 2015, 2.2.61–64)

In other words, purgation and purification are hoped for but never achieved as the very waters, which should cleanse the stain and do away with it will then turn red, blood being thicker than water as the proverb goes. So, after taking a look at a possible historical parallel or precedent, I will analyse the place and function of water and wells, before considering the tentative idea that the baths are presented as a source of female emancipation and pleasure.

1 Historical Precedents

Besides its obvious links to the tradition of the revenge tragedy inaugurated by Thomas Kyd in *The Spanish Tragedy* (probably written in the late 1580 s) and plays like *Titus Andronicus*, *Hamlet* or *Macbeth*, such an obsession with blood in *The Duchess of Malfi* may also have taken its cue from a contemporary and particularly gory *fait divers*, namely the discovery by the Hungarian prince Palatine György Thurzo and his men (at the request of king Mathias Ist), of the gruesome blood baths which countess Elizabeth Báthory (1560–1614) used to take at her castle of Čachtice (part of today's Slovakia) in the hope of acquiring eternal youth. The blood was that of hundreds of young virgins, either servants of the castle or from the nearby villages. Indeed, '[s]he believed [...] that in a maiden's blood she possessed the elixir vitae, the source of never-failing youth and beauty' (Paget 1839, 68). The bloody Countess was arrested and she died in prison in 1614, at the time when Webster was writing his play.[2] But, in *The Duchess of Malfi*, it is of course not the title part but her two brothers, Ferdinand and the Cardinal who, metaphorically, but no less sadistically, 'bathe' themselves in their victims' blood.

Ironically, in the play, the Duchess's servant, Cariola, alludes to the baths in Spa or Lucca (3.2.301–302) in order to avoid making what she calls a 'feigned pilgrimage' (3.2.304) at the suggestion of Bosola who has just been made privy to the Duchess's secret marriage to her steward Antonio. Now, since the average temperature of the warm springs at Villa di Lucca by and large corresponds to the temperature of human blood (37–42° Celsius), there is a possible analogy with the Transylvanian countess (who was to inspire Bram Stoker's *Dracula* by way of the Jesuit scholar Laszlo Turoczi's *Tragica Historia* published in 1729), all the more so as Webster's Duchess also seems anxious to keep her youthful appearance when she expresses her fear that her hair ''gin to change' and that it will 'wax gray' (3.2.58–59). But the comparison between the two is of course only accidental as the Duchess, like her maid Cariola, is one of the main victims in the play. And, in contrast to the evil Countess, who was believed to be an adept of witchcraft and a black arts practitioner, Cariola is a simple, superstitious young woman for whom a progress to the baths at Lucca, a thermal station which, in the sixteenth century, was well known for its curative effects, is certainly to be preferred to the idea of committing a sacrilege ('this jesting with religion', 3.2.305). She had rather rely on lay and medical practices since, in her eyes, religion is a serious matter not to be tampered with. But, if one must identify a character in this play who is a representative of the dark forces of Satanism, it is certainly Ferdinand, the Duchess's brother, the future spectacular and grotesque werewolf in the last act. And naturally, against this radical and

[2] I have unfortunately been unable to find contemporary English documents (by way of pamphlets, ballads or broadsides) referring to the infamous countess. The first book that mentions the case is indeed the anonymous *The Present State of Hungary*, London, 1687. So, short of finding any evidence showing that Webster may have been aware of the case, I can only draw here a conjectural historical parallel between his play and the then much talked about *fait divers*.

absolute incarnation of evil, neither holy water nor the warm waters of the wells prove of any avail.

Still, one may wonder what the exact function of the various allusions to water, wells and baths in *The Duchess of Malfi* is, and whether they provide the expected purification in a play in which the simple idea of purgation remains at best a very distant illusion and, at worst, a dazzling mirage.

2 The Role of Wells and Water

For Aristotle, tragedy is a form of therapy, supposed to achieve a catharsis at the end meant to purge passions through the arousal of terror and pity. Oddly enough, the first permanent playhouse in London, the Theatre, was built outside the City walls on land known as Holy Well:

> [The Theatre] was located in the ancient land of Halliwell or Holy Well, so named from a holy well harboured within a Benedictine nunnery in the vicinity [...] It marks an interesting association, since other theatrical sites have sprung up beside holy wells. The first miracle plays in London were performed at Clerkenwell beside the clerks' well, for example, and the Sadlers Well theatre was erected beside a healing well of the same name. The association has never been properly examined, but it suggests that the theatre was still in a subliminal sense seen as a sacred or ritual activity. (Ackroyd 2005, 126)

In *The Duchess of Malfi*, a play performed at the private theatre of the Blackfriars, an ancient Dominican monastery in the precincts of the City, the Duchess swears by St Winfred (1.1.381), or Winifred, a saint whose shrine was in Holywell, Flintshire, 'a place of pilgrimage for the wealthier Catholic families of Warwickshire', according to the same historian (Ackroyd 2005, 23). Such an association between drama and a place known as an ancient sacred well, to which pilgrimages were probably made in pre-Reformation times, is indeed an intriguing one. According to Sophie Lemercier-Goddard, the pilgrimage to Loreto is evoked in the last act and it may have suggested to an English audience 'the popular shrine of Walsingham, Norfolk, which was then known as England's Nazareth' (Lemercier-Goddard 2019, 130). This association of playhouses with former places of pilgrimage and sacred wells indirectly suggests a connection between drama and holy waters as both places and institutions were meant to cleanse, purge, and purify on the physical, mental and spiritual levels.

In what he calls his 'meditation' (2.1.44), Bosola presents Castruccio and the Old Lady with a vision of the human body as a succession of the ugliest skin diseases:

> Man stands amazed to see his deformity
> In any other creature but himself.
> But in our own flesh, though we bear diseases
> Which have their true names only ta'en from beasts,
> As the most ulcerous wolf and swinish measle,
> Though we are eaten up of lice and worms,
> And though continually we bear about us
> A rotten and dead body, we delight
> To hide it in rich tissue [...]
> [*To Castruchio*] Your wife's gone to Rome: you two couple,
> and get you to the wells at Lucca to recover your aches.
> (2.1.50–62)

A cynic and a malcontent, he presents man's moral deformity in terms of medical imagery and it is thus logical that he should recommend the old couple to resort to 'the wells at Lucca' to try and cure their various ills and aches. What's more, as a former university student, he may indeed have heard from the works of Gabriele Falloppio, who was at the time a renowned Italian physician who believed in the curative powers of the wells (Moss 2012, 61–82).[3] As Valerie Finucci notes, '[t]he acqua di Villa [at Bagni di Lucca] was recommended, among other things, for dermatological problems [...] Earlier, another doctor [different from Falloppio] had given this same recommendation to his great grand-father, Francesco, who needed to address facial skin complications most likely caused by syphilis' (Finucci 2015, 110).

Melancholy is another disease, a mental and moral one this time, the runs deep in the Amalfitan court and it seems to affect almost all the characters in the play. According to Antonio who draws the following portrait of Bosola,

[3] The Italian physician was well known in England and is mentioned, for example, in the following (anonymous) title: *The true and perfect order to distill oyles out of al maner of spices seedes, rootes, and gummes with their perfect taste, smel, and sauour* (1575).

[t]his foul melancholy
Will poison all his goodness, for I'll tell you,
If too immoderate sleep be truly said
To be an inward rust unto the soul,
It then doth follow want of action
Breeds all black malcontents.
(1.1.72–78)

Bosola describes Ferdinand and the Cardinal 'as plum trees that grow crooked over standing pools' (1.1.48–49), while Ferdinand warns his sister, the Duchess, in those terms:

Now, hear me—
You live in a rank pasture here i'th'court
There is a kind of honeydew that's deadly;
'Twill poison your fame [...].
(1.1.297–300)

'Deadly honeydew', 'standing pools' or 'inward rust' are all varieties of stagnant waters that are associated with poison as they seem to spread forms of contagion that contaminate the body or endanger mental health, an idea which metaphorically stands for corruption.

Retrospectively, one sees the importance of the following passage, probably added for the revival of the play in 1617–1618, and directly lifted, in Webster's magpie style of writing, from Thomas Elyot's *The Image of Governance* (1541):

Antonio
In seeking to reduce both state and people
To a fixed order, their judicious king
Begins at home, quits first his royal palace
Of flatt'ring sycophants, of dissolute
And infamous persons—which he sweetly terms
His master's masterpiece, the work of heaven,
Consid'ring duly that a prince's court
Is like a common fountain, whence should flow
Pure silver drops in general; but if't chance
Some cursed example poison't near the head,
Death and diseases through the whole land spread.
(1.1.5–15)

This allusion to the Concino Concini affair (Louis XIII had then secretly encouraged the assassination of the Maréchal d'Ancre in April 1617 to purge the court of the Spanish influence) and the trope of the 'common fountain' serve as an overarching image which calls for a general purification of the court at Amalfi as well as for a veiled criticism of the corruption at the court of James I in the wake of the Howard–Carr scandal (Marcus 2009, 95; Laroque 2018, 41–44). The important words in the quotation are 'fountain', 'flow' (as opposed to 'rust' and 'standing pools'), 'silver drops', which right from the start emphasize the importance of resorting to cleansing waters in order to get rid of corruption, whether physical, mental, moral or political. In *The Duchess of Malfi*, the world is indeed presented as a great hospital—'places in the court are but like beds in the hospital' (1.1.65), Bosola exclaims in the first half of the play—and as a lunatic asylum in the second. In this desacralized context where religion is used as a source of power with no real spiritual mission or ambition, the sacred seems to have been replaced by a form of vague medical lore which is itself unable to cure the deep-seated evils the Duchy is a prey to. Instead of the 'pure silver drops' of the fountain of good government, the poison of rumour, of mad sexual fantasies and sadistic cruelty has turned Amalfi into a claustrophobic universe which becomes just another name for hell on earth. So, the purgation or purification process which is normally expected towards the denouement of a tragedy here fails to take place. At the end of the play, during which the Duchess and Antonio, their children (except one), Cariola, Bosola and the two Aragonian brothers all die poisoned, strangled or bled to death, the impression that prevails is one of absurdity and general confusion:

> *Bosola*
> Oh, this gloomy world!
> In what a shadow, or deep pit of darkness,
> Doth womanish and fearful mankind live!
> (5.5.98–100)

However, at this rather desperate and pessimistic juncture, it still remains possible to give another interpretation of the role of baths and thermal waters in the play, a role which will lead me to present the Duchess and her servant Cariola in a fairly different light, i.e. less as victims of the brothers' mad fury and jealousy, and rather as women with their own agenda in a world dominated by men.

3 The Baths as a Means of Female Emancipation and Autonomous Pleasure

The domestic scene in which the Duchess, Antonio and Cariola are indulging in apparently innocent jesting and merry-making, before the sinister arrival of Ferdinand, dagger in hand, represents one of the rare moments of happiness in a world always in danger of being destroyed because of the brothers' opposition to the idea of a possible remarriage on the part of their sister:

Duchess
To what use will you put me?
Antonio
We'll sleep together.
Duchess
Alas, what pleasure can two lovers find in sleep?
Cariola
My lord, I lie with her often, and I know
She'll much disquiet you—
Antonio [To the Duchess]
See you are complained of!
Cariola
For she's the sprawling'st bedfellow!
Antonio
I shall like her
The better for that.
Cariola
Sir, shall I ask you a question?
Antonio
I pray thee, Cariola.
Cariola
Wherefore still when you lie with my lady
Do you rise so early?
Antonio
Labouring men
Count the clock oftenest, Cariola,
Are glad when their task's ended.
Duchess
I'll stop your mouth.
[Kisses him]
Antonio
Nay, that's but one. Venus had two soft doves

> To draw her chariot; I must have another. [Kisses her].
> (3.2.9–22)

As Judith Haber puts it, 'here the three characters engage in a playful, erotic "chafing" (3.2.56) aimed not at the phallic orgasm/death that is constitutive of conventional tragedy, but at the feminine sexual excitement that was associated with pregnancy [...]. [T]hroughout this scene, the sexual innuendo circulates freely between [the three of] them' (Haber 1997, 138–139). Haber then associates this kind of erotic speech with 'gossip' and a specifically feminine kind of talk:

> [...] one must note that 'gossip' is associated with speech – and with a particular kind of speech, both feared and disdained by men: a chattering, frivolous, 'sportive' speech [...]. In early modern contexts [...] 'to gossip' seems to imply 'to speak as a woman'; loosely flowing like women's bodies, similarly lacking in control and closure, 'gossiping' was the activity of all-female gatherings, and was often connected with explicit hostility to males. (Haber 1997, 143)

Pascale Aebischer goes even further when she claims that Mike Figgis's *Hotel*, a 2001 film loosely adapted from *The Duchess of Malfi*, allows us to 'embody and sexualize the implicit causal link in Webster's play between the mutual affection of mistress and maid, which creates 'a secret space in the midst of male society' and 'a haven where the normal modes of subjection are cancelled', and the Duchess's ability to express her autonomous identity and desires. It is the homosocial (and potentially homoerotic) egalitarian intimacy between the Duchess and her female bedfellow that is exposed in *Hotel* as the unacknowledged origin of the Duchess's preposterous heterosexual transgression of class and gender boundaries (Aebischer 2009, 279–305).

As I have already pointed out above, in act 3, scene 2, the Duchess is also worried by the idea that she is beginning to age (3.2.58–95), something which may suggest a latent desire to resort to the baths in order to rejuvenate her figure as in the myth of the Fountain of Youth painted by Lucas Cranach the Elder in 1546. What's more, bearing in mind this idea of female gossip and of complicity between women, one may propose a new reading of the passage when Cariola says that it were better for the Duchess 'to progress to the baths/At Lucca, or go visit the Spa/In Germany' (3.3.301–303). Indeed, the situation of the

Duchess, as a woman locked up by her brothers in her palace, is somewhat reminiscent of the Turkish women who, according to Nicolas de Nicolay (1517–1583), delight to go to the baths 'as an honest excuse to go abroad of their houses':

> The Turks wiues by ordinary custome & auncient obseruation, which they do reserue of the old custome of Asia and Graecia do delight et al. times to haunt the bathes, aswel for the continuaunce of their health, as beautifiyng of their persons which is not to be reputed as spoken of the women of base estate or condition, but likewise of the great and notable dames, which ordinarily doe frequent the bathes 2. or 3. times in the weeke, not the publike but their priuate bathes, which for the most part they haue very fair within their houses or Sarails, [...] to haue good occasion and honest excuse too goe abroade out of their houses, within the whiche they are continually closed vppe for the greate ielousie of theyr husbandes [...] so as the Turky women being shut vp without permission to go abroad, nor to appeare in the streets openly, except it be going to the bathes, [...] for that to those bathes no men do frequent, so long as the women are there very great amity proceding only through the frequentation & resort to the bathes: yea & somtimes become so feruently in loue the one of the other as if it were with men, in such sort that perceiuing some maiden, or woman· of excellent beauty, they wil not ceasse vntil they haue found means to bath with them, & to handle & grope them euery where at their pleasures, so ful they are of luxuriousnes & feminine wantonnes. (de Nicolay 1585, Book II, chap. 22, fols. $59^{r\text{-}v}$)[4]

Speaking of Antonio, Bosola had indeed alluded to the Turks in his wild hypocritical flattery of the Duchess: 'Should you want/Soldiers, 'twould make the very Turks and Moors/Turn Christians and serve you for this act' (3.2.276–278). The Turkish baths that Nicolas de Nicolay depicts in his 'Oriental peregrinations' is not represented in any of the many engravings which richly illustrate the book but they will later inspire the French orientalists as may be seen on the famous 'Turkish bath', a painting by Jean-Auguste-Dominique Ingres (1852–1859).

Since the pressure put by the two Aragonian brothers on the Duchess amounts to what Turkish women were then being subject to, it is tempting to read Cariola's allusion to the 'baths at Lucca' and to 'the Spa in Germany' as an occasion for maid and mistress to release the tension

[4] The book was originally published in French in 1563.

and find an outlet, a space of liberty for gossip and erotic 'chafing', away from the stifling, despotic authority of patriarchy. As a matter of fact, going to the baths at Lucca for the Duchess and Cariola would produce a result exactly contrary to what Bosola's false encomium announces, as it would amount to making the two Christian women literally turn Turk!

But, like the false pilgrimage to Ancona, going to the baths in Lucca is bound to prove a total illusion as any sort of escape is de facto made impossible in the play; the two women will be brought back to their Amalfitan palace, then transformed into a prison and a site of excruciating moral and physical torment. The prospect of sensual baths in the warm springs of Villa di Lucca—the equivalent for Cariola and the Duchess of the Turkish delights described by the French traveller and geographer—finally take us back to the dark no-exit place where the grotesque horrors perpetrated by Ferdinand against the Duchess and her maid turn the wish-fulfilment of rejuvenation at the baths into a frail fantasy rapidly annihilated by the frightening nightmare of persecution and torture.

4 Conclusion: Dirty Waters

So, even though the allusions to water, wells, baths and thermal waters in Webster's tragedy certainly work as tentative efforts to achieve some sort of physical and moral purification, a role which, up to a point, was also that of the public playhouses in London which were supposed to provide the spectator with a form of *catharsis*. But in the tragedy, they all prove powerless and fail to reverse the tragic course of events and provide the spectator with the expected purgation at the end. However, in a play where women are represented as women on top who challenge patriarchy and take the initiative in love and marriage, but who, on the other hand, are being victimized by sick and sadistic brothers embodying a form of repressive patriarchy, the allusion to the 'baths at Lucca' may well have referred, albeit unconsciously, to a vague and vain hope of rejuvenation popularized by the old myth of the Fountain of Youth. Indeed, rather than achieve a general purification and moral cure, the recurrent allusions to fountains, pure water drops, bubbles and baths in the play all actually seem to point to a tentative chance to enjoy an all-female company far from the constant male harassment at Amalfi. Sadly, such an illusion is only brought forth in order to be later blown to pieces, not by the mad jealousy of a husband, as in the case of the Turks, but by the morbid sexual fantasies of the two Spanish brothers who, to the eyes of a Puritan like John Webster, both stand for the radical evil of a perverted Catholicism and, more topically, for the vices and corruption at the court of James I, which this particular tragedy proves so anxious to expose. Ultimately, the play leaves us with a vision of melting snow and dirty waters.

Works Cited

Primary Sources

An. 1575. *The true and perfect order to distill oyles out of al maner of spices seedes, rootes, and gummes with their perfect taste, smel, and sauour: where vnto is added some of their ver[t]ues gathered out of sundry aucthors. As Gualterius, Rissius, Guinthery Andernaty, Phillipus, Hermanus, Leonardo, Phirauante, Phallopius, Cardanus*. London: Printed by J. Charlewood, STC (2nd ed.)/ 19181.3.

Nicolay, Nicolas de. 1585. *The Nauigations, Peregrinations and Voyages, Made Into Turkie by Nicholas Nicholay*, Trans. Thomas Washington. London: Printed by Thomas Dawson, STC (2nd ed.) 18574.

Shakespeare, William. 2015. *Macbeth*. eds. Sandra Clark and Pamela Mason. London: Bloomsbury (The Arden Shakespeare).

Webster, John. 2009. *The Duchess of Malfi* (1612). ed. Leah S. Marcus. London: Methuen (Arden Early Modern Drama).

Webster, John. 2015. *The Duchess of Malfi* (1612). ed. Michael Neill. New York and London: W.W. Norton & Company.

Secondary Sources

Ackroyd, Peter. 2005. *Shakespeare, the Biography*. London: Chatto and Windus.

Aebischer, Pascale. 2009. Shakespearean Heritage and the Preposterous 'Contemporary Jacobean' Film: Mike Figgis's Hotel. *Shakespeare Quarterly* 60: 279–303.

Finucci, Valerie. 2015. *The Prince's Body. Vincenzo Gonzaga and Renaissance Medicine*. Cambridge: Harvard University Press.

Haber, Judith. 1997. "My Body Bestow upon My Women": The Space of the Feminine in *The Duchess of Malfi*. *Renaissance Drama*, New Series, vol. 28, The Space of the Stage, 133–159.

Laroque, François. 2018. *John Webster. The Duchess of Malfi*. Paris: Éditions Ellipses.

Lemercier-Goddard, Sophie. 2019. Going Places. Hauntings and Mobilities in *The Duchess of Malfi*. In *John Webster's 'Dismal Tragedy'*. The Duchess of Malfi

Reconsidered, eds. Sophie Chiari and Sophie Lemercier-Goddard, 121–136. Clermont-Ferrand, Presses Universitaires Blaise Pascal.

Moss, Jean Dietz. 2012. The Promotion of Bath Waters by Physicians in the Renaissance. In *Rhetoric and Medicine in Early Modern Europe*. eds. Stephen Pender and Nancy S. Struever, 61–82. Routledge, London and New York.

Paget, John. 1839. *Hungary and Transylvania: With Remarks on her Condition: Social, Political, Economical*. 2 vols. London: John Murray.

Wicker, Tom. *The Duchess of Malfi*. *The Stage*, 8 March 2018. https://www.thestage.co.uk/reviews/the-duchess-of-malfi-review-at-swan-theatre-stratford-upon-avon–blood-soaked-and gut-wrenching. Accessed October 26, 2020.

CHAPTER 3

Taking the Cure: Mineral Waters and Love's Folly in Lady Mary Wroth's *The Countess of Montgomery's Urania*

Tiffany Jo Werth

Plunges into icy cold salty water from sea cliffs, immersive warm water baths underground, draughts drunk from healing springs—characters throughout Lady Mary Wroth's English romance, *The Countess of Montgomery's Urania* (1621), engage a variety of hydrotherapeutic cures to erase or enflame love's afflictions. Even Melissea, the narrative's revered source of counsel and enchantress, operates what appears to be a kind of curative spa on the island of Delos. In multiple episodes, the newly revived interest in the healing properties of mineral waters infiltrate the imaginative landscape. Self-consciously writing within a narrative template of classical and continental romances where miraculous water cures eradicate love's folly, Wroth subtly nuances how her characters take the water. This chapter demonstrates how *Urania*'s imagined cures speak to evolving

T. J. Werth (✉)
Department of English, University of California, Davis, CA, USA
e-mail: tjwerth@ucdavis.edu

S. Chiari and S. Cuisinier-Delorme (eds.), *Spa Culture and Literature in England, 1500–1800*, Early Modern Literature in History,
https://doi.org/10.1007/978-3-030-66568-5_3

understanding of the world's natural wonders, changing medical practice, and shifting religious belief. They foreground, moreover, a coterie of women who practise the efficacious ministration of healing water for both physical and mental health. Wroth's early seventeenth-century romance offers *avant la lettre* a fascinating perspective on how the literary imagination might be both responsive to, but also proleptic of, an emergent spa culture.

I argue that the early modern literary imagination was conversant with an emerging bath culture. The focus will be the late sixteenth- and early seventeenth century, when the medicinal powers of mineral waters regained popularity in England but before spa culture became fashionable. Three questions drive the argument. First, how, or does, the vogue for 'taking the water' infiltrate the literary imagination? Second, how might imaginative episodes of water cures within literary texts herald the later development of spa cultures? And third, what correlations can be drawn between literature and formative cultural processes? As early modern historian Amanda E. Herbert shows, urban spas at notable cities such as Bath, Tunbridge, and Epsom were vibrant spaces in England by the Restoration in 1660 (Herbert 2014, 118). *The Countess of Montgomery's Urania*, the first prose romance written in English by a woman, Lady Mary Wroth, is published almost half a century earlier, in 1621, and yet it shows a marked fascination with water cures.

Lady Mary Wroth's *Urania* offers an imaginative perspective on this volume's focus on early modern English bath and spa culture because it centres around a network of women who inhabit a chivalric romance landscape and who undergo, at critical narrative junctures, a variety of prescribed water cures. *Urania*'s plot centres around two major pairs of brothers and sisters, Pamphilia and Parselius (children to the King of Morea) and Urania and Amphilanthus (children to the King of Naples), and a network of kin, whose star-crossed and unrequited loves complicate—and drive—the story. The narrative revives the fantasy of the Holy Roman Empire in the West that had been given new life with King James' ascension to the throne, which brought Britain under one rule. Pamphilia, one of several avatars within the fiction for Lady Mary Wroth herself, pursues the love of Amphilanthus, an emperor who seeks to unify the Christian world, but who is also a coded reference to Wroth's cousin and lover, William Herbert. Their story provides the basis for one of the text's key *questioni d'amore*: constancy in love. Other characters who figure in this essay include Amphilanthus's sister, the eponymous Urania, a close friend and confidant to Pamphilia and cipher for Mary Sidney Herbert, the Countess of Pembroke; Parselius, Pamphilia's brother who loves Urania; a wise woman and seer named Melissea, who dwells on the island of Delos; and a shepherdess, Alarina, rejected by her lover. These characters inhabit a two-volume narrative of interpolated chivalric romance adventure and pastoral interludes.

Although *Urania* features many of the stock conventions of the romance and pastoral modes, Wroth's frequently satirical perspective renders it a highly self-conscious narrative. The characters as well as many of the story's episodes are metanarratives of contemporary Jacobean characters and incidents—so much so that one contemporary, Sir Edward Denny, cried foul over what he believed was a slanderous portrayal of his family. He subsequently wrote and circulated a vicious verse attack on Lady Mary Wroth.[1] Sir Edward Denny's impassioned attack reveals what a large body of criticism interprets as an all too real interpenetration of the imaginative romance and its pastoral modes with Jacobean court life and culture. Thus, although imaginative fiction, *Urania's* depiction of historical events and people puts its portrayal of water cures in dialogue with the kinds of historical shifts in bath and spa culture at the heart of this volume.

1 Literary Contexts for Taking the Waters

In this chapter, I examine three critical episodes within *Urania*'s two-volume story when characters 'take the water' to cure their love melancholy. These episodes happen at the so-called Lover's Leap at Santa Maura, at a remote medicinal mountain spring, and deep inside what Wroth describes as a 'Very curious Vault' at the heart of Melissea's palace on Delos (Wroth 1999, 2.52).

In the first, mariners guide a boat to 'the white Rocke' where a brother, Amphilanthus, and his lovesick sister, Urania, land and climb to stand atop a high 'Rocke' overlooking the sea near Santa Maura, a fort located on the northern coast of Leucas, an Ionian island off the western coast of Greece (Wroth 1995, 1.181). Standing atop the cliff, Amphilanthus holds his sister Urania close as he explains an earlier directive given to him by the text's wise woman and counsellor Melissea: 'I must throw thee

[1] Edward Denny's attack is reprinted in (L.M. Wroth 1983) 34.

into the Sea; pardon me, Heaven appoints it so' (Wroth 1995, 1.230). '[K]inde teares proceeded from them both' when he lets her slip from his arms to plummet into the sea below (Wroth 1995, 1.230). As 'shee fell, so fell his heart in woe, drownd in as deep an Ocean of despaire' but before Urania can sink below the waves, a third figure 'who lay in a craggy part of the Rocke, furiously threw himself unto her,' amidst the churning waves (Wroth 1995, 1.230). Rather than a tragic drowning, however, Amphilanthus and the reader are immediately called to 'wonder and all joy' as 'two men in a boate came rowing' who 'spared not danger, or life it selfe' to rescue both Urania, and the character Parselius who dove off the cliff after her for love, from the 'Deepes' that were 'ambitious of such a prize' (Wroth 1995, 1.230).

The second episode features a shepherdess named Alarina who, despairing from an unrequited love, wanders alone with her sheep into 'a countrie hilly' with 'rocks which were both steepe yet easie to ascend' atop a ragged hill 'crownd with milke white rocks, in bignesse strange' (Wroth 1995, 1.223). She 'sat downe in a stone of mighty height' and from this lofty perch spies below 'as it were a Spring' where 'folks below' 'did drinke' (Wroth 1999, 1.223). Descending to the plain below, she 'civilly demanded if that spring were medicinable, or what made them with so much affectionate ceremony to drinke, and as it were, adore it;' one man 'made answere' that it was 'divine and sacred water, which did cure all harmes' and recounted 'many strange works that water had perfomd' (Wroth 1999, 1.223). The shepherdess learns that she must drink of it 'seven times and thrice seven dayes' and so she 'resolv'd the task, and dranke' and soon found herself 'alterd in al things [...] my whole condition alterd, I grew free, and free from love, to which I late was slave' (Wroth 1999, 1.223). To reflect her altered state of mind, she changes her name from Alarina to Silviana. In the third and most arresting episode, the reader must imagine a young noblewoman, named Antissia, wearing what the narrator describes as a strange attire and acting with 'too high wrought' folly and 'frantick tricks' (Wroth 1999, 2.52) arriving at Delos, home to the text's seer and wise woman, Melissea. Melissea possesses skill in the 'Art of Astrologie' (Wroth 1995, 1.139), administers prophecies of love, and, most important for this reading, prescribes a variety of water cures to love-afflicted characters. It is her directions that Amphilanthus follows when he 'lets slip' Urania from Santa Maura's cliff into the sea. Antissia, like all the characters thus far discussed, suffers from unrequited love (despite having been married to another). The 'frantick' Antissia sails to seek cure from Melissea in her 'faire Pallace of Alabaster' (Wroth 1999, 1.139).

Deep inside a cave, far below her alabaster palace, Melissea brings Antissia to a 'stately roome' where music plays softly. In a fit of fury, Antissia flings herself on a 'rich bed' (Wroth 1999, 2.52). Then, the bed 'pleasingly and quietly sunck with her into a Very curious Vault' where if she waked, she'd discover 'extreame darck' and should she move suddenly, 'she showld fallinto a deepe Lake of water, luke warme onely and made by Melisseas skill' (Wroth 1999, 2.52). She remains submerged in this 'Vault' for 'four and tweny howers;' when one day later she awakes, her 'colour rose in her cheeks, shame in her hart' at her 'apparel, soe strange, soe phantastick' and at the remembrance of her 'extreame passion' (Wroth 1999, 2.53). The narrator describes her as 'perfectly recovered from all her follys and frantick tricks, receaving her right spirits againe about her' (Wroth 1999, 2.52). To ensure 'misfortunes' and 'phantesie perish' and are 'never more appeere,' Melissea also gives her a 'rich cup of Gold wherin was most pleasing drinke' (Wroth 1999, 2.53). Lest Antissia's husband also remember all that had passed, he too is given a drink 'his owne health in Leathe' and so too 'love, and all civility remained' while all 'fancies ore the thoughts of phantasies being cleane lost' (Wroth 1999, 2.53). The newly happy couple stay some days with Melissea in 'great content' (Wroth 1999, 2.53).

This essay examines only three such episodes, but water cures recur as a motif with various forms of hydrotherapy administered throughout *Urania*. These three episodes exemplify the larger textual patterns that depict external as well as internal methods of taking the water: the first external method at Santa Maura plunges the patient into salty cold water; the second and third entail an internal cure by drinking a draught from a spring or a cup; and the third appears to operate along external principles familiar to modern audiences who might visit a float house.[2] All three incidents of taking the waters aim to cure erotic passions, to lift

[2] Contemporary examples of similar flotation therapy are on offer at Float house (Canada). The web page (http://www.floathouse.ca. Accessed October 26, 2020) advertises how clients might visit the Float House in Vancouver, BC where they might experience 'extreme positive buoyancy' and a sensory deprivation where the client doesn't 'feel, see or hear anything;' the website claims that such sensory deprivation has a 'plethora of benefits' for health and wellbeing. These modern-day float houses promise similar cures to that which Melissea provides for the lovesick Antissia.

spirits burdened by unrequited love, and to sooth an enflamed, overactive memory—that is, to put it in modern terms, they promise a form of affective, or what we might term mental or emotional healing, a plethora of benefits cued especially to women, but also salubrious for men.

To understand how Wroth's *Urania* enters into dialogue with cultural and historical attitudes for taking the waters, her hydrotherapeutic treatments need to be read first against literary precedents. The first episode, Urania's plunge from Santa Maura's cliff into the turbulent sea, revisits a famous legend told in both classical and continental sources. A geographic as well as mythological place, Santa Maura was a fort along the high promontory of Leucas, one of the Ionian islands off the western coast of Greece. Its earliest myths recorded tell how, to appease the gods' fury, sacrificial victims were hurled annually into the waves below.[3] But another legend also sprang up via Ovid that Wroth adopts. In the likely source story of Ovid's *Heroides*, which was translated into English by George Turberville, Sappho's unrequited love prompts her to ponder Leucadia's lofty cliff. Sappho recalls how Deucalion, inflamed with love for Pyrra, 'did fall/Of purpose' and 'sustained no hurt at all. /And straight conuersed loue forsook his swelting breast/That was ydrencht' (Ovid 1567, Sig. Piii^{v}). The Ovidean tale marvels that Deucalion 'sustained no hurt at all' but, unlike Wroth, the story provides no rescue boat; rather its 'power' is a 'hidden force by kind' (Ovid 1567, Sig. Piii^{v}).[4] The reader is called to wonder how the immersive drenching 'straight' cured 'his swelting breast' of its afflictive melancholy, 'conversed love' (Ovid 1567, Sig. Piii^{v}). In Ovid's account the immersion in the waters below Santa Maura cure by 'hidden force' immediately, miraculously and conclusively.

The classical account of Leucadia also appears in Wroth's near-contemporary Italian predecessor Jacobo Sannazaro in his *Arcadia*. In the Ninth eclogue, a shepherd company meets the lovesick character Clonico; they counsel him to travel to Leucadia's cliff. They tell Clonico that one night a sparrow advised a weeping nightingale to find a cure 'in Leucadia' where 'stands a lofty cliff, such that whoever should leap from it into the

[3] See L.M. Wroth (1995, 733). In the *Commentary* accompanying her edition of *Urania*, Josephine Roberts cites as sources for this legend Strabo's *Geography* (10.452), Ovid's *Fasti* (5.630) and Aelion *On the Characteristics of Animals* (11.8–10).

[4] According to Josephine Roberts, Joan de Jean traces the process by which Ovid's tales became a part of Sappho's biography (L.M. Wroth 1995). See Joan de Jean, *Fictions of Sappho 1546–1937* (Chicago: University of Chicago Press, 1989), 69–70, 104–105.

sea would be, without any injury, free from his sorrow' (Sannazaro 1966, 92). A lark chimes in that this lofty cliff lies 'in the territory of Greece' (Sannazaro 1966, 92). The nightingale protests that 'there was no virtue in the water' but a black merle, a grosbeak, and a siskin reprove him for his folly in not believing in 'the heavenly powers [that] were infused in sacred springs' wherewith they reassure him of all the 'virtues' of various water sources (Sannazaro 1966, 92). Sannazaro's story of the lover's leap from Santa Maura abounds with wondrous details that firmly align Leucadia's water with miraculous 'heavenly' powers, and whose promised cure, like that in Ovid, is conclusively transformative.

Wroth follows the literary precedent of the Leucadian lover's leap from Ovid and Sannazaro and allots healing powers to the waters below Santa Maura. But her description, while retaining elements of wonder, complicates 'heavenly' or miraculous powers as being the source for the characters' sudden change of heart. Instead, Wroth's narrative renders the healing agency, or 'virtues,' in the waters ambiguous. A few small, critical alterations bear notice. First, Wroth's characters act on the instructions of *Urania's* wise woman, Melissea, who counsels those suffering from love melancholy to be plunged into its waters. Second, her characters are not miraculously saved from drowning, but are instead rescued by a nearby boat who hazards its own safety to deliver them to shore. The rescue boat provides a plausible rationale for how those who leap do not drown but are safely brought back to shore.

Finally, and perhaps most crucially, the leap from Santa Maura only appears as efficacious as that in Ovid or Sannazaro; Urania and Parselius arrive safely on shore 'soundly washed' (Wroth 1995, 1.230). All their friends on shore witness 'the operation of that water:' both characters find their former passions quite forgotten, Parselius 'knew nothing of his former love to her,' and Urania can without 'jealousie, or anger' wish Parselius happiness with his new bride, Dalinea (Wroth 1995, 1.230–231). As the narrative progresses, however, it becomes evident that the cure itself is deceptive, or at least short-lived. As I have argued elsewhere, a melancholy guilt and sense of loss haunts the characters and taints their future relationships.[5] Sad dreams will haunt Parselius wherein Urania appears and 'furiously revild me for my change' and sends 'revenge

[5] In the introduction to Volume 1, Josephine Roberts calls attention to Wroth's seeming wariness of miraculous water cures (see L.M. Wroth 1995, xxvii). See also my discussion in Werth 2011, 146.

in scorne, and worst contempt' (Wroth 1995, 1.243). Late in the second volume, Urania remembers her 'Olde passions' with 'hunny, with Gall, with pleasure, with torture, with injoying, with flatt laments for never obtaining' (Wroth 1999, 2.32). Taking the waters might alleviate love's melancholy, but the drenching does not erase the 'flatt laments' of unrequited love, whose feelings linger and flare years later. Wroth thus subtly nuances the earlier literary accounts, rendering the operation of the water less wholly miraculous and more contingent on strategic interventions by close friends and alliances.

A similarly reversible outcome results from the internal ministration of taking the waters in *Urania*. The second exemplary episode, in which the shepherdess Alarina discovers a remote mountain spring, appropriates a water cure motif from another continental romance, Jorge de Montemayor's *Diana* (1559). Like *Urania*, much of *Diana's* trajectory seeks relief from unrequited love. As rendered into English in 1598 by Bartholomew Yong, two love melancholic characters seek an enchantress, Felicia, who, similar to Wroth's Melissea, works 'to cure and remedie the passions of love' (Montemayor 1968, 160). In this version of the story, Felicia prescribes that the afflicted characters drink from 'two cruets of fine crystal' filled with a miraculous water. Drinking the waters transforms the lovers into a sleepy oblivion. 'Thou shalt marvell yet more, after they awake,' Felicia promises the anxiously waiting friends, 'because the water hath by this time wrought those operations it should do' (Montemayor 1968, 187). As promised, the former lovers soon awake with 'perfect wits and judgement' (Montemayor 1968, 187). In Montemayor's story, the water's effects are comprehensive and long term, for later in the narrative when one character, Syrenus, encounters his former beloved, the titular Diana, it makes such a 'forcible motion in his minde' that 'if the virtue of the water, which sage Felicia had given him, had not made him forget his olde love; it might well have beene, that there was nothing else in the worlde that coulde have let him from renewing it againe' (Montemayor 1968, 220). The 'virtue' of the water is such that it works lasting wonders, but in Wroth's reworking of the motif, the cure is less miraculous.

Wroth's shepherdess Alarina, who also takes the curative spring water internally by drinking, experiences a later narrative regression similar to that of Urania and the 'soundly washed' lovers who leapt from Santa Maura. When Pamphilia first meets Alarina, Alarina tells of her 'cure' that resulted from drinking the mineral waters bubbling from the remote mountain stream. After taking the prescribed cure, her love melancholy evaporates and prompts her to adopt a new identity as Silviana, a chaste nymph devoted to the virgin huntress Diana. Although the administration of drinking the waters limns that of Montemayor's story, Wroth departs from the narrative template in critical ways. Montemayor's Felicea administers the miraculous water via 'two cruets of fine crystal' (Montemayor 1968, 187). Bartholomew Yong's translation from the original Spanish into the English word 'cruet' points to a sacramental reading.[6] The *Oxford English Dictionary*, for instance, defines 'cruet' to be a small container specifically for the water or wine used in the Eucharistic service. Montemayor's delivery method for taking the waters, then, suggests a miraculous transformation, undergirded by religious undertones that might justify the virtue of the water as being holy or blessed. By contrast, in Wroth, Alarina 'civilly demands' of the local inhabitants if the spring is 'medicinable' and receives answer that 'it was divine and sacred,' but that a regimen must be followed that entails drinking of the waters from the stream seven times and 'thrice seven dayes' (Wroth 1995, 1.223). The cure, in other words, is not instant and miraculous. It entails a regimen of drinking the waters according to a prescribed formula. As detailed in the next section, prescriptions for taking the waters were gaining ground in contemporary discourse, including medical treatises as well as Robert Burton's *The Anatomy of Melancholy*, also published the same year as Wroth's *Urania* in 1621.

Given the nature of Alarina's tasked course for taking the waters, the reader may understandably share Pamphilia's bewilderment when, only a couple of hundred pages later, she again meets Silviana aka Alarina, who is bedecked for her marriage to her previously scornful lover. She has abandoned her chastity and service to Diana. Alarina, as she again calls herself, hastens to explain the resumption of her former passion. She recounts how, upon sight of her beloved, she 'hung downe' her head that she thought to deceive herself that she was otherwise than a 'poore miserable captive to love' (Wroth 1995, 1.483). Unlike in Montemayor's story, taking the water does not provide a lasting cure. The only miracle in *Urania* is that the lover who previously scorned Alarina now, inexplicably, adores her. Alarina herself seems blithely untroubled by her return to love. But the reader may well share Pamphilia's scepticism that such a reversal is inconstant and troubling.

[6] For a reading of this episode within a larger discussion of romance's Catholic taint for many English readers, see Werth (2011, 148).

Finally, in one of the most spectacular immersive water cures portrayed in *Urania*, Antissia's twenty-four-hour submersion in Melissea's early seventeenth-century version of a float house, a similar pattern emerges, although there does not appear to be a literary precedent for comparison. In the first two cases of taking the waters, Urania and Alarina suffer unrequited love melancholy; they are not, however, mad. Antissia, the third case study, becomes so by Volume 2. The narrator describes how her eventual husband, Dolorindus, is a 'loving husband tormented with a mad wife; a discreet man brought to bee accompany[i]ed onely with frenzeis and distempers' that bring him nothing but 'perpetuall vexation' and 'never ceasing torments for ungratefullnes (Wroth 1999, 2.50). In what one must imagine is desperation, he sails with his frantic wife Antissia to 'the Coste of Delos, wher the sage Melissea remain'd' (Wroth 1999, 2.51). '[C]onveied' as 'secretly as they cowld to the pallace' they consult Melissea who administers the 24-hour immersion below the alabaster palace within a 'deep Lake of water, luke warme onely' (Wroth 1999, 2.52). Like the previous episodes, the immersive cure appears efficacious. Antissia seemingly recovers herself and the couple leave in 'great content' (Wroth 1999, 2.53). But, as with the other water cures, a couple of hundred pages later, the reader encounters Antissia again slipping into madness. She confesses that she is 'nott soe perfectly recovered in my owne opinion' and fears she will entertain her 'olde whimsies again' (Wroth 1999, 2.252, 253, and 255).

All three examples of taking the waters in Wroth's *Urania* show subtle but critical revisions to existing literary motifs. In what follows, the essay explores how Wroth's revisions correspond to epistemological and religious shifts around bath culture in late sixteenth- and early seventeenth-century England. While Wroth does not entirely dismiss the water's miraculous powers, she includes a variety of non-miraculous details and delivery methods that work to enhance the natural, rather than supernatural, explanations for their power. She does so in dialogue with new knowledge about the natural world, specifically about mineral waters and healing, that were shaping medical practice. These epistemological shifts, moreover, made taking the waters more congenial to a reformed, and reforming, English religious culture.

2 Historical Interloquators: Aqueous Mineral Genesis, Medical Practice, and Religious Belief

A little noticed, but crucial, descriptive textual detail of the landscapes wherein Wroth's water cures occur merits attention. Wroth does not designate her curative water as explicitly mineral nor are the waters taken at a designated spa town or well. However, she supplies a critical descriptive detail that speaks to emerging knowledge about natural landscape elements that were believed to indicate the likelihood of healing water. In each of the above three case studies, the curative waters flow in proximity to rather unusual, notable, rocky formations. In the first, Santa Maura, familiar from classical as well as continental literature as 'the lover's leap' or 'the Leucadian leap,' is recognizable as a geographic as well as a fictive location on account of its distinctive rocky white cliff jutting above a choppy, briny sea; in the second, Alarina discovers the curious healing spring amidst a jumbled crown of unusual white rocks; in the third, Antissia floats for twenty-four hours deep within the vault of an alabaster palace on the island of Delos. These seemingly incidental landscape details matter because they adduce evidence of healing waters differed from 'common' waters in that they possessed a mineral content.

The rocky mineralized settings of *Urania*'s healing waters engage them in conversation with the emerging scientific pursuit to understand mineral water sources and their virtues. When Wroth publishes *Urania* in 1621, it was still impossible to ascertain what constituted mineral waters. As Noel G. Coley writes, as late as the early 1700s, 'an accurate analysis of waters was one of the most difficult problems;' the first attempt to systematize mineral water analysis in England didn't occur until the 1730 s and, even then, it was not very successful (Coley 1990, 58). But even although the precise mineral or metallic content of waters could not be defined, they were believed to differ from common water in their medicinal effects on the body and writers relied on sense perception and external observation to gauge—or discover—their mineral composition.

As a 1587 treatise by Walter Baley on 'medicinall waters' in Warwickshire in England explains, 'no doubt many and rare vertues and qualities are in them far beyond common waters, as will appeere by diligent search of their minerals' (Baley 1587, Sig. A^r).[7] Baley undertakes a 'diligent search' to uncover the 'minerals' from 'which the water' took their virtues by first distilling them, after which he concludes that a 'certaine residence, in color whitish, and in taste somewhat salt' remains (Baley 1587, Sig. B3^v). This property, Baley writes, is common to 'limestone, plaister, and alabaster' but mostly indicative of limestone, ordinarily white in colour, which might be discerned by a certain 'stonie crust' around the water source that indicates the presence of Nitre or Allum (Baley 1587, Sig. B4^r). Baley's treatise shows that as the lay English public became interested in identifying natural causes for the healing waters, they often looked for evidence of its mineral qualities—whether in the external presence of the whitish stone crust or in its quality of what Baley will call 'stone juice' (Baley 1587, Sig.A4^v). Baley's treatise offers one example for how despite deficiencies in contemporary chemical analysis, the popularity of mineral waters rose steadily, if sporadically, from the late 1580's onwards in England.[8]

Baley's interest in uncovering the mineral source for healing waters was likely influenced by the Italian physician Francesco Frigimelica, who published *De balneis omania quae extant* in 1552. Medical historian Roy Porter, in fact, regards this 1552 publication as a 'chronological watershed' in the perception and use of water as therapy as this influential treatise rehabilitated the medicinal use of spa waters (Porter 1990, x). In England, the medicinal rehabilitation of healing waters relied on identifying the properties from which the healing waters 'draw their vertues,' which were frequently observed to reside in a mineral content (Baley 1587, Sig. B2^v). Baley stresses the importance to 'better understand the secret faculties of these waters' by examining their mineral quality or 'stone juice' (Baley 1587, Sig.B2^v).

[7] For a discussion of mineral waters in a Scottish context, which similarly sought to dampen the miraculous while retaining the therapeutic virtues, see Jillings, Karen (2013). 'Scotland's 'naturall elixirs' and 'sacred liquors': Explaining the Medicinal Power of Mineral Waters'. *Parergon* 30 (2): 59–79.

[8] While this essay focuses on Baley's treatise, other examples can be found in the following late sixteenth-century English texts: Jones, John. 1572. *The Bathes of Bathes Ayde: Wonderfull and most excellent, agaynst very many sicknesses approued by authoritie, confirmed by reason, and dayly tryed by experience*. London; Lesse, Robert. 1580. *A brief view of all baths*. London; Turner, William. 1562. *A Booke of the natures and properties as well of the bathes in England as of other bathes in Germany and Italy/very necessary for all seik persones that can not be healed without the helpe of natural bathes*. London.

Baley's 'stone juice' likely references the earlier seminal 1541 work of Georgius Agricola, *De Re Mettalica*. As historian of science John Norris argues, Agricola was one of three influential figures, including Paracelsus and the French ceramicist Bernard Palissy, who over the course of the sixteenth century developed theories that detailed how mineral substances arise from aqueous processes (Norris 2007, 69). Their ideas grew from observation in mining areas of a concurrence of water and minerals. Crucially, these thinkers contravened prevailing theory to argue that water, rather than a 'vapour' (usually understood as a spiritual form of Sulphur or quicksilver), is the 'mobilizing factor in the emplacement of all minerals and as necessary for generating their compositions' (Norris 2007, 73).[9] I summarize briefly Norris's conclusions about these important theoretical developments because their work casts light on the increased interest in the natural—as opposed to supernatural—curative qualities of mineral waters and of the perceived essential relation between rocks and water for healing.

Agricola, humanist scholar, physician and author of *De Re Metallica*, drew from his knowledge of classical and Arabic authorities such as Pliny, Dioscorides, Galen, and Avicenna, but, importantly, supplemented them with his own experiential knowledge 'taken from his observation of mining practices' (Norris 2007, 73). Agricola observes that the 'quantity of water involved and the relative hardness of the rock' determined 'the size, amount and straightness of the fissures formed' that, in turn, he reasoned, 'over long periods of time such waters would absorb some of the mineral matter through which they flowed, thus creating liquids or mineral 'juices,' or in the Latin, *Succi* so *succi concreti* (solidified juice) (quoted in Norris 2007, 74).[10] Through a process of absorption, transport, and mixing, his theory of mineral juices made possible 'an immense variety of mineral assemblages' (quoted in Norris 2007, 75). According to Agricola, 'the generation of minerals by a heated juice' produced a variety of minerals, including 'vitriol, alum, and various other salts' (Agricola

[9] Geber (thirteenth century) and other alchemists propounded the idea that meals were composted of 'spiritual' Sulphur and quicksilver. The planets were also thought to be involved. See notes on earlier theories of ore deposits in Agricola 1950, n.1 43–53.

[10] For the translator's notes, see Agricola 1950, n.3: '*Succi* – "juice", or *succi concreti* – "solidified juice". Ger. Trans., *saffte*. The old English translators and mineralogists often use the word juices in the same sense, and we have adopted it'. The words 'solutions' and 'salts' convey a chemical significance not warranted by the state of knowledge in Agricola's time.

1950, n. 3). It was these minerals that were thought, in turn, to produce a variety of healing effects. The medicinable benefits were believed to be gained through drinking, bathing, or being applied topically. The mineral or 'stone juices', for instance, are key, in the English Bayley's account, to the water's 'virtues' or healing properties.

Around the same time as Agricola, Norris argues, the French ceramicist and natural philosopher, Bernard Palissy, was also formulating an influential theory of aqueous mineral generation from what he thought of as mineral seeds (Norris 2007, 80). Palissy posits that the generation of minerals must be connected to moisture or water and regarded salt as the 'generative matter of minerals' by observing the formation of crystals from solutions (Palissy 1957, 86).[11] Palissy recognized that waters containing mineral seeds might be visually unidentifiable from pure, or common water, and recommends discerning their presence either by taste or by 'observing the eventual congelation of mineral matter' (quoted in Norris 2007, 81). Palissy, like Agricola, seeks to explain the process by which mineral water comes into existence and transforms ordinary or 'common' water into 'congelative' water, indicative of a mineral presence. His theory of mineral seeds, like that of Agricola's mineral juices, advances the understanding of the natural questions asked by influential ancient authorities such as Plutarch.

Plutarch, in his *Natural Questions* discusses springs of hot water as sites where it 'seemeth that nature would have us to woonder heereat' and that 'we should enquire for some secret cause, and demand how that may be, which is but seldome observed' (Plutarch 1603, 1013).[12] The 'secret cause,' Agricola and Palissy later propose, can be revealed by study of natural processes at work, rather than a 'secret cause' whose source might be heavenly or divine power. As Norris documents, these early modern attempts to explain the 'secret causes' of mineral water's virtues eschew supernatural explanations, whether of divine or other 'astral influences'. Instead, they focus on the 'nature of the physical processes by which minerals' were generated (Norris 2007, 85).

[11] see *Discours admirables de la nature des eaux et fontaines, tant naturelles qu'artificielles, des métaux, des sels et salines, des pierres, des terres, du feu et des émaux*. Paris: Martin le jeune, 1580. The translation is that of Aurèle La Rocque from The Admirable Discourses of Bernard Palissy (1580).

[12] I thank Vin Nardizzi for alerting me to this reference.

The nature of the physical processes which led to aqueous mineral generation was further explored—and most widely diffused—by Theophrastus von Hohenheim, known as Paracelsus, primarily a physician, but also an alchemist with a long and well-documented interest in minerals. For Paracelsus, 'it has seemed good to God to create water as an element, and that from it should be everyday produced minerals for the use of men' (quoted in Norris 2007, 77). Unique to Paracelsus's understanding of mineral generation was his correlation of their physical processes with the spiritual entities of the *tria prima*. An influential aspect of his theory correlated physical as well as spiritual or mental curative property to mineral waters.

The emergent medical practices of hydrotherapy advocated by Paracelsian and later by Helmontian practice helped to erode the prevailing 'humoral theory and Galenic medicine' (Wear 2000, 39). Because they based their thinking on chemical principles including salt, sulphur, mercury, but also water, medical historian Andrew Wear sees their work as instrumental to promoting the mineral content of water as critical to healing (Wear 2000, 39). Their advocation of new philosophical methods of empirical observation and an experimental methodology align with the interest in the natural sources for mineral generation that English writers like Bayley seeks to understand as operative to healing waters.

The sixteenth-century theories of aqueous mineral generation, which in turn influenced medical practice, regarded rocks as jumbled masses 'amongst which certain recognizable minerals occur' (Norris 2007, 84). While they could not at the time 'relate the underlying crystal form' that gave rise to minerals, they nonetheless recognized the presence of rocks and water as necessary precursor conditions and materials for the generation of mineral juices within curative water (Norris 2007, 84). Whether or not Wroth was familiar with theories of aqueous mineral generation or the principles of Paracelsian medicine, her allusive descriptions for the sites of healing waters underscore their proximity to unusual rocky formations thought to be indicative of curative, and mineral, waters. Wroth's contemporary, Richard Burton, who wrote extensively on cures for love melancholy, includes a section on springs and baths, and cites various sources that specify bathes with a mineral content, a 'mixture of brasse, Iron, Allum, Sulphur' as being preferable to those without, but nonetheless urges that melancholy lovers 'warily' frequent them, and when they do so, to do so as part of a larger holistic healing regimen (Burton 1621,

314). Wroth's healing water sources all flow from distinctive rock formations, often whitish in colour, a colour believed to be a telltale sign of limestone, the stone Bayley identifies as the most likely source for the generation of healing waters. Wroth's inclusion of such specific, naturalistic landscape details furthers other naturalistic and non-miraculous aspects of her account for how *Urania*'s characters take the water.

Despite the proliferation of aqueous mineral theories and interest in hydrotherapy by physicians like Paracelsus, or more popular treatises such as Baley's that detail the medicinal benefits of mineral wells, the adoption of hydrotherapeutic practice across the continent and the British Isles remained contentious, dependent on local practice and varying religious beliefs. For instance, according to the French historian Laurence Brockliss, the practice of taking the water did not reach Vichy until the last two decades of the sixteenth century when it finally became socially respectable (Brockliss 1990, 23). As early modern English historian Alexandra Walsham notes, the developments being made in Paracelsian (as well as Helmontian) medicine were implicated in and stimulated by the religious upheavals of the sixteenth century, a context of particular relevance for the long reformation in England and Lady Mary Wroth's *Urania* (Walsham 2008, 209).

Lady Mary Wroth wrote from within a circle of, if not quite hot, then certainly warmly cosmopolitan Protestant-inflected godliness. It is not incidental that she proudly reminds readers on *Urania*'s title page that she is niece to 'the ever famous, and ever renowned' Sir Philip Sidney (Wroth 1995, title page). Sidney's untimely death abroad fighting for the Protestant cause in Zutphen rendered him a religious *cause celebre* at court, and a figurehead for Protestant literary endeavours. Wroth's imaginative taking of the waters adapts and modifies the medieval and Catholic accounts of holy wells. She does not reject the curative potential of water, but her modifications align with the historical image drawn by Alexandra Walsham.

In her research on 'Sacred Spas' in the English context, Alexandra Walsham argues that the 'old certainties about Protestantism's role in [...] [a] processes of desacralization have eroded in the face of nuanced accounts'. Scholars now reject 'any simply link between the demise of medieval holy wells and the apotheosis of fashionable resorts renowned for their sanative water' (Walsham 2008, 209). Instead, Walsham details 'the more subtle processes of adaptation and modification that accompanied the entrenchment of the Reformation between 1550 and 1700'

(Walsham 2008, 209–210). As she writes, healing springs and holy wells already, in the late medieval period, hovered 'on the fringes of both religious and medical respectability' (Walsham 2008, 212). Protestantism increased that scepticism with 'sustained assault on the assumptions that underpinned the practice of pilgrimage to sacred healing springs' (Walsham 2008, 213). Some wells, as a result, were the target of iconoclasm such as Sadler's Well at Islington which was defaced in the early phases of the Reformation. Yet despite the protracted crusade, many outlying springs remained 'the destination of a steady stream of sick patients' (Walsham 2008, 214).

Likely in response to this demand, some wells reinvented themselves; those that did, Walsham notes, usually did so by 'demonstrating that their waters possessed a mineral content' (Walsham 2008, 215). That is, they displaced the curative power from a supernatural cult of saints to a natural cause. Protestant commentators saw 'mineral springs which cured through natural causes as a means of counteracting clerical efforts to restore the nation to obedience to Rome' (Walsham 2008, 217). Bayley's 1587 treatise again affords an example. In the preface, Bayley writes that a 'superstition hath creped in amongst Christians' in 'the late ignorant age' when men have 'dedicated some bathe waters to S. Anne, others to S. Gregorie, others to S. Nicolas, others to S. Wynefride, others to S. Rumboll, and so others to diuers other saints, through ignorance vnskilfull of the causes of the faculties of such waters, they supposing the effects doone by them to come by the grace of som saint' (Bayley 1587, Sig. B2^{r}). He hopes that his little 'pamphlet' might 'sufficietly explane the true minerals of these bathes' (Bayley 1587, Sig. B2^{r}). As Walsham summarizes, the cultural process of reclaiming 'former holy wells which bore traces of vitriol, alum, bitumen, chalybeate, and nitre gathered momentum and pace in the seventeenth century' (Walsham 2008, 217). The attempt to understand the mineral content of waters as a natural process within natural philosophy and medicine was further catalyzed by the changing religious culture which sought to dampen the more miraculous, and therefore more Catholic, element of former holy wells.

As medical practice paid attention to forms of mineral and iatrochemical healing, they relied on new theories for an aqueous mineral generation. These developments, coupled with the Protestant emphasis on natural causes for holy wells and healing springs, lent new vigour to developing a cultural framework responsive to the lay population's ongoing desire to access sites that might alleviate stress and disease. These historical forces inflect Wroth's imaginative depiction of taking the waters and nuance the miraculous aspects more apparent in her literary precedents. Wroth does not discard wholesale the literary motif. Her characters conspicuously and repeatedly take the waters. But she adapts their doing so by playing up their mineralized origins and by making their cure only one part of a larger, holistic, network of healing.

3 Conclusion: Literary Prolepsis of an Emergent Spa Culture

Thus far this essay has tracked Wroth's seeming responsiveness to changing epistemological and religious attitudes, but she also sets a precedent for later developments within spa culture, namely the importance of forging female alliances as part of an ongoing curative labour taken in conjunction with water cures. As these three episodes show, taking the waters in the *Urania*, finally, offers an inconclusive cure; yet, again and again, characters return to Melissea or find water sources that they believe might give them respite from their erotic torments. This fictional pattern of demand despite unproven results aligns with Amanda E. Herbert's finding that in the later seventeenth century, spa popularity persists despite evidence that the health 'results of the spa visit' were often 'inconclusive' (Herbert 2014, 129). Wroth's literary text thus highlights a seeming gap between the character's knowledge and their ongoing practice, a gap that aligns this imaginative world with historical trends. The allure of taking the waters in this fictional account extends beyond its inconclusive miraculous—or even natural—ability to heal. Although *Urania* questions the efficacy of taking the waters, it nonetheless repeatedly features them in ways that highlight their centrality to cultural habits, and especially, their place within a healing network of female alliances. Wroth's water cures may not be conclusively efficacious in erasing love's melancholy from her afflicted characters, but they nonetheless compose one critical method that, when used in conjunction with other strategies, facilitates her characters' living what we might now want to term functional, fully social lives. Urania and Parselius both go on to marry, have children, go on adventures, and remain friends; Alarina marries, happily, and disappears from the narrative; even the worst case, the 'frantick' Antissia threatens, but never fully, relapses into her lovesick madness.

Wroth's characters anticipate a development that Amanda E. Herbert traces in her recent monograph *Female Alliances* that devotes a chapter to

'Hot Spring Sociability'. Herbert argues that in late seventeenth-century England, the social diversions at the spas show them to be places where feminine identity might be created and where 'the provision of health care at spas' might be read as enriching 'their female alliances' (Herbert 2014, 141). In other words, the efficacy of taking the waters may not be the most important factor in their popularity, rather it was the social practices—and alliances—they facilitated.

Wroth's *Urania* anticipates these later cultural developments by highlighting the central role of the wise woman, Melissea, who both prescribes water cures and administers them. Her role as both an authoritative healer and as a counsellor combines the taking of the waters with long expositive sections where she advises the characters how to best navigate love's turbulent affective torment. In its long format, moreover, Wroth's storylines unfold as embedded, narrated storytelling, usually between female characters. They spotlight the critical nature of female alliances and the importance of storytelling as its own mode of affective healing. Finally, and perhaps most conspicuously, the titular character, Urania, hones her skills as a counsellor after the water cure fails to fully erase the pain of her former love. As Aurélie Griffin argues, Wroth's engagement with the 'revival of interest in melancholy', in both medical and psychological treatises, and the experience of the unrequited female lover, show her establishing a connection between the expression and treatment of love melancholy as part of a creative license to tell—and listen to—stories (Griffin 2015, 159). By ascribing ongoing natural labour as critical to the water's therapeutic potential, Wroth highlights the importance of learned advice and sound counsel. Wroth's characers are not simply passive in the face of a miraculous water cure; rather they exhibit active engagement and an ongoing effort. Clare R. Kinney aruges that one of ways that Wroth refigures Ovidean complaint entails replacing an 'anonymous and uncaring lover' with sympathetic listeners (Kinney 2018, 250). All of these narrative details show Wroth building an imaginative world where female alliances are bolstered by their ongoing conversations around and experience with taking the waters.

Taking the waters in Wroth's 1621 *Urania* proleptically enacts the spa sociability that would emerge almost half a century later in cultural practice. It highlights the water cures as being one palliative element within a larger holistic program of healing. Although the waters do not work a comprehensive miracle, they do catalyse recovery, and perhaps most crucially, they generate stories. The stories, in turn, offer an equally critical component to bearing erotic torment and to healing love's melancholy. In the imaginative realm of Wroth's *Urania* literature converses with emergent scientific theories around hydrotherapy but, also, anticipates and shapes social practice, making storytelling a central pillar of the bath and spa water experience. Wroth's romance thus provides evidence for how science, literature, and social practice were understood to be mutually informing and sustaining in the bath and spa waters culture of early modern England.

Works Cited

Primary Sources

Agricola, Georg. 1950. *De Re Metallica*. Trans. Herbert Hoover. New York: Dover.

Baley, Walter. 1587. *A Briefe Discours of Certain Bathes or Medicinall Waters in the Countie of Warwicke neere vnto a Village called Newnam Regis*. London.

Burton, Robert. 1621. *The Anatomy of Melancholy*. Oxford: Printed by Iohn Lichfield and Iames Short, for Henry Cripps.

Montemayor, George. 1968. *A Critical Edition of Yong's Translation of George of Montemayor's Diana and Gil Polo's Enamoured Diana*. Ed. Judith M. Kennedy. Oxford: Clarendon Press.

Ovid. 1567. *The Heroycall Epistles of the Learned Poet Publius Ouidius Naso*. Trans. George Turberville. London: Printed by Henry Denham.

Palissy, Bernard. 1957. *The Admirable Discourses of Bernard Palissy* (1580). Trans. Aurèle La Rocque. Urbana: University of Illinois Press.

Plutarch. 1603. *The Philosophie, Commonlie Called, the Morals Vvritten by the Learned Philosopher Plutarch of Chæronea. Translated Out of Greeke into English, and Conferred with the Latine Translations and the French*. Trans. Philemon Holland. London: Printed by Arnold Hatfield.

Sannazaro, Jacopo. 1966. *Arcadia*. Trans. Ralph Nash. Detroit, MI: Wayne University Press.

Wroth, Lady Mary. 1983. *The Poems of Lady Mary Wroth*. Ed. Josephine A. Roberts. Baton Rouge: Louisiana State University Press.

Wroth, Lady Mary. 1995. *The First Part of the Countess of Montgomery's Urania*. Ed. Josephine A. Roberts. Binghamton, New York: Medieval & Renaissance Texts & Studies.

Wroth, Lady Mary. 1999. *The Second Part of the Countess of Montgomery's Urania*. Eds. Josephine A. Roberts, Suzanne Gossett and Janel M. Mueller. Tempe, AZ: Renaissance English Text Society in conjunction with Arizona Center for Medieval and Renaissance Studies.

Secondary Sources

Brockliss, L.W.B. 1990. The Development of the Spa in Seventeenth-century France. In *The Medical History of Waters and Spas*. ed. Roy Porter, 23–47. London: Wellcome Institute for the History of Medicine.

Coley, Noel G. 1990. Physicians, Chemists, and the Analysis of Mineral Waters: "The most difficult part of chemistry". In *The Medical History of Waters and Spas*. ed. Roy Porter, 56–66. London: Wellcome Institute for the History of Medicine.

Griffin, Aurélie. 2015. Love Melancholy and the Senses in Mary Wroth's Works. In *The Senses in Early Modern England*. eds. Simon Smith, Amy Kenny and Jackie Watson, 148–164. Manchester: Manchester Univeristy Press.

Herbert, Amanda E. 2014. *Female Alliances: Gender, Identiy, and Friendship in Early Modern Britain*. Yale: Yale University Press.

Kinney, Clare R. 2018. Mary Wroth Romances Ovid: Refiguring Metamorphosis and Complaint in *The Countess of Montgomery's Urania*. In *A History of Early Modern Women's Writing*. ed. Patricia Phillippy, 241–256. Cambridge: Cambridge University Press.

Norris, John A. 2007. Early Theories of Aqueous Mineral Genesis in the Sixteenth Century. *Ambix* 54 (1): 69–86.

Porter, Roy. 1990. Introduction. In *Medical History of Waters and Spas,* i–xii. London, Wellcome Institute for the History of Medicine.

Walsham, Alexandra. 2008. Sacred Spas? Healing Springs and Religion in Post-Reformation Britain. In *The Impact of the European Reformation*. eds. Bridget Heal and Ole Peter Grell, 209–230. Burlington, Ashgate.

Wear, Andrew. 2000. *Knowledge and Practice in English Medicine, 1500–1680*. Cambridge: Cambridge University Press.

Werth, Tiffany. 2011. *The Fabulous Dark Cloister: Romance in England after the Reformation*. Baltimore, MD: Johns Hopkins University Press.

Website

'Float House'. http://www.floathouse.ca. Accessed October 26, 2020.

CHAPTER 4

Bristol and Bath in Frances Burney's *Evelina*

Anne Rouhette

Over a third of Frances Burney's first novel *Evelina* (1778, three volumes) takes place at Bristol Hotwells,[1] a spa which was less fashionable than Bath but nevertheless well-known in the eighteenth century. Evelina experiences a severe psychological shock which causes 'depression of [...] spirits', 'heaviness of heart', a profound 'melancholy' perceptible in her 'altered' looks and her 'pale and ill' appearance (Burney 2008, 256 and 259). Her concerned guardian, Mr Villars, convinces her to 'try the effects of the Bristol waters' (Burney 2008, 269), effects so powerful that she recovers her estranged father as well as her health when in Bristol, where she also acquires a husband, a brother, and a sister. The fairy-tale outcome achieved in the Bristol section of *Evelina* represents something of an exception in the literary context of its time. For instance, the image conveyed of spa towns in the other well-known novel of the 1770s, Smollett's *The Expedition of Humphry Clinker* (1771), is far from being

[1]The spa is referred to as 'Bristol Hotwells' or 'Bristol Hotwell' in *Evelina*. It is also known as The Hot Wells or The Hot-Wells.

A. Rouhette (✉)
Département d'Etudes Anglophones, Université Clermont Auvergne, Clermont-Ferrand, France
e-mail: anne.rouhette@uca.fr

S. Chiari and S. Cuisinier-Delorme (eds.), *Spa Culture and Literature in England, 1500–1800*, Early Modern Literature in History,
https://doi.org/10.1007/978-3-030-66568-5_4

altogether positive, especially when they are seen through the eyes of Matthew Bramble, who criticises their society as well as their therapeutic value. This satirical dimension is echoed in other works of the second half of the eighteenth century such as *The New Bath Guide*, a verse satire by Christopher Anstey (1766),[2] or Sheridan's *The Rivals* (1775), 'one of many social comedies not only set in, but about, the way society is shaped by and to Bath' (Stern 2004, 21).

In this respect and in others, *Evelina* enters into a dialogue with these works, either directly, as *The New Bath Guide* is mentioned by the heroine within the narrative, or indirectly,[3] which leads me to consider the role played by spas in *Evelina* in the light of Emily Allen's view of the novel's place in the generic struggles of the late eighteenth century. Allen convincingly analyses Burney's work as the site of a tension between the novel and other forms, mostly drama, a tension which echoes the difficult striving after female identity which constitutes the thematic core of the novel, especially in spatial terms:

> In *Evelina* we have a narrative that thematizes the triumph of the novel as a struggle between a newly emergent genre and the residual forms it must displace and, on some level, embrace. So, too, we have in the novel's construction of the private domain of female subjectivity a thematics of struggle, struggle between the public and the private spheres whose supposed separation would later come to undergird middle-class domestic ideology. (Allen 1998, 435)

This comes to a head in the Bristol section, where, after spending two volumes in the social limbo to which her mysterious origins condemned her, Evelina gains two identities in quick succession, first as daughter, then as wife. As I will examine in the first part of this chapter, the paradoxical blend of fixity and change that defines the heroine's status is perfectly paralleled by her relationship to Bristol. I will then turn to the properly novelistic dimension of this spa in *Evelina*, before focusing on the questions of genre and gender raised by the depictions of Bristol and of Bath.

[2] For a detailed analysis of the depiction of spas in *Humphry Clinker* and in *The New Bath Guide*, see Cossic-Péricarpin (2017).

[3] For Burney's debt to Smollett and more particularly to *Humphry Clinker*, see Anderson (1980) and Paulson (1988), which focuses on the two authors' use of satire.

Table 1 The Structure of *Evelina*

Volume I	*Volume II*	*Volume III*
March–May Letters I–IX: Evelina in the countryside: Berry Hill (Dorset) and Howard Grove (Kent) Letters X–XXIV: Evelina in London Letters XXV–XXXI: Evelina in the countryside (Howard Grove)	May–August Letters I–VIII: Evelina in the countryside (Howard Grove) Letters IX–XXV: Evelina in London Letters XXVI–XXIX: Evelina in the countryside (Berry Hill) Letter XXX: Evelina at Bristol Hotwell	August–October Letters I–XXII: Evelina at Bristol Hotwell then in Clifton. Excursion to Bath related in Letter XXI (5 pages).

1 Bristol Hotwells, Between Permanence and Transience

Spas in the eighteenth century were of course mostly seasonal places, where the sick or the fashionable would set up residence for a few weeks or a few months. As Phyllis Hembry notes, '[b]y the 1750s the Clifton Hotwells [at Bristol] was a crowded, fashionable resort attracting people of rank' by the beauty of its landscape and the various entertainments provided, for instance in the two assembly rooms operating (Hembry 1990, 246).[4] In *Evelina*, this transitory character is granted an almost permanent dimension. Table 1 below charts the movements of Burney's heroine as she makes her 'entrance into the world', according to the subtitle of this epistolary novel:

Evelina goes from a fictional estate in Dorset, in the countryside, to another fictional estate in Kent, also in the countryside, then to London and back to Kent in the first volume. The second volume follows a similar pattern from the countryside to London and back to the countryside but with a slight twist at the end as Evelina leaves again, this time for Bristol, a move related in a letter dated August 28 (Burney 2008, 269). There is probably a deeper, more literary reason for Burney's choice of Bristol over Bath as a spa to send her heroine to, as I will argue further down, but it must have been at least partly motivated by this date; the season for

[4] For details regarding the rise and decline of the Bristol Howells as a thermal resort, see Hembry (1990, 245–250).

taking the waters at Bristol ran from May to September while what the foppish Mr Lovel calls the 'right season' for Bath (Burney 2008, 395) was the spring, as Vivien Jones explains in her notes (Burney 2008, 454). Indeed, 'Bath and [Bristol] were complementary rather than competing spas' (Hembry 1990, 246).

And then, strikingly, after so much travelling back and forth, Evelina remains more or less static in the third volume, only moving once her health has improved from the vicinity of the Hotwells to Clifton, the fashionable area of Bristol where Matthew Bramble also resides, and going on a one-day outing to Bath. Her last letter, which closes the novel, announces her return to Berry Hill and Dorset but it is still written from Clifton (Burney 2008, 406), leaving Burney's heroine in transit, poised in-between two permanent homes and two statuses, that of a poor, orphaned girl at the beginning and that of a rich and married heiress at the end. The place of transit that is Bristol becomes paradoxically the location where she spends the longest uninterrupted time narratively speaking, over a volume, and which, narratively again, she never leaves, unlike Matthew Bramble and his family in *Humphry Clinker*. By having Evelina remain in a place supposed to afford only temporary residence, Burney questions the very idea of permanence, which arguably reinforces one of the aspects of her novel as her heroine resists meeting with her father for as long as she can, while presumably this encounter would at last endow her with the name and identity she has supposedly been in quest of since the beginning. Likewise, in spite of her professed love for Orville, Evelina tries her utmost to delay their wedding and the moment when she will receive a fixed position, to remain 'in transit' and not be settled, which explains why, in a highly significant pun, she does not want to hear about any marriage 'settlements' (Burney 2008, 379)—this Bristol echoes in a way that London or the fictional countryside estates could not, precisely because of its transitory nature. In the economy of the novel, being 'settled' means that Evelina will lose her voice as she stops writing: as the site of a tension between permanence and transience, the setting of this last volume thus mirrors the heroine's conflicting desires while leaving ever so slightly open the very possibility of her writing.

2 Bristol, a Literary Place

And yet this permanent transitory home receives very little descriptive attention, if any, in a section which has been considered as 'the most complicated, the best-written part of the book' (Montague and Martz 1949, 174). Evelina goes to the pump-room across the Avon, finds shelter from the rain in a milliner's shop, goes to several balls in the assembly room, but none of those places is depicted. She does not mention 'the dirt, the stench, the chilling blasts, and perpetual rains, that render this place [...] intolerable' to Matthew Bramble when he visits it in April for instance (Smollett 2009, 24), and she is far more allusive than Bramble's niece Lydia Melford, who waxes lyrical when she refers to the Hotwells as 'a charming romantic place' with

> mountains covered with flocks of sheep, and tender bleating wanton lambkins playing, frisking and skipping from side to side; the groves resound with the notes of blackbird, thrush, and linnet; and all night long sweet Philomel pours forth her ravishingly delightful song. Then, for variety, we go down to the nymph of Bristol spring, where the company is assembled before dinner; so good-natured, so free, so easy; and there we drink the water so clear, so pure, so mild, so charmingly maukish. There the sun is so chearful and reviving; the weather so soft; the walk so agreeable; the prospect so amusing; and the ships and boats going up and down the river, close under the windows of the Pump-room, afford such an enchanting variety of moving pictures, as require a much abler pen than mine to describe. (Smollett 2009, 27)

Evelina merely remarks: 'We are situated upon a most delightful spot; the prospect is beautiful, the air pure, and the weather very favourable to invalids. I am already better' (Burney 2008, 269), without specifying what 'spot' or what 'prospect' she is referring to or what she finds 'delightful' and 'beautiful' about them. She never alludes to 'the scenic beauty' of the gorge of the Avon which forms the place's 'main attraction', according to Phyllis Hembry (Hembry 1990, 245). This absence of details contrasts with the rest of the novel when it comes to referential places like those she visits in London, Pall Mall, the Ranelagh, Vauxhall Gardens etc., to which Evelina usually devotes a few descriptive lines. For instance, 'St. James's Park [...] by no means answered [her] expectations: it is a long straight walk, of dirty gravel, very uneasy to the feet; and at each end, instead of an open prospect, nothing is to be seen but houses built of bricks' (Burney 2008, 28). Burney herself advertised the documentary aspect of her novel when she contacted a potential publisher. Her first volume, she writes, includes 'a round of the most fashionable Spring Diversions of London', while the second volume, she adds a month later, sees the heroine '[partake] of a round of Summer Diversions' (Burney 2008, xiii) in much less elegant circles. Describing the various places of entertainment or the London sites she visits, Evelina sends to her guardian sketches which Vivien Jones likens to 'notes from a guidebook for the discriminating tourist' (Jones 2008, xvii), offering a subjective and lively counterpart to the impersonal tourist guides which were contemporary with Burney's novel (e.g. *A Brief Description of the Cities of London and Westminster*, 1778). This might have led us to expect that in the last volume of the novel, Bristol Hotwells, another referential place, should be dealt with in the same manner as London in the previous ones. Such is not the case, as we saw, and in this respect, the treatment which Bristol receives is much closer to that bestowed upon the fictional places of the novel, Howard Grove and Berry Hill, which are never described.

The fictionality of Bristol is brought out in an important passage which contains a direct reference to Christopher Anstey's *The New Bath Guide*.[5] Towards the beginning of the volume, after Evelina has moved to Clifton, to a house where, by a lucky coincidence, the young man she loves also happens to be staying, she relates the following episode:

> [Lord Orville] took up the New Bath Guide, and read it with me till supper-time. In our way down stairs, Lady Louisa said, 'I thought, Brother, you were engaged this evening?'
>
> 'Yes, Sister,' answered he, 'and I have been engaged.' And he bowed to me with an air of gallantry that rather confused me. (Burney 2008, 295)

This short vignette pictures two characters in a largely satirical epistolary novel, temporarily residing in a spa, engaged in reading a satirical epistolary poem whose characters are temporarily residing in another spa which Orville and Evelina will visit near the end of the novel, once they are properly engaged. This reading of *The New Bath Guide* is not only proleptic; it also serves a narrative function, revealing the growing intimacy between the two protagonists whose relationship, so far, has been fraught with misunderstanding, as they learn to know each other through the mediation of a work of fiction that resembles, at least in some aspects, the one they are in. It also signals the literariness of a novel whose characters are repeatedly compared to other fictional characters,

[5] For an analysis of Anstey's satirical description of Bath in *The New Bath Guide*, see Cossic-Péricarpin (2017) and Shaun Regan's chapter in this volume.

either specific (Don Quixote for instance for Lord Orville, Burney 2008, 369) or generic as Evelina and Orville are thus suspected of 'planning some pastoral dialogue' (Burney 2008, 368), reminding the reader of the pastoral dimension of the names given to the two fictional country estates, Berry Hill and Howard Grove, and again taking Bristol out of 'reality' and into fiction. It is perhaps worth noting that *The New Bath Guide* concludes with a satirical plan for a novel '[f]it for modest young Ladies' (Anstey 2010, 173) which Burney seems to have taken literally:

> Why if thou must write, thou hadst better compose
> Some Novels, or elegant Letters in Prose.
> Take a Subject that's grave, with a Moral that's good,
> Throw in all the Temptations that Virtue withstood
> In Epistles like PAMELA's chaste and devout [...]
> O! pray let your Hero be handsome and young,
> Taste, Wit, and fine Sentiment, flow from his Tongue,
> His delicate Feelings be sure to improve
> With Passion, with tender soft Rapture and Love.
> (Anstey 2010, 173)

Advocating the writing of a sentimental epistolary novel with a moral intent, a chaste heroine and a dashing hero, this passage sounds like a blueprint for *Evelina*—and, to be fair, for countless other novels of the late eighteenth century.[6] This literariness brought out in the last volume partly explains, in my view, the vagueness of the setting: Burney would thus be emphasising the fictionality of what she is writing, moving decidedly away from the 'guidebook' aspect by discarding any pretence at referentiality.

3 Bath, Genre and Gender in *Evelina*

Indeed, Evelina's relation of her visit to Bath, 'that celebrated city' (Burney 2008, 390), is far more reminiscent, at least to some extent, of

[6] To give a few examples from the 1760s and 1770s which follow this pattern more or less closely: *The Faithful Fugitives; Or, Adventures of Miss Teresa. In a Series of Letters to a Friend* (anon., 1766); *The History of Miss Pittborough. In a Series of Letters* (By a Lady, 1767); *The Mistakes of the Heart: Or, Memoirs of Lady Carolina Pelham and Lady Victoria Nevil. In a Series of Letters.* (Pierre-Henri Treyssac de Vergy, 1770); *The Delicate Distress: A Novel. In Letters.* ('Frances', 1775); *The Maiden Aunt* (By a Lady, 1776), etc.

the tone and contents of some of her letters sent from London, to which she compares the famous spa:

> The charming city of Bath answered all my expectations. The Crescent, the prospect from it, and the elegant symmetry of the Circus, delighted me. The Parades, I own, rather disappointed me; one of them is scarce preferable to some of the best paved streets in London; and the other, though it affords a beautiful prospect, a charming view of Prior Park and of the Avon, yet wanted something in itself of more striking elegance than a mere broad pavement, to satisfy the ideas I had formed of it. (Burney 2008, 392)

This time, the reader knows what prospects Evelina alludes to and what it is exactly that she finds delightful—or ridiculous, and in this matter, Burney's use of satire belongs to a particular literary tradition. Unlike the social satire which pervades the London volumes and targets general moral flaws and human behaviour such as greed (the Branghtons) and hypocrisy (Sir Clement Willoughby), in Bath, the satirical passage which follows up on these referential remarks remains topically relevant, much more so than in the rest of the third volume, which does, however, concern itself briefly with 'fashionable diseases' (Cossic-Péricarpin 2017) when Lady Louisa parades her 'weak nerves' at Clifton (Burney 2008, 361). This passage deals with vanity and excesses in matters of fashion, with a dialogue between the would-be fashion-setter Mr Lovel and the affected Lady Louisa—spas and Bath in particular were famous for the luxury clothes sold and worn there by the fashionable élite.[7] Lovel and his eulogy of the *bon ton* are then made fun of by the blunt Captain Mirvan, who threatens to throw Lovel into the vat below the pump-room. In this respect, the Bath passage is reminiscent of the satire found in *Humphry Clinker* or in *The New Bath Guide*, except for one important detail: *Evelina*'s satire is not directed against fashionable medicine or medical practice. As Annick Cossic-Péricarpin explains,

> In *The New Bath Guide*, as in *Humphry Clinker*, the butt of satire is not just the nature of the treatment but also the therapeutic infrastructure, the

[7] Jenny W-D-R thus devotes an ode to 'The Birth of Fashion' in *The New Bath Guide* (Letter III), exclaiming: 'Dress be our care in this gay Scene /Of Pleasure's blest abode, /Enchanting Dress!' (Anstey 2010, 95). Shaun Regan addresses this topic at greater length in the present volume.

> new spa attributes. The two books expose an architecture of disease, the inadequacy of the Pump Room and of the bathing establishment. Smollett, through satire, makes the same contention already to be found in his Essay on the External Use of Water, namely that Bath creates disease and does not cure it. (Cossic-Péricarpin 2017, 542)

Not so in *Evelina*, if only because the heroine does recover her health in Bristol, more on account on the weather apparently than because of the waters, whose effects or 'charmingly maukish' flavour she never mentions, unlike Lydia Melford—another instance of the vagueness that characterises her stay at the Hotwells. The one medical character in the novel, an apothecary, is not depicted as a greedy charlatan, and in fact fulfils no medical function at all; he proves himself to be a valuable source of information by his knowledge of who's who and where at the Hotwells, playing a part similar to Nurse Rooke's in Austen's *Persuasion*.

This visit to Bath also allows the heroine to display her refined sensibility, as she does repeatedly throughout the novel: 'At the pump-room, I was amazed at the public exhibition of the ladies in the bath; it is true, their heads are covered with bonnets; but the very idea of being seen, in such a situation, by whoever pleases to look, is indelicate' (Burney 2008, 393). However, the phrase 'public exhibition' also harks back to the theatrical dimension of the London volumes, in contrast with the passages set in Bristol. As Emily Allen notes, 'geographically, the London world of public theatrical pleasures that dominates the first two books of the novel is replaced by Bristol's privatized realm of drawing-room intrigue' (Allen 1998, 438), which aligns the novel with novelistic conventions rather than with the theatrical paradigms on which the London and Bath episodes rely. What Evelina objects to, more precisely, is the confusion that occurs at the pump-room as what should remain private in her view is here made public; on the contrary, she expressed great pleasure at the London theatres, because they are places meant for public entertainment. Evelina's reluctance to witness such spectacles in Bath testifies to a valorisation of the private life, to a move inwards which her activities corroborate. While her visits to the theatre or the opera were given pride of place in London, in Bristol she is associated with reading: 'the young Lady *reads*', explains Mrs Selwyn to an importunate suitor who wants to know what Evelina does with herself in Bristol (Burney 2008, 275), and of course she pictures herself reading *The New Bath Guide* in the passage discussed above. Here lies probably the greatest difference between the roles played by Bath and Bristol in *Evelina*, a distinction which is both generic and gendered: if the Bath passage possesses a theatrical dimension reminiscent of the earlier part of the novel, it also offers a satirical viewpoint evocative of some of its predecessors, be they verse satires like *The New Bath Guide* or men's novels like *Humphry Clinker*—or men's plays, like Sheridan's *The Rivals*. The Bristol section, on the other hand, if it does not entirely repudiate other literary forms or its great novelistic precursor, situates the novel in the inward space with which it is associated, a space which is properly gendered feminine,[8] paving the way for Austen's works.

4 Conclusion: From Fiction to Life

Unlike her experience of London, which was first-hand as she lived there and knew well the places of entertainment Evelina visits, Burney's knowledge of Bristol and Bath was imaginary and largely based on her readings, as her first visit to Bath came after *Evelina* was published, from March to June 1780 (Burney 2001, x). But it also came from family lore, as Bristol and Bath were places 'privately associated by the author to the mother', as Margaret Anne Doody notes (Doody 1988, 46). Burney's mother, Esther Sleepe Burney,[9] died in late September 1762 of a sudden illness, possibly tuberculosis or cancer, which the waters of Bath and Bristol Hotwells could not cure. Evelina's stay in Bristol, also in September, partly reverses Burney's loss since her heroine finds both health and family there. It is during this stay, almost at the heart of this volume (Letter XIII out of 23), that Evelina, who is 'the lovely resemblance of her lovely [and deceased] mother' (Burney 2008, 133), receives the posthumous letter of Caroline Evelyn, the mother whose name is inscribed in hers; she then brings her back to life, as it were, in the eyes of her father who exclaims: 'does Caroline Evelyn still live!' (Burney 2008, 372). The ghost-like presence of Evelina's mother discreetly haunts this last volume, as the loss of Burney's own mother haunted her daughter for a long time, as many critics have observed. Maybe, in its turn, Burney's ghost may be said to haunt Bath,

[8] The link between novel-writing and the privatisation of female subjectivity lies outside the scope of this chapter; see Armstrong (1987).

[9] On Burney's mother, see Erickson (2018).

where she died in 1840 and where she is buried beside her husband and her son.

Works Cited

Primary Sources

Anstey, Christopher. 2010. *The New Bath Guide* (1766), ed. Annick Cossic. Bern: Peter Lang.

Burney, Frances. 2001. *Journals and Letters*. Selected with an introduction by Peter Sabor and Lars E. Troide. London: Penguin.

Burney, Frances. 2008. *Evelina; or, A Young Lady's Entrance into the World* (1778), ed. Edward A. Bloom. Introduction and notes by Vivien Jones. Oxford: Oxford University Press.

Smollett, Tobias. 2009. *The Expedition of Humphry Clinker* (1771), ed. Lewis M. Knapp. Revised by Paul-Gabriel Boucé. Oxford: Oxford University Press.

Secondary Sources

Allen, Emily. 1998. Staging Identity: Frances Burney's Allegory of Genre. *Eighteenth-Century Studies* 31 (4): 433–451.

Anderson, Earl R. 1980. Footnotes More Pedestrian than Sublime: A Historical Background for the Foot-Races in *Evelina* and *Humphry Clinker*. *Eighteenth-Century Studies* 14: 56–68.

Armstrong, Nancy. 1987. *Desire and Domestic Fiction. A Political History of the Novel.* Oxford: Oxford University Press.

Cossic-Péricarpin, Annick. 2017. Fashionable Diseases in Georgian Bath: Fiction and the Emergence of a British Model of Spa Sociability. *Journal for Eighteenth-Century Studies* 40 (4): 537–553.

Doody, Margaret Anne. 1988. *Frances Burney. The Life in the Works.* Cambridge: Cambridge University Press.

Erickson, Amy Louise. 2018. Esther Sleepe, Fan-Maker, and her Family. *Eighteenth-Century Life* 42 (2): 15–37.

Hembry, Phyllis. 1990. *The English Spa, 1560-1815: A Social History*. London: Athlone Press.

Jones, Vivien. 2008. Introduction. In *Evelina; or, A Young Lady's Entrance into the World* (1778), by Frances Burney, ed. Edward A. Bloom. Oxford: Oxford University Press.

Montague, Edwine, and Louis L. Martz (eds). 1949. Fanny Burney's *Evelina*. In *The Age of Johnson, Essays Presented to Chaundy Brewster Tinker*, ed. Frederick W. Hilles, 171–182. New Haven: Yale University Press.

Paulson, Ronald. 1988. Evelina: Cinderella and Society (1967). *Fanny Burney's* Evelina, ed. Harold Bloom, 5–12. New York, Chelsea House Publishers.
Stern, Tiffany. 2004. Introduction. In *The Rivals*, by Richard Brinsley Sheridan, ed. Tiffany Stern. London: Bloomsbury.

CHAPTER 5

'Oh! Who Can Ever Be Tired of Bath?' The Sense of Place in Jane Austen's *Northanger Abbey* and *Persuasion*

Marie-Laure Massei-Chamayou

> Geography is not an inert container, is not a box where cultural history 'happens', but an active force, that pervades the literary field and shapes it in depth. Making the connection between geography and literature explicit, then—mapping it: because a map is precisely that, a connection made visible—will allow us to see some significant relationships that have so far escaped us. (Moretti, 3)

If Bath became a world heritage site in 1987 thanks to its Roman remains and outstanding eighteenth-century architecture, the elegant Georgian city now also largely thrives upon its particular connection with Jane Austen, which has become synonymous with a highly profitable industry. This 'Austen connection' is not merely due to the fact that Jane Austen lived there between 1801 and 1806 (Le Faye 1995, 592–594), or that Bath features as a major setting both in *Northanger Abbey* and *Persuasion*

M.-L. Massei-Chamayou (✉)
Université Paris 1 Panthéon-Sorbonne, Paris, France
e-mail: marie-laure.massei-chamayou@univ-paris1.fr

S. Chiari and S. Cuisinier-Delorme (eds.), *Spa Culture and Literature in England, 1500–1800*, Early Modern Literature in History,
https://doi.org/10.1007/978-3-030-66568-5_5

and in their adaptations, it is also embedded, so to speak, in the city's architecture: the Duke of Chandos, who, thanks to his impressive wealth, commissioned John Wood to rebuild part of St John's Court Hospital in the first half of the eighteenth century, happened to be Mrs. Austen's great-uncle.

Bath now therefore boasts an annual Jane Austen Festival, and a Jane Austen Centre located on Gay Street (at No.40), next to the house where Jane, her mother and her sister Cassandra rented rooms for a few months after the death of the Reverend George Austen in January 1805. This Jane Austen Centre is 'a must-see' for any Jane Austen fan: besides its cosy Regency tearooms where 'Janeites' can treat themselves to a cream tea served by costumed staff while admiring a portrait of Colin Firth as Mr. Darcy, it features Jane Austen's striking waxwork. Part of this attractive heritage industry is the Regency tour of Bath which also enables visitors to take a walk in Jane's own footsteps and discover the places mentioned in her novels: from Sidney Place—where No.4 is the only house in Bath to have a plaque informing us of Jane Austen's residency—to Gay Street, down to Green Park buildings and Trim Street—the Austen women's final lodging located in a less fashionable part of the city at the time.[1] Bath is the city where you can definitely be 'en bons thermes'[2] with Jane Austen—a relevant pun coined by the French magazine *Télérama* (Crom 2016, online), which testifies to Austen's crossover status as a classic and popular figure.

With so many fascinating activities on offer, 'who can ever be tired of Bath?', to quote Catherine Morland as she dances with Henry Tilney in the Assembly Rooms. If this enthusiastic reaction may convey what Jane Austen may have initially thought before her first recorded stay there in 1797, her letters, novels and some biographical elements all point to more nuanced views of Bath, which are ironically at odds with the city's 'nostalgic, reassuring and escapist image' of Austen (Ballingher 2013, online).

[1] The Austen family first lived at 4 Sidney Place, between 1801 and 1804, then at 3 Green Park buildings East in 1804–1805. Following George Austen's death, Mrs. Austen and her daughters lodged temporarily at 25 Gay Street, then in Trim Street, one of the first streets built outside the city walls, between January and June 1806.

[2] This phrase is a pun on the French words *thermes* (thermae) and *termes* (on good terms with).

This chapter thus considers the various representations and metaphors that Jane Austen associated with Bath, both in her letters and two novels, *Northanger Abbey* and *Persuasion,* which partially use the city as a dramatic stage, to illustrate her ambivalent connection with the place and shifting sense of place.[3] While her letters betray her growing disappointment in Bath, her fictional depiction of the city actually allows for more nuanced representations. Even though *Northanger Abbey* and *Persuasion* were published together posthumously with a 'Biographical Notice of the Author' drafted by Henry Austen in December 1817—revealing, for the first time, Jane Austen's authorship—their respective atmospheres testify to their author's changing perceptions of Bath, especially as they were written some fourteen years apart.[4]

If *Northanger Abbey*'s representation of the city is shaped by Austen's literary project to at once parody and experiment with fiction, *Persuasion* explores more fully the complex emotional potential of such a dramatic setting: even though Bath appears as a site of ironic dislocation, synonymous with alienation and social competition, its urban space nonetheless enables the blissful reunion of Anne Elliot and Captain Wentworth.

[3] In *Jane Austen in Bath*, Laura M. Ragg aptly remarks that 'Jane Austen could not keep a mention of Bath out of her novels' (Ragg 1938, 12). Indeed, in *Sense and Sensibility*, Colonel Brandon regrets having allowed his ward, Eliza, to go to Bath 'at her earnest desire'; in *Pride and Prejudice*, Wickham is sent off to Bath 'to enjoy himself'; in *Emma*, Mr. Elton makes the most of Bath's famous marriage market to seek a wife; and in *Mansfield Park*, while Mr. Rushworth goes down to Bath to fetch his mother, the Rev. Dr. Grant chooses the spa town to be cured of the gouty symptoms induced by gluttony.

[4] According to Cassandra Austen's Memorandum, *Northanger Abbey* (or 'Susan') was probably drafted in 1798-99, after Jane Austen's visit to Bath in November 1797. As mentioned in the 'advertisement, by the authoress, to *Northanger Abbey*' written in 1816, the novel was 'intended for immediate publication, in 1803', since the London firm of Crosby and Co. paid £10 for the manuscript, but 'the business proceeded no farther'. In 1809, Jane Austen personally wrote to Crosby under the pseudonym of Mrs. Ashton Dennis (which enabled her to sign the letter with the evocative initials 'MAD.-') to both offer to send another copy of the manuscript if it had been lost, and warn Crosby that she would approach another publisher if he failed to answer. While threatening to take legal proceedings against the rival publisher, Crosby proposed to return the manuscript for the original price, but Jane Austen could not afford such expenditure. In the spring of 1816, she asked Henry to buy the manuscript of 'Susan' back from Crosby. She revised it in August 1816. In December 1817, *Northanger Abbey* and *Persuasion* were eventually published together posthumously, by John Murray, with a 'Biographical Notice' added by Henry Austen (given as 1818 on the title page).

1 'Examining Some of These Putrifying Houses'

The first surviving letter that explicitly conveys Jane Austen's personal reaction to Bath dates from May 1799 when she was invited there by her wealthy brother Edward, who had been ill for some months, and his wife Elizabeth. As Edward's complaints were believed to have a gouty origin, he had been advised to go to Bath to try a new medical treatment, including electricity. Jane relates their arrival to Cassandra in the following terms:

> Our first view of Bath has been just as gloomy as it was last November twelvemonth. [...] We stopt in Paragon as we came along, but [...] it was too wet & dirty for us to get out [...]. There was a very long list of Arrivals here, in the Newspaper yesterday, so that we need not immediately dread absolute Solitude—and there is a public Breakfast in Sydney Gardens every morning, so that we shall not be wholly starved. (*Letters* 19, Friday 17, May 1799; Le Faye 1995, 40–41)

Despite the typically humorous and ironic Austen style, we can feel some slight disappointment in her account, mainly due to the lack of acquaintance in Bath, whereas the long visitors' list testified to the importance of the city as a pleasure resort, fuelled by increasing geographical and social mobility. Her four surviving letters are variously concerned with Bath's shops and fashion or with Edward's health, but Jane feels sceptical about the perceived benefits of the waters:

> As the Waters have never *dis*agreed with him in any respect, We are inclined to hope that he will derive advantage from them in the end;– everybody encourages us in this expectation, for they all say that the effects of the Waters cannot be negative. (*Letters* 21, Tuesday 11, June 1799; Le Faye 1995, 44)

Apart from the beautiful fireworks in Sidney Gardens which surpassed her expectations, Jane notes that they 'have not been to any public place lately, nor performed anything out of the common daily routine of N°13, Queen Square' (Le Faye 1995, 45).

It is in a letter dated January 1801 that Bath really becomes a 'hot topic' after Mr. Austen had decided to retire as rector of Steventon in favour of his son James, and settle permanently in the Georgian city on account of Mrs. Austen's poor health—but also probably because

Cassandra and Jane were still both single. Bath was where George and Cassandra Austen had married in 1764, at the medieval church of St Swithin's Walcot, and, in the first years of the nineteenth century, the city was still famous for its 'proper' marriage market. As Roy Porter notes, 'unlike Restoration Tunbridge Wells, Bath was not a hotbed of sexual debauchery, possibly because Beau Nash was heedful to preserve Bath's reputation' (Porter 1991, 227). Jane, moreover, had expressed her disappointment with the latest balls at Deane, in Hampshire, as evidenced by a letter dated November 1, 1800: 'There was a scarcity of Men in general, & a still greater scarcity of any that were good for much' (Le Faye 1995, 53). As a country-dance was 'an emblem of marriage', to take up Henry Tilney's famous comparison in *Northanger Abbey* (Austen 1998b, vol. 1, Chapter 10, 56), the lack of dancing partners simply did not bode well for spinsters. Now, if 'the advantages of Bath to the young are pretty generally understood' (Austen 2002, *Emma* vol. 2, Chapter 14, 223), Jane's immediate reaction to the news that they would soon be leaving Steventon for Bath was not one of relief at all, since, according to the family story, she 'fainted'. Her letters to Cassandra between November 1800 and January 1801 reflect the sense of upheaval she felt at having to move, especially as the family discussions were fraught with nervousness about the trouble and expense of removal: Jane, in particular, was neither satisfied with the projected domestic arrangements, nor with the disappointing valuation and sale of live-stock and furniture. By January 1801, however, she seemed to have accepted the idea:

> I get more & more reconciled to the idea of our removal. We have lived long enough in this Neighbourhood, the Basingstoke Balls are certainly on the decline, there is something interesting in the bustle of going away, & the prospect of spending future summers by the Sea or in Wales is very delightful.—For a time we shall now possess many of the advantages which I have often thought of with Envy in the wives of Sailors or Soldiers.—It must not be generally known however that I am not sacrificing a great deal in quitting the Country - or I can expect to inspire no tenderness, no interest in those we leave behind. (*Letters* 29, Monday 5, January 1801; Le Faye 1995, 68–69)

In May 1801, Jane writes to Cassandra from their uncle Leigh-Perrot's home at the Paragon, but once more, she can barely hide her disappointment: 'The first view of Bath in fine weather does not answer my expectations; I think I see more distinctly thro' Rain.—The Sun was got behind everything, and the appearance of the place from the top of Kingsdown, was all vapour, shadow, smoke & confusion' (Le Faye 1995, 82). As the Austens were actively looking for a house, the main problem was to find suitable accommodation. Jane's remarks stress her father's anxiousness to get a respectable address despite strained finances: 'He grows quite ambitious & actually requires now a comfortable & creditable looking house' (Le Faye 1995, 73). Even though George Austen had tried to raise his tithes in order to get six hundred a year ahead of the removal (Le Faye 1995, 69), such an income was hardly sufficient to afford a truly respectable address in the fashionable city. David Nokes aptly comments on Jane Austen's acute awareness of her family's finances: 'What she found chiefly depressing was a constant preoccupation with money. As they trudged along the dusty streets of Bath in search of their new home, it was impossible to ignore the reality of their strict financial constraints' (Nokes 1997, 236). Bath, moreover, was 'socially brittle' and so 'fragmented by class privilege and money and snobbery' that 'the intercourse of the social classes was more difficult and improbable than at Steventon' (Honan 1987, 170–171)—a remark in line with Jane's own account of their tiny parties:

> I dressed myself as well as I could, & had all my finery much admired at home. [...] Before tea, it was rather a dull affair. [...] Another stupid party last night; perhaps if larger they might be less intolerable, but here there were only just enough to make one card table, with six people to look over, & talk nonsense to each other. (*Letters* 36, 12–13 May, 1801; Le Faye 1995, 84–85)

As renting a house had turned into a challenge, Jane kept bemoaning the price of food—although the Duchess of York's removal was expected to make the price of salmon more reasonable!—and the dampness of the buildings they were visiting: 'The apartment [...] pleased me particularly. [...] The only doubt is about the Dampness of the Offices, of which there were symptoms' (*Letters* 35, 5–6 May 1801; Le Faye, 1995, 85–87). A few weeks later, her remarks to Cassandra were even bitterer:

> Our views on G.P. Buildings seem all at an end; the observation of the damps still remaining in the offices of an house which has been only vacated a week, with reports of discontented families & putrid fevers, has given the coup the grace.—We have now nothing in view. When you arrive, we will at least have the pleasure of examining some of these putrifying

> Houses again;—they are so very desirable in size & situation, that there is some satisfaction in spending ten minutes within them. (*Letters* 37, 21–22 May, 1801; Le Faye 1995, 86–87)

While Bath was famous for the curative virtues of its waters, theoretically synonymous with purity and purification, Jane's letters thus point to other metaphors: in a city whose economy flourished on illness and sickness, even the houses, ironically enough, seemed contaminated.

The Austens finally settled in Sydney Place, a newly developed area across the river Avon, between 1801 and 1804. Although the lively social life of Bath could still prove an exciting scene for the novelist, it led neither to marriage nor to the publication of novels. In January 1805, George Austen's death left his widow and two single daughters in even more straitened circumstances. Not only were the three women forced to move to smaller and cheaper lodgings where they would probably be 'unwelcome to everybody', they were also forced to rely on the voluntary contributions of the Austen brothers to avoid their 'sinking in poverty'.[5] As David Nokes remarks, 'to be poor in the country was one thing; to be poor in a place like Bath where an unfashionable address might mean all the difference between acceptability and exclusion, was quite a different matter' (Nokes 1997, 223). Jane's description of their shrinking social circle in the spring of 1805 conveys her grief, anger and bitterness: 'There was a monstrous deal of stupid quizzing, & common-place nonsense talked, but scarcely any Wit' (Le Faye 1995, 104). Whereas Bath offered a brilliant circle of pleasant company indulging in conspicuous consumption, it was, for Jane Austen, synonymous with frustration, deprivation and isolation, although their acquaintances were still inviting her and her mother to quiet tea parties, in keeping with their mourning status and reduced financial means.

In 1806, Jane Austen finally left Bath for Clifton, 'with what happy feelings of Escape!' from a city where she could never be free of 'vulgar economy', as she called her nagging concern with the necessity of managing the domestic budget (Le Faye 1995, 138). It was only in the tranquillity of Chawton Cottage, however, that, thanks to her brother Edward, she could enjoy the necessary peace of mind to start revising her novels, far from the clamour of the town and free from the fear of

[5] In a letter to Cassandra dated 24 August 1805, Jane Austen actually describes herself as 'a Sister sunk in poverty' (Le Faye 1995, 108).

spiralling rents. As her memories of Bath thus turned into a literary material, the 'sense of place' Jane Austen felt evolved over time, as evidenced in *Northanger Abbey* and *Persuasion*.

2 *Northanger Abbey*: Bath as a Place of Adventures

In *Northanger Abbey*, Jane Austen's choice of Bath as a fictional setting is chiefly linked to her literary project and fictional agenda:

> Charming as were all Mrs. Radcliffe's works, and charming even as were the works of all her imitators, it was not in them perhaps that human nature, at least in the midland counties of England, was to be looked for. Of the Alps and Pyrenees, with their pine forests and their vices, they might give a faithful delineation; and Italy, Switzerland, and the South of France, might be as fruitful in horrors as they were there represented. [...] But in the central part of England there was surely some security for the existence even of a wife not beloved, in the laws of the land, and the manners of the age. (Austen 1998b, vol. 2, Chapter 10, 161)

In this audacious burlesque of contemporary popular fiction which begins with a plain heroine and 'a resounding no',[6] Jane Austen obviously intended to distance herself from such sublime landscapes and Gothic clichés as characterised the sensational works of Mrs. Radcliffe or Eliza Parsons, full of haunted castles, secret passages, murdered wives and cruel *banditti*. Terry Castle rightly argues that 'in telling a story of 'no's' and 'not's', the novelist was making a statement about her own art—about what it would *not* be, what it would *not* describe, what it would *not* endorse' (Austen 1998b, x). Instead of relying on supernatural horror or on exotic scenery, Austen chose to draw upon the mundane, urban and realistic setting of Bath, to bring together her main characters, show the usual distractions available to young girls, and advance her marriage plot:

> Every body acquainted with Bath may remember the difficulties of crossing Cheap-street [...] It is indeed a street [...] so unfortunately connected with the great London and Oxford roads [...] that a day never passes in which parties of ladies, however important their business, whether in quest of

[6] See Terry Castle's 'Introduction' to *Northanger Abbey* (Castle 1998b, vii).

> pastry, millinery or even (as in the present case) of young men, are not detained on one side or other by carriages, horsemen, or carts. (Austen 1998b, vol. 1, Chapter 7, 27)

In a self-consciously literary and referential novel, the narrator highlights that daily incidents, authentic places and a particular relationship between literature and experience would thus be the subject of her fiction, far from the sensational doings of romance. Yet, the narrator's description of the heroine's arrival in Bath stands in stark contrast with Austen's own discovery of the city: 'They arrived in Bath. Catherine was all eager delight [...] as they approached its fine and striking environs. [...] She was come to be happy, and she felt happy already' (Austen 1998b, vol. 1, Chapter 2, 6). In *Northanger Abbey*, Bath appears as 'the resort of the sound rather than the sick' to take up Daniel Defoe's words,[7] especially as leisure and the pursuit of pleasure had become more respectable in the eighteenth century (Porter 1991, 227). Henry Tilney's description of his daily activities in Bath—'here, you are in pursuit only of amusement all day long' (Austen 1998b, vol. 1, Chapter 10, 59)—seems to echo Lord Chesterfield's advice to his son: 'Pleasure is now, and ought to be, your business' (Porter 1991, 227). *Northanger Abbey* is unique among Austen's novels in depicting at length the public world of a well-known city, conveying its smart allure 'with its crowds of people passing in and out, up the steps and down', its Pump-Room where 'every creature in Bath was to be seen at different periods of the fashionable hours' (Austen 1998b, vol. 1, Chapter 4, 16). Such descriptions are in keeping with the *New Bath Guide* of 1801 where the city is compared to a 'vortex of amusement' (*The New Bath Guide*, 26) filled with noise and bustle, pandering to the whims of real and imaginary invalids.

In this society bent on pleasure and acquisition, Bath's 'good shops' and public places foreground consumer signs as so many powerful markers of taste, status and income—hence Mrs. Allen's 'consolation' in finding that 'the lace on Mrs. Thorpe's pelisse was not half so handsome as that on her own' (Austen 1998b, vol. 1, Chapter 4, 17). Although the narrator here refrains from becoming judgemental, things and commodities are subtly used to mark out the characters' motivations in order to guide

[7]'Now we may say it [Bath] is the resort of the sound, rather than the sick; the bathing is made more a sport and diversion, than a physical prescription for health' (*A Tour Through the Whole Island of Great Britain*, Defoe 1971, 360).

the readers' assessment of their reliability. From that perspective, Isabella Thorpe's knowledge of 'dress, balls, flirtations, quizzes and news items' (Austen 1998b, vol. 1, Chapter 4, 18), which is typical both of Bath's pleasure-seeking society and of a feverish search for novelty and status, is exposed by the narrator who favours other moral and polite qualities.

Beyond the referential allusions to the city streets, Bath's main public attractions—the Upper and Lower Rooms, the Pump-room, theatre and concert hall—are also used in a symbolic way, both as literary spaces and as a dramatic stage fit for a naive 'heroine's entrée into life'—as in Frances Burney's *Evelina* (1778), which is partly set in Bath. Catherine Morland thus makes her entrance into the world in the Assembly Rooms, which form the perfect matrimonial background for the swift development of a pretty love story between young people under the eyes of their parents, chaperons or the master of ceremonies. But the narrator also manages to defamiliarise this referential setting by hinting at 'all the difficulties and dangers of a six weeks' residence in Bath' (Austen 1998b, vol. 1, Chapter 2, 5). Although Mr. Allen is ordered there merely 'for the benefit of a gouty constitution' (Austen 1998b, vol. 1, Chapter 1, 5), Austen's narrator repeatedly plays on the contrast between her readers' Gothic and sentimental expectations, and her own more down-to-earth agenda, as 'Mrs. Morland knew so little of lords and baronets that she was wholly unsuspicious of danger to her daughter from their machinations' (Austen 1998b, vol. 1, Chapter 2, 6). We can see here Austen's technique of both capitalising on and parodying well-known plots—already showcasing 'the anxieties of common life' over 'the alarms of romance' (Austen 1998b, vol. 2, Chapter 10, 161)—in order to suggest what she would not endorse artistically.

Ironically enough, Bath comes to represent Austen's 'sense of abroad', where the heroine is conveniently sent off to accompany Mrs. Allen, 'a good-humoured woman, [...] probably aware that if adventures will not befall a young lady in her own village, she must seek them abroad' (Austen 1998b, vol. 1, Chapter 1, 5). Catherine's progress as a heroine will thus consist in learning to navigate the actual and symbolic dangers associated with the spa town. In a work concerned with the reading of novels and of other people's words and actions, the Bath marriage market appears as a transactional space filled with potential dangers, scandals, seducers, speculators and would-be consumers, a place both associated with fiction, and with the need to create fictions about an heiress's dowry. As Tamara S. Wagner aptly argues,

> the Bath scenes contain a social Gothic that manifests itself in oppressive crowds, deceitful would-be suitors, and social embarrassments as painful as the supernatural horrors delineated in the novels Catherine consumes. [...] Bath's social Gothic anticipates the reinvestigation of traditional Gothic trappings that Catherine more literally embarks on at Northanger Abbey'. (Wagner 2012, 260)

Even though, ironically enough, the 'dangers' are not exactly those that Catherine anticipates, the ball rooms are actually packed with such cunning women as Isabella Thorpe, whose malevolent influence on Catherine definitely has sinister overtones. And a fortune hunter like John Thorpe leads her into a constant train of mortifying social blunders: 'To escape, so narrowly escape John Thorpe' becomes her main concern, to put an end to her Gothic-like 'agony' and 'fright' (Austen 1998, vol. 1, Chapter 10, 55) after the mock abduction scene. But as Thorpe takes her away from his main rival in the Bath streets, the whole scene amounts to a symbolic rape: 'Catherine, angry and vexed as she was, was obliged to give up the point and submit' (Austen 1998, vol. 1, Chapter 11, 65). If such stratagems recall the eighteenth-century character of the rake, they indeed foreshadow Catherine's encounter with an actual gothic villain within the abbey. By juxtaposing Thorpe's comments about the sale of a horse—'Tilney, does he want a horse? Here is a friend of mine, Sam Fletcher, has got one to sell that would suit anybody. A famous clever animal for the road—only 40 guineas!' (Austen 1998, vol. 1, Chapter 10, 56)—and Henry Tilney's remarks on marriage, Austen sets out to question and deconstruct the very workings of the marriage market. On this actual and symbolic market, both women and beasts are commodified and can be bought, despite the prevalence of a standard polite conversation, veneer of good manners and highly codified rituals. As Porter recalls, 'the rules of etiquette laid down by Beau Nash, the master of ceremonies, ensured that, once arrived there, all ranks had to behave alike' (Porter 1991, 233). If these strict rules of dancing and etiquette were meant to educate the gentry and middle classes, they also contributed to the impression that Bath could be 'dull', thereby echoing Elizabeth Montagu's cynical statement of the city where 'the only thing one can do one day, one did not do the day before, is to die' (Porter 1991, 227). This ironic representation actually enables Austen to criticise the social values associated with the spa town, notably its gregarious socialising—a relevant enterprise in a novel which not only interrogates literary constructs and genres, but also deconstructs the social rituals and false sociability characteristic of Bath: 'For a fine Sunday in Bath empties every house of its inhabitants, and all the world appears on such an occasion to walk about and tell their acquaintance what a charming day it is' (Austen 1998, vol. 1, Chapter 5, 19). While the master of ceremonies introduces Catherine to Henry, the heroine repeatedly fails to understand the city's codes, leading to much misunderstanding, misreading and misinterpreting. This constrained sociability precludes any sincere and private conversation, all the more so when such trivial topics as lace and muslin are foregrounded in female speeches as their main quality criterion. In this vortex of shallow amusement, vanity and superficiality, where genuine exchanges are blocked, interior spaces may also easily turn into traps, since 'the season was full, the room crowded, and the two ladies squeezed in as well as they could' (Austen 1998, vol. 1, Chapter 2, 7). A stifling crowd may not only prevent genuine social encountering, it can also turn into a dangerous mob, symbolising women's powerlessness, passivity and utter plight on the marriage market.

As the Bath social comedy is both staged and discussed, the narrator hints at another possible 'danger' inherent in a six-week residence in the spa town: ruin or bankruptcy, when all passions are spent along with the money, forcing people to leave. If visitors 'ought to be tired at the end of six weeks', after which Bath becomes 'the most tiresome place in the world', it is also probably because most 'people can afford to stay no longer' (Austen 1998, vol. 1, Chapter 10, 58). Whereas people flocked to Bath to be *cured*, Isabella Thorpe's somewhat ironical exclamation—'I get so immoderately *sick* of Bath [...] though it is vastly well to be here for a few weeks, we would not live here for millions [...] preferring the country to every other place' (Austen 1998, vol. 1, Chapter 10, 51)—was undoubtedly endorsed by Jane Austen who well knew that 'we do not look in great cities for our best morality' (Austen 1998, *Mansfield Park*, vol. 1, Chapter 9, 66). In *Northanger Abbey*, however, there is no escaping Bath since it forms an intermediate space and construct allowing for much irony, parody and social unmasking. Such a conventional, animated and comic backdrop enables the heroine to go through the necessary public trials and 'persecutions' before she can eventually reach a capacity for female enlightenment and domestic happiness. Austen's reconstructed Bath thus partakes of her literary goal to combine a rewriting of generic and narrative conventions with an entertaining criticism of an emerging consumer society.

While Bath, according to an eighteenth-century observer, provided the same 'specimen of company as usual, "widows wanting husbands, old men wanting health, and misses wanting partners"' (Porter 1991, 227), Austen succeeds in varying both her approach to the city and her depiction of its space in *Persuasion*. Far from the hybrid text of *Northanger Abbey*, which at once parodies and reshapes Gothic and sentimental fiction, *Persuasion* showcases a more complex representation of the city, more alert to the changing social nuance of location and to the breaking up of a society hardly aware of its derelictions.

3 *Persuasion*: Between Ironic Dislocation and Blissful Reunion

The early chapters of *Persuasion* draw a striking parallel between the fate of Jane Austen and that of her heroine, Anne Elliot, forced to remove to Bath because of her father's straitened circumstances. Although a small house 'in the country' was 'the object of her ambition', 'the usual fate of Anne attended her [...] she disliked Bath, and did not think it agreed with her—and Bath was to be her home' (Austen 1995, Chapter 2, 10). This forced relocation is mainly due to Sir Walter Elliot's extravagance and debt, which require both a change of abode and radical financial measures as suggested by the prevailing metaphor of retrenchment: 'They must retrench [...] Bath was a much safer place for a gentleman in his predicament—he might there be important at comparatively little expense' (Austen 1995, Chapter 2, 10). The Bath economy does not merely thrive on physical illness, but also on the moral flaws of the bankrupt members of the upper gentry. Contrary to Catherine Morland's 'eager delight' as they approached Bath's 'fine and striking environs', Anne's first view of the city conveys her melancholic sense of estrangement, loneliness and alienation:

> She persisted in a very determined, though very silent, disinclination for Bath; caught the first dim view of the extensive buildings, smoking in rain, without any wish of seeing them better; felt their progress through the streets to be, however disagreeable, yet too rapid; for who would be glad to see her when she arrived? And looked back, with fond regret, to the bustles of Uppercross and the seclusion of Kellynch. (Austen 1995, Chapter 14, 89)

Anne's blurred vision of the cityscape, underlined by the shift to free indirect discourse, not only suggests the painful loss of her familiar rural world with its reassuring bearings, it also intimates a sense of dislocation, the erosion of traditional landmarks and values. This impressionistic visual approach stands in stark contrast with Lady Russell's enthusiastic aural response to the city:

> When Lady Russell was entering Bath on a wet afternoon [...] amidst the dash of other carriages, the heavy rumble of carts and drays, the bawling of newsmen, muffin-men and milk-men, and the ceaseless clink of pattens, she made no complaint. These were noises which belonged to the winter pleasures. (Austen 1995, Chapter 14, 89)

But Anne has not come to Bath of her own free will to participate in its festivities and merely 'be happy', especially as she dreads 'the possible heats of September in all the white glare of Bath' (Austen 1995, Chapter 5, 23). She enters her father's rented house 'with a sinking heart, anticipating an imprisonment of many months' as she resumes her unenviable position as a 'nobody' in a family hit by social, financial and moral decline (Austen 1995, Chapter 15, 90). In *Persuasion*, the representation of Bath mainly serves to expose the vanity, stupidity and improper pride of Sir Walter Elliot and of his eldest daughter Elizabeth, who, impervious to their degradation, choose to take 'a very good house in Camden-place, a lofty, dignified situation, such as becomes a man of consequence' (Austen 1995, Chapter 15, 90). As had been the case for the Austens, the 'credit' (Austen 1995, Chapter 2, 8) and 'consequence' (Austen 1995, Chapter 2, 9) of the Elliot family definitely depend on a fashionable address in Bath—although this relocation can never equal the whole series of obligations and responsibilities implied in the initial juxtaposition of 'Sir Walter Elliot, of Kellynch-hall, in Somersetshire' (Austen 1995, Chapter 1, 3). The free indirect style gives even more poignancy to Anne's disappointment at her father's self-delusion: 'She must sigh that her father should feel no degradation in his change; should see nothing to regret in the duties and dignity of the resident land-holder; should find so much to be vain of in the littleness of a town' (Austen 1995, Chapter 15, 91). Camden Place had less impressive views than the Royal Crescent, but this classical crescent built in 1787-8 on the northern heights of the city was a site for the new money to stage their social achievement. David Selwyn notes that Camden Place perfectly reflects the vanity of the baronet, since, 'grand as it was, it was never actually finished: landslips had prevented further building, with the consequence that the imposing pediment was awkwardly off-centre' (Selwyn 1999, 41). In her last completed novel, Austen significantly relies on the symbolism of place to emphasise the shifting social nuances of location characteristic of Bath at a time of momentous change, in 1815. While Lady Dalrymple and her daughter station themselves in Laura-place where they 'would be living in style' (Austen 1995, Chapter 16, 98), Queen Square is not considered as fashionable enough by the Musgrove girls, since the Musgroves, 'like their houses, were in a state of alteration, perhaps of improvement' (Austen 1995, Chapter 5, 27). Rising into social consequence thanks to naval prize money at the end of the Napoleonic wars, the Crofts confidently settle in the city centre in Gay Street, 'perfectly to Sir Walter's satisfaction', for the admiral will be mainly known in Bath as the renter of Kellynch-hall (Austen 1995, Chapter 18, 111). While Jane Austen draws on real locations to help readers grasp her characters' respective values and social aspirations, this geographical distribution also dramatises the hierarchisation of space and increasing social competition in the novel. The Elliots, who 'move in the first circle of Bath' in order to get only 'great acquaintance' and 'make use of the relationship', look down upon their 'social inferiors' (Austen 1995, Chapter 16, 99), particularly if they happen to live in a less fashionable part of the city. Hence Sir Walter's indignation at Anne's going to Westgate buildings:

> And who is Miss Anne Elliot to be visiting in Westgate-buildings?—A Mrs. Smith. A widow Mrs. Smith,—and who was her husband? One of the five thousand Mr. Smiths whose names are to be met with every where. And what is her attraction? That she is old and sickly.—Upon my word, Miss Anne Elliot, you have the most extraordinary taste! Every thing that revolts other people, low company, paltry rooms, foul air, disgusting associations are inviting to you. (Austen 1995, Chapter 17, 104)

Through the baronet's scornful remarks, Austen draws attention, much more satirically than in *Northanger Abbey*, to the social compartmentalisation and fragmentation of the 'fashionable' spa, where social classes are estranged: *Persuasion* depicts a town of both want and plenty, attracting 'nouveaux riches' and 'nouveaux pauvres' alike, but with hardly any connection between the social circles. As the text's geography is as referential as it is symbolic, the Elliots' ambition and social pretension lead them to prefer 'the elegant stupidity of private parties', too numerous for intimacy, too small for variety, and leading to a 'state of stagnation' (Austen 1995, Chapter 19, 119). Contrary to *Northanger Abbey*, the 'theatre and the rooms are deemed not fashionable enough' for the elite (Austen 1995, Chapter 19, 119), thus precluding any social mixing. If Bath had become 'the cynosure of elegance' (Porter 1991, 227), the harmonious architecture of the city actually jars with the poor manners of the elite, whose appreciation of 'inferior people' merely depends on outward signs and appearances, as with Captain Wentworth: 'A very fine young man indeed!', said Lady Dalrymple, 'more air than one often sees in Bath' (Austen 1995, Chapter 20, 125). As the bankrupt elite is forced to come to terms with the social dilution characteristic of a time which may bring 'persons of obscure birth into undue distinction' (Austen 1995, Chapter 3, 14), the Captain's distinguished bearing and enviable fortune in prize money mark him out as a new asset in such a compressed social milieu. In a novel where 'good company requires only birth, education and manners' (Austen 1995, Chapter 16, 99), the social elite draws on such empty mottos as 'rank is rank', a tautology which reflects their utter snobbery and vanity, now that good manners have degenerated into meaningless signifiers. As in *Northanger Abbey*, genuine communication is blocked, especially for Anne who, 'sick of knowing nothing', 'so surrounded and shut in' by her own circle, cannot communicate with Captain Wentworth 'standing among a cluster of men at a little distance' (Austen 1995, Chapter 20, 125). In *Persuasion*, the spa town is a place for the sick, physically and morally, where leisure degenerates into boredom and vanity.

Whereas most characters go to Bath to be cured physically and emotionally—its waters symbolising a smooth circulation and flow—the representation of Bath in *Persuasion* thus ironically conveys a sense of social competition and disunion. Worse, with the trading of landed values for financial and speculative ventures, Bath appears as a city full of intrigues and scandals where characters like Mrs. Clay and Mr. Elliot prosper. Roger Sales aptly notes that the values and mores associated with such watering places produce as much sickness as they cure—in *Emma*, it is actually in the 'idlest haunts in the kingdom' that Frank Churchill has acquired manners that threaten to disrupt the rural community (Sales 1994, 170).

If Bath is used as a revealing stage to dramatise the tensions between the assertion of modern values and the preservation of former customs, it is Anne, who, as an 'in-between', allows for a more harmonious circulation between people and social classes, whether with 'the gentlemen of the navy' or with Mrs. Smith. Anne visits her 'poor, infirm, helpless' friend in lodgings near the hot baths, but ironically enough, it is in the latter's 'noisy parlour and dark bed-room behind' that she gets the most enlightening information: thanks to Nurse Rooke's truly 'profitable gossip' (Austen 1995, Chapter 17, 103)—this powerful parallel female economy—the murky business dealings and despicable behaviour of Mr. Elliot are exposed, shedding new light on the most prominent members of Bath society. Thanks to their mobility, gossip and resilience, women defeat social compartmentalisation. While Anne bemoans her father's seeing 'funds of enjoyment' (Austen 1995, Chapter 15, 90) in the company of such stupid nonentities as Lady Dalrymple and her daughter, she conversely appreciates her female connections' 'fund of good sense and observation' (Austen 1995, Chapter 17, 102), which ultimately lead her to reject Mr. Elliot's proposal. As the fate of this heroine was 'to learn romance as she grew older' (Austen 1995, Chapter 4, 21), she is rewarded for bringing back fluidity between the different economies at work. Bath's 'Union Street' is thus aptly used as a symbolically privileged site to enable Anne's blissful reunion with Captain Wentworth:

> In half a minute Charles was at the bottom of Union-street[8] again, and the other two proceeding together: and soon words enough had passed between them to decide their direction towards the comparatively quiet and retired gravel walk, where the power of conversation would make the present hour a blessing indeed; and prepare for it all the immortality which the happiest recollections of their own future lives could bestow. There they exchanged again those feelings and those promises which had once before seemed to secure everything, but which had been followed by so many, many years of division and estrangement. There they returned again into the past, more exquisitely happy, perhaps, in their re-union, than when it had been first projected; more tender, more tried, more fixed in a knowledge of each other's character, truth, and attachment; more equal to act, more justified in acting. And there, as they slowly paced the gradual ascent, heedless of every group around them, seeing neither sauntering politicians, bustling house-keepers, flirting girls, nor nursery maids

[8] 'Union Street – i.e. the union of Milsom and Stall Streets – was projected as early as 1789, but it was not completed till the close of 1806' (Ragg 1938, 59).

> and children, they could indulge in those retrospections and acknowledgments, and especially in those explanations of what had directly preceded the present moment, which were so poignant and so ceaseless in interest. (Austen 1995, Chapter 23, 160)

The Bath topography is here symbolically significant, as the scene takes place on 'the quiet and retired gravel walk' behind *Gay* Street and The *Circus*, protected by the city bustle, in an in-between space, half-private, half-public. This blissfully climactic scene, heightened by Austen's choice of an actual street-name endowed with strong symbolism, stages antithetical moments and movements: whereas this reunion is of the highest significance for the couple after years of estrangement, their feeling of intimacy and privacy is paradoxically emphasised by placing them alongside anonymous strollers. While the three present participles, 'sauntering', 'bustling' and 'flirting' epitomise transience and superficiality, we notice that Austen's style blends prose and poetry to mark the fact that two lives and souls are joined again. The cityscape is subtly used because the sense of completion, achievement and meaningful conversation is brought forward against a background of vagueness and general noise, allowing emotional barriers to break down. While Bath's oppressive public places had prevented the lovers' conversation, its outer space fosters their reunion by protecting their intimacy and genuine communication. Austen uses Bath as more than just a stage: its humdrum surroundings are infused with movement, dynamic motion, radiating positive energy as if the world was bursting into new life. In this moment of supreme harmony, far from the former 'division' and 'estrangement' both characteristic of the lovers' former relationship and of the social functioning of Bath, the verb 'exchange' conveys reciprocal giving and receiving. In this scene, Jane Austen is undertaking a radical reassessment of her system of values and view on her art, in keeping with her narrator's description of Anne: 'She had been forced into prudence in her youth, she learnt romance as she grew older' (Austen 1995, Chapter 4, 21). After Bath's various public places were synonymous with disillusion, conflict, misunderstanding or misreading, its outer space eventually allows the lovers to overcome past tensions and achieve a true union of hearts and minds. The ascending street becomes a metaphor to represent life as a journey into the future, epitomising the lovers' increasing comprehension and upward progress in life, as they 'slowly paced the gradual ascent': while the verb conveys a measured movement, the adjective 'gradual' suggests a progressive process, taking place by degrees. Space and time thus seem to be fused in this particularly expressive line. Austen's realism here dissolves into symbolism, as Bath's outer referential space becomes an ultimate moment and place, in time.

4 Conclusion: Opening up New Vistas

Despite Catherine Morland's enthusiastic exclamation, 'Oh! Who can ever be tired of Bath?', the most recurrent metaphors that run through the two novels reveal disturbing undercurrents, probably accounting for the fact that Jane Austen herself did grow tired of Bath, tired of watching people 'in pursuit only of amusement all day long'—especially when *she* could not afford all the pleasures the fashionable city had to offer, or simply could not stand the intellectual poverty of its tiny parties.

While Franco Moretti contends that Austen's novels represent a 'small, homogeneous England' (Moretti 1998, 14), their reconstruction of Bath as a literary space rather epitomises conflicting values, especially as it draws contradictory sensations and responses from characters. If both *Northanger Abbey* and *Persuasion* use Bath as a theatrical stage and play on the social, cultural and literary imaginary associated with the spa town, they offer nuanced representations inherent in their respective generic affiliations. While *Northanger Abbey* is tinged with Gothic and sentimental parody, *Persuasion* explores a wider spectrum, from a realistic portrayal of Bath society's moral vacuity to a romantic and idealised representation of its outer space, enabling the lovers' reunion. In both novels, however, the interdependent economies of health, sickness, marriage and gossip work to uncover what actually lies beneath the genteel surface of harmonious architecture, polite manners and civilised conventions.

Significantly, Austen's last completed novel enacts a transition in her oeuvre, from the representation of the spa town to that of the seaside resort, as Bath was losing its high society glamour in the first decades of the century. With its references to the navy and its scenes set by the seaside in Lyme Regis, *Persuasion* foreshadows both the development of the nineteenth-century seaside pleasure resort with sea-bathing as the newly fashionable health treatment, and the emergence of a new kind of novel, *Sanditon*. Austen's last work features a family of 'helpless invalids' who abdicate their responsibility as landlords to turn 'a quiet village of no pretensions' into a fashionable bathing place' (Austen 1998b,

Sanditon, 328), thereby becoming greedy property speculators.[9] If, in terms of social mobility, *Sanditon* appears as the logical sequel of *Persuasion* where the social pretension of such unreliable characters as Mrs 'Clay' already thrived despite their shaky foundations, it also definitely represents a radically new thematic, fictional and stylistic departure. Kathryn Sutherland rightly argues that 'with its cliffs and downs and immense skies, its company of misfits and idlers, and its air of restless anxiety, *Sanditon* might just be the first English seaside novel', foregrounding the prevalence of new metaphors in Austen's work:

> What [seaside novels share] is an understanding of the sea and shore as a place of flux. Where land dissolves into sea, where romantic scenery is the consequence of landslips and cataclysm, the seaside is a space between, a place of transformation and transcendence—especially of human reality in the face of nature's great unaccountability. Here the mind responds to limitless views of sea and sky, intimating new beginnings or something darker: dissolution and death. Either way, as the term 'sea change' suggests, the effect is powerful and mysterious. (Sutherland 2019, online)

Leaving behind the security of green rural England with its quiet villages 'of no pretensions' (Austen 1998b, *Sanditon,* 328) and its inherited values, Jane Austen was definitely treading uncertain ground in her last work, left incomplete by her declining health and death. As, 'a little higher up, the Modern began' (Austen 1998b, *Sanditon,* 339), *Sanditon* or 'sand-eaten', is definitely concerned about the transformative powers of inflation, speculation and 'activity run mad!' overtaking communities in such bathing places (Austen 1998b, *Sanditon*, 363). But as Austen was exploring the shifting values of this hectic, eccentric and unstable world, her style paradoxically gained a compelling sense of vista, her heroine 'looking over the miscellaneous foreground of unfinished building, waving linen, and tops of houses, to the sea, dancing and sparkling in sunshine and freshness' (Austen 1998b, *Sanditon*, 340)—a far cry, indeed, from Bath's 'putrifying houses'.

[9] See Massei-Chamayou (2012, 230–240).

Works Cited

Primary Sources

An. *The New Bath Guide; or, Useful Pocket Companion For all Persons residing at or resorting to this Antient City*. 1801. Bath: R. Cruttwell.

Austen, Jane. 1995. *Persuasion (1818)*. London, New York: Norton.

Austen, Jane. 1998a. *Mansfield Park (1814)*. London, New York: Norton.

Austen, Jane. 1998b. *Northanger Abbey, Lady Susan, The Watsons, Sanditon (1818)*. Oxford: Oxford University Press.

Austen, Jane. 2002. *Emma (1816)*. New York: Bedford/ St Martin's Press.

Defoe, Daniel. 1971. *A Tour Through the Whole Island of Great Britain (1724–1726)*. London, New York: Penguin.

Le Faye, Deirdre (ed.). 1995. *Jane Austen's Letters*. Oxford: Oxford University Press.

Secondary Sources

Ballinger, Gill. 2013. Austen's Bath and Bath's Jane: Austen Writing the City and Its Twenty-first Century Marketing of Heritage Jane. In *Persuasions On-line*, v. 34, N°1 (Winter). http://jasna.org/persuasions/on-line/vol34no1/ballinger.html. Accessed October 26, 2020.

Crom, Nathalie. Bath, une ville en bons thermes avec Jane Austen (May 8, 2016). *Télérama*. https://www.telerama.fr/livre/bath-une-ville-en-bons-thermes-avec-jane-austen,141756.php.

Honan, Park. 1987. *Jane Austen: Her Life*. London: Weidenfeld & Nicolson.

Massei-Chamayou, Marie-Laure. 2012. *La Représentation de l'argent dans les romans de Jane Austen*. Coll. Des Idées et des femmes. Paris: L'Harmattan.

Moretti, Franco. 1998. *Atlas of the European Novel, 1800–1900*. London, New York: Verso.

Nokes, David. 1997. *Jane Austen: A Life*. London: Fourth Estate.

Porter, Roy. 1991. *English Society in the Eighteenth Century*. London: Penguin.

Ragg, Laura M. 1938. *Jane Austen in Bath*. London: Alexander Moring.

Sales, Roger. 1994. *Jane Austen and Representations of Regency England*. London, New York: Routledge.

Selwyn, David. 1999. *Jane Austen and Leisure*. London: Hambledon Press.

Sutherland, Kathryn. Did Jane Austen Write the First Seaside Novel? (July 22, 2019). *The Guardian*. URL: https://www.theguardian.com/books/2019/jul/22/austen-at-seaside-new-resorts-novel. Accessed October 26, 2020.

Wagner, Tamara S. 2012. 'Would you have us laughed out of Bath?': Shopping Around for Fashion and Fashionable Fiction in Jane Austen Adaptations. In *Women, Popular Culture, and the Eighteenth Century*, ed. Tiffany Potter, 257–273. Toronto, University of Toronto Press.

PART II

Taking the Waters: Myth, Recreation and Satire

CHAPTER 6

Bath and Bladud: The Progress of a Wayward Myth

Tiffany Stern

Mention King Bladud, and most people look, first, bemused, then, amused: to the British ear, 'Bladud' sounds like 'bladdered', a slang term for having a full bladder, i.e. being drunk. It is an unfortunate name for the great and mythical king who founded Bath. But Bladud's mythical story is just as bemusing and amusing: it is muddled (did Bladud find Bath or create it?), unfixed (how and when did Bladud lose his magical skills and gain leprosy?) and partially—as when Bladud attempts to fly to the sun and dies—borrowed from other, better-known, legends.

This chapter is on the legend of King Bladud, 'maker' of the baths of Bath. It is in two parts. Part one tells the tale of Bladud, as first related by Monmouth in the eleventh century, up until now, showing the changes and permutations it underwent over time. Part two tells the story of Bath over the same period, revealing how Bladud's founding myth was reconceived whenever beliefs about the hot water changed. Both parts consider what an unfixed foundation mythology reveals about its spa city. To what

T. Stern (✉)
The Shakespeare Institute, University of Birmingham, Birmingham, UK
e-mail: t.stern@bham.ac.uk

S. Chiari and S. Cuisinier-Delorme (eds.), *Spa Culture and Literature in England, 1500–1800*, Early Modern Literature in History,
https://doi.org/10.1007/978-3-030-66568-5_6

extent has Bladud's story shaped Bath and its baths, and to what extent has Bath and its baths shaped what is, in more than one sense, the fluid tale of Bladud?

1 The Bladud Myth

The myth of King Bladud was first related by Geoffrey of Monmouth in his powerful, and largely fictional, *Historia regum Britanniae* (*The History of the Kings of Britain*) of c. 1136. That book, written in Latin, was designed to suggest that Britain was founded at roughly the same time as Ancient Rome, its culture thus representing another version of the Golden Age. In Monmouth's pseudo-history, which muddled together classical stories and Celtic ones, 'Brutus' or 'Brute' the Trojan, great grandson of Aeneas of Troy, left his land for 'Albion'. Having killed off Albion's native giants, Brute gave the land on which he now settled a version of his own name, 'Britain'. He sired, there, a line of legendary kings (and queens): Locrinus, Gwendolen, Madden, Mempricius, Ebraucus, Brutus Greenshield, Leil, Rud Hud Hudibras, Bladud, Lear…

Monmouth's work was extremely popular, both in itself, and as a source for literary narratives. Rud Hud Hudibras, Bladud's father, gives his name to the title character of Samuel Butler's *Hudibras*, 1684 (via Spenser's *Faerie Queene*), for instance, while Bladud's son Lear is the subject of one of Shakespeare's most famous plays. The story of Bladud, however, has made far less of an impact on literature. That is partly because, in Monmouth's book, Bladud's myth is sandwiched between that of two more intriguing mythical kings; and partly because his actual story in itself lacks logic and drive.

As Monmouth tells it, 'Bladud […] built Kaerbadus, now Bath, and made hot baths in it for the benefit of the public'. From the first, then, what Bladud actually did is unclear: did he create the baths through magic or skill, or did he erect structures for waters that were already there? Bladud then, continues Monmouth, 'dedicated' his baths 'to the goddess Minerva': but was this a humble 'thank you' because the goddess was responsible for the Baths; or a nod from one variety of godhead to another?

Undoubtedly King Bladud was 'very ingenious' for, as Monmouth relates it, he 'taught necromancy in his kingdom': so suggesting Bladud's magical skills are ultimately behind the baths. Yet the unfortunate death that Bladud met undercuts the idea that he was a tremendous magician or even an insightful man. He wanted to fly, relays Monmouth, and fashioned some wings for the purpose. But he crashed 'upon the temple of Apollo, in the city of Trinovantum, where he was dashed to pieces' (Monmouth 1999, 28). That abortive flight, away from Bath (Trinovantum is thought to be London) oddly concludes the life Bath's founder—but odder still is the fact that it is, seemingly, borrowed from the more famous legend of Daedalus and Icarus.[1] Why did Bath get its very own king, but not its own original narrative?

Many other questions are raised by the confusions set out in this originary story. Was Bladud a king or a god; an artful man or a skilful magician; notably smart or obstinately stupid? Behind these ambiguities are what this tale says—or leaves conflicted—about the hot waters that Bladud 'made'. In that they reflect him, are they to be understood as magical, natural or supernatural? More importantly, are they in their origin and use, good or bad?

Bladud's Myth in Time

After Monmouth, the King Bladud story is repeatedly retold, sometimes as legend, sometimes as pseudo-history. Up to the early modern period, it is nearly always an aspect of a bigger narrative, for no specific individual writer chose to 'own' it, as Shakespeare did Lear. Instead, many, perhaps including Shakespeare himself, touched on Bladud while telling more weighty tales.

By the time John Hardyng comes to relate King Bladud's life, in rhyme and some 400 years after Monmouth, the king's scholastic credentials have been firmly established. Bladud 'makes' the Baths using his ability in magic, which he hones academically by studying abroad at the best university, Athens. He returns home from Athens with four educators in tow:

> He made anone ye hote bathes there [Bath] infere
>
> When at Athenes he had studied clere
>
> He brought with hym. iiii. philosophiers wise

[1] Clark 1994, 43, points out that there are several tales about men attempting to fly to the sun, including Simon Magus, the German Volund/Weland, and the prophet Elijah, which might lie behind the Bladud story. The Daedalus one is the best known, however.

Schole to holde in Brytayne and exercyse.
(Hardyng 1543, C6^{r})

Bladud, with his scholars, then founds Britain's first university in Stamford, Lincolnshire:

Sta[m]forde he made yt Sa[m]forde hight this daye
In whiche he made an universitee
His philosophiers as Merlyn doth saye
Had scolers fele of greate habilitee
Studyng ever alwaye in unitee
In all the seven liberall science
For to purchace wysedome and sapience.
(Hardyng 1543, C6^{r})

Yet despite bringing 'Athenian' learning to Britain—thus indeed making Britain a triumphant continuation of the classical world—Bladud remains lumbered with the same foolish 'death', which sits particularly poorly on this version of the story. Hardyng does his best to explain that Bladud wants 'to flye with winges' because of his eternal quest for 'doctrine' or knowledge, his downfall thus being a tragic example of hubris: 'He flyed on high to the temple Apolyne/And ther brake his necke for al his great doctrine' (Hardyng 1543, C6v). The result, however, is that the mythical founder of Britain's university system is, awkwardly, brought down by his desire for knowledge—raising questions about the connection between intelligence and universities; and whether we should trust the waters, or anything else, that Bladud had made.

Over the next couple of centuries, the King Bladud story was further embellished. Bladud's 'magic', a sticking point for Christians, was roundly condemned by some; given an authoritative, scientific grounding by others. There were those who 'dare not attribute [the baths'] original' to '*Art-Magick*' (Camden 1695, 70); those who let Minerva ultimately take the credit ('Bladud [...] kindle[d] the sulphurous veines, of purpose to burne continually [...] in the honour of *Minerva*', Holinshed 1577, 88); and those who left the role of Bladud in the foundation myth open to question: 'Some affirme that King *Bladud* [...] by his cunning in Magick did frame [Bath]; or rather by his search did finde it, or at least with his cost did first found it' (Harington 1653, F1v). Elucidating Bladud's part in the existence of the hot waters was one way of 'explaining' them, and hence the myth was continually worried at. Working up from medieval manuscript 'scientific' accounts that described the way Bladud's baths were made by heating 'tunnes of bras' (quoted in Fisher 2004, 79-80), John Higgins has his Bladud say:

> I made the holesome Baths at Bathe,
> And made therefore two Tunnes of burning brasse:
> And other twaine seven kinds of salts that have
> In them in closde, but these be made of glasse,
> With sulphur fil'd, wilde fire emixt there was,
> And in foure welles these Tunnes I did assay,
> To place by arte that they might last of aye.
> (Higgins 1619, $F4^{r}$)

This explanation gives a logical rationale to the hot waters that also explicates their sulphurous smell; it exalts Bladud as a brilliant man rather than a creepy magician; and allows the baths to be '[w]holesome'. But the disadvantage is that it renders the source of the baths' heat now dangerously close to gunpowder. Even attempts to give Bladud and his baths a scientific rationale, then, were destabilised, by the water itself, its smell, and its surprising heat, none of which seemed truly 'natural' and all of which hinted at a destructiveness that undercut what might otherwise seem positive in Bladud's narrative.

King Bladud's unfortunate end, the most troubled bit of the story, acquired a range of explanations dependant on whether he himself was seen as good or bad. Often, he remained a tragic, hubristic archetype. In the *Mirour for Magistrates*, Bladud explains how 'God gave grate', but 'Presumption proude, deprivde my breath' (Higgins 1574, $F5^{r}$-$F5^{v}$): the waters are the result of a good God; Bladud's fall was the product of his flaws. In book 2 of Spenser's *Faerie Queene*, meanwhile, where a series of cantos run through the story of the ancient kings of Britain, Bladud is also praised for baths which 'wealth [...] well' (pour out wealth) to 'her people [...] And health to every forreyne nation'. Here, too, the baths are good, but Bladud 'contending to excell/The reach of men, through flight into fond mischief fell' (Spenser 1590, 332).

Other writers see the end of the story as appropriate, given the dangerous 'magic' King Bladud used throughout his life:

> [Bladud] presuming to flye over the towne of *Bathe* broke his neck by falling upon the Temple which he there had built. A fit rewarde for all such as use *Nigromancie* or any such unlawfull acts. (T.I. 1595, $D1^{v}$)

> [Bladud] addicted himselfe so much to the devilish arte of Necromancie, that he wrought wonders thereby: in so much that hee made himselfe wings, and attempted to flie like *Dedalus:* but the devill (as ever, like a false knave) forsooke him in his journey, so that he fell downe and brake his necke. (de Chassanion 1597, I1^{v})

In both of these instances, the baths themselves are 'bad' because Bladud is; that Bladud dies on the very temple that he had built, in the first account, makes the entire tragedy a Bath-centric one. One 'bad Bladud' narrative even suggested that the term 'black art', an Anglification of 'necromancy', descended etymologically from Bladud's name, so that his title enclosed his wickedness and inevitable fall: 'a far fetch'd Etymology, but perhaps as well *Black Art* from *Bladud*, as *Magick* from *Magus* King of *Brittaine*' (Baron 1647, Q3^{v}).

King Bladud's two most significant literary outings of this period reflect the ambiguity of his story. In Marlowe's *Doctor Faustus,* a prologue summarises the play to come explaining how Faustus took 'sweete delight':

> In heavenly matters of *Theologie*,
> Till swolne with cunning of a selfe conceit,
> His waxen wings did mount above his reach,
> And melting heavens conspirde his overthrow.
> (Marlowe 1604, A2^{r})

Though generally glossed as a Daedalus and Icarus analogy, Faustus here is compared to one flying man, not two, and one, moreover with a dangerous quantity of aggrandising self-conceit. And, as Faustus and Bladud were both necromancers who delighted in academic pursuits and were brought down by a desire for knowledge that exceeded its bounds, 'Bladud' in fact seems to infuse the entire play. Yet if this is a direct Bladud reference it is simultaneously his most and least famous literary outing: as he is not actually named here, most readers fail to spot the reference.[2]

[2] Possibly this reference was more recognisable in the period; it may have gestured towards a now-lost play, *The Conquest of Brute, with the first finding of the Bath*, or *Brute Greenshield*, performed by the Admiral's Men in 1598. For further links between the *Conquest of Brute* and *Doctor Faustus*, see Borlik, 2016, 3. For a conjecture as to the story of this lost play, see Wiggins, 2014, 4:78–79.

Marlowe's comparison, however, puts Bladud firmly in the 'bad' camp: he is a magician who over-reaches just as Faustus does.

Other 'hidden' King Bladud references are, or may be, in Shakespeare's *King Lear*. When mad Lear, obsessed with 'poor Tom', declares 'I will keepe still with my Philosopher [...] Come, good Athenian' (Shakespeare 1968, TLN 1659–1664), he shows a knowledge of Athenian philosophy unexpected in an ancient British king, but explicable, as Guy Butler notes, if we recall that his father founded a university made up of such (Butler 1985, 29). Gloucester's 'false fall' from what he believes to be Dover Cliff, also recalls Bladud, and the 'implied human vainglory' of his flight, suggests William Poole (2012, 536–538). These potential Bladud references, to someone who relishes thinkers yet is brought down by bad judgement, provide a mirror for Lear himself. The comparison reminds us that Shakespeare will have to have been familiar with the Bladud tale, which precedes Lear's in most chronicle accounts. But, as ever, Bladud is in danger of undermining the literature he touches upon. The fact that Lear never knew his aging father—his father never reached old age—or had to wait impatiently to inherit his crown, because his dad died ... flying into the sun, provides a problematic subtext to Lear's story.

In the seventeenth century, however, King Bladud's tale received a much-needed overhaul. In 1673, Henry Chapman, mayor of Bath and promoter of the city, printed a rhyming appendix to his book *Thermae redivivae* that replaced the 500-plus-year-old Bladud story. In 'Somerset' dialect the poem related how Bladud, when a prince, contracted leprosy and was expelled from his father's palace. An outcast, he was reduced to working as a swineherd, where his disease even spread to his pigs. One day, however, Bladud's pigs found some natural hot water, bathed in it—and were cured. Bladud immersed himself in the same hot water, and was also cured. He returned home to triumph and rejoicing, and founded Bath on the site of his recovery:

> Then *Bladud* did the Pigs invect [infect], who grunting ran away
> And vound whot [found hot] waters prezently, which made um vresh [them fresh] and gay.
> *Bladud* was not so grote a Vool [great a fool], but zeeing [seeing] what Pig nid [need?] doe,
> He beath'd [bathed] and wash'd and rins'd and beath'd from Noddle [head] down to toe.
> *Bladud* was now (Gramercy [thanks] Pig) a delicate Vine [fine] boy,

> So whome [home] he trudges to his Dad, to be his only Joy.
> And then he bilt this gawdy Town.
> (Chapman 1673, 17)

Every single aspect of the tale has changed, here, apart from King Bladud's name. And, with no conclusion given (the story stops at the happy foundation of Bath) Bladud is spared an awkward death. Here, Bladud is no longer a potentially creepy magician, or even an over-educated man. Instead, he suffers like, and works as, a common man, and learns his greatest lesson when humbled to the level of his pigs. The baths, meanwhile, are not magical but a natural wonder, so wonderfully curative that they bring beast and king equally back to health. It is clear why this story is 'better' for Bath than the old one. But how did it come about? And did Chapman, who printed the poem, create its narrative?

The King Bladud poem is, Chapman maintains, not actually by him, but from the pen of 'Tom Coriat'. As Thomas Coryate lived from 1577 to 1617, but spent his last years abroad, that would date this poem to before 1612 when Coryate left the country. It would mean that the 'new' Bladud tale was around when Shakespeare and others were dealing with the complexities of the 'old' one.[3] Yet if Coryate wrote the poem, why did he not publish it himself, and why did he and others never mention it? Why is the piece in-jokey dialect? And how, so many years later, did Chapman acquire the text? As the poem itself claims to tell a tale from 'Two Thowsand and vive hundred years, and thirty vive to that', and as Bladud's date of birth is typically said to be 863, the poem seems in fact to be from 1672: Strachan concludes it is by Chapman himself (1962, 301), and Clark calls it 'fakelore'—though all versions of the Bladud tale have a right to that title. Most likely to be a Restoration joke poem by Chapman, the claim that the piece is much older may be intended to lend historic authority—or to enhance it with the adventure, satire or exoticism of one of Somerset's most famous sons, Coryate, the noted traveller.

[3] Coryate did have links with the Bladud story that makes his authorship just—remotely—possible. His friend Joannes Jackson attributed his ability to travel to having Fortunatus' magic hat, given that 'wings since Bladuds time/Were out of date'. The reference suggests a shared Bladud knowledge: not surprising for Coryate, who hailed from Somerset. See Coryate 1611, N1^{r}.

Yet the poem also gestures to a source for the tale itself that is worth considering. It claims its narrative is to be found in a 'table'—an inscription—hanging in the King's Bath: 'O Invidels if yee woon [believe] not me, yet chee [I] pray believe the Table' (Chapman 1673, 17). And, as slightly earlier versions of the 'new' tale do seem to have been making the rounds, there may be some truth to the one-time existence of the now-lost 'table'. A manuscript, later published as anonymous, but seemingly by Robert Gay in c.1666, supplies a version of the Bladud/pig story which, it says, comes from 'tradition':

> Bladud [...] became a swineherd near *Bathe*, which was then a bogg [...] of hot water, in which his swine often wallowed, and one of them [...] was thereby cured, whereupon Bladon [sic] [...] was also cured, whereupon he built a Temple, and consecrated it to the sun, as God of the heat of the Bath-water. (Langtoft 1725, 2: 489)

Other accounts too tell of a 'table' that related the pig narrative and that was replaced in the Restoration:

> the famous *John* Earl of Rochester coming to *Bath*, the story of *Bladud* and his Pigs became a Subject for his Wit, and this proved the Cause of striking it out of the Inscription placed against one of the Walls of the King's Bath. (Wood 1749, 1: 76)

This anecdote, while coyly avoiding what precisely the wit, satirist and rake John Wilmot, Earl of Rochester (1647–1680), actually said, seems to date from the 1670s, when Rochester, whose wife's father lived in Bath, visited the city with some regularity (Greer 2000, 21). He, with his interest in grotesque sex—and pigs—apparently teased the narrative out of the inscription.

Yet though the 'new' King Bladud/pig tale was something of a joke in first publication, and the butt of a joke when twitted by Rochester, it took over from the old. In 1704, when the new Pump Room was erected in Bath, a song was 'handed about, and greatly admir'd' which placed Bladud's illness and miraculous recovery at the heart of Bath—though, perhaps for Rochester reasons, it did not mention the pigs:

> Great BLADUD born a Sov'reign Prince,
>   But from the Court was Banish'd thence,
>   His dire Disease to shun,

> The Muses do his Fame record,
> That when the Bath his Health restor'd,
> Great *Bladud* did return.
> (Wood 1749, 1:223–224)

A Bladud puppet-show by Martin Powell, of around the same time, also created to celebrate the new Pump Room, likewise celebrated Bladud (and once again appears to have erased the pigs). Recorded in an advertisement of 1711, the show depicted:

> the History of King Bladud, Founder of the Bath. The Figures being drest after the manner of Ancient Britains. With the Walks, Groves, and Representation of the King's Bath and new Pump-house. The Figures of Ladies and Gentlemen all moving in real Water. (*Daily Courant* 1711)

The focus of the puppet-show is, it seems, the contrast between ancient Britain and the new pump room; the constant is the curative water that joins 'then' to 'now', and King Bladud with 'Ladies and Gentlemen'.

Yet the pigs did not stay out of King Bladud's new tale for long. They were homely, domestic and 'British', and they led easily to satire, giving them obvious appeal. Their return, however, did not bring about a much-needed updating of Bladud's death, still stuck in its 'old' form. So, in 1728 Captain Thomas Goulding of Bath published scene descriptions of his pageant, *The transformation, or the fall of Bladud as he assumed the seat of Jupiter*:

> Scene 1—Pastoral, representing a grove of oaks with a herd of swine masting.
> Scene 2—A discovery of the Bath waters by a breeding sow's bathing in her extrane [sic] poverty, after which she raises her young.
> Scene 3—The swineherds recommending their virtues.
> Scene 4—Bladud plum'd on the mount of Beckon Hill ready for flight.
> Scene 5—Dissuaded from any such attempt.
> Scene 6—A magnificent entertainment for all his nobles.
> Scene 7—His flight and fall.
> (Green 1902, 1: 214)

With the new Bladud, who is not a magician or academic or over-reacher, a death by flying makes less sense than ever. Many versions of his tale carefully stopped at the moment of his triumphant cure.

The new tale, provided the 'death' were not part of it, had another advantage over the old: it was not reliant on magic, and so was 'believable'. Over time, the people of Bath started to think that their king had been real—making Bath a 'royal' seat, of course. A 1741 manuscript, drawn up by prominent Bathonians, declared their utter belief in the Bladud/pig tradition: 'We whose names are hereunder written, natives of the city of Bath, having perused the above tradition, do think it very truly and faithfully related' (Warner 1801, 13). They became so proud of their story that, wrote Warner in 1801, they taught 'the history of [Bladud] and his pigs' to their children 'to instil into them a proper sense of that supposed dignity which attached to them […] from drawing their first breath in a city that made so respectable a figure in ancient British story' (Warner 1801, 12). The pride was, of course, as much in the water as it was in Bladud. He had been the first to be 'cured' by the baths; and his humility, wisdom and gratefulness reflected upon, perhaps even seemed to emanate from, the hot water itself.

King Bladud's new myth, however, still appears to have struck writers as lacking. Dickens, who took up the tale as an inset account in the middle of his *Pickwick Papers* (1836), provided both the pig version and an alternative. First, he gave a new twist to Bladud's death in the pig narrative: Bladud, he relates, took a bath in waters that were too hot, and was killed—presumably cooked—as a result; the waters that had healed him also brought about his demise. He also supplied an entirely different narrative which, he declares, is the 'real' tale of Bladud. In the new tale, Bladud, while in Athens for educational reasons (from the 'old' story), fell in love with an Athenian woman, and determined to marry her. Returning home, he told his father of his love, but his father, who wanted to bring about a different, political, match of his own, had him imprisoned. Escaping his bonds, Bladud returned to Athens, only to discover that his beloved had married someone else. He returned to England where he wept so much that he was swallowed into the earth; his tears created the waters of Bath. Intriguingly, then, Dickens reacts against the 'pig' tale, here the product of waters that are both curative and killing, in favour of baths created from grief. Perhaps he was illustrating 'the absurdity and pretence of Bath' (Levy and Ruff 1967, 125), now a place for the young to make matches in: according to him, the baths really have at their source unhappiness and love that is misbegotten.

But the pig narrative stuck: and, indeed, the pigs came to ever more prominence. In 1908 the Bath Amateurs performed a Gilbert-and-Sullivan-style comic opera, *Bladud*, in which the pigs took central stage:

> 'My lot is truly hard,' I said,
> 'My troubles are fair corkers,'
> The cuticle complaint I'd caught
> Broke out among the porkers.
> (quoted in Hammond 2012, 36)

The following year, a Bath Historical Pageant was mounted by the city in Victoria Park, the fifth episode of which was a self-contained 'masque of Prince Bladud' ('Bath Historical Pageant', online). Here a Bladud actor, wearing furs, performed in the park's pond accompanied by some bemused children and a team of real swine: an occasion lovingly recorded on surviving postcards and slides (Fig. 1).

Twentieth-century writers liked the pigs, too. They, however, returned with renewed vigour to the 'flying' episode from the earlier tale. Ambrose

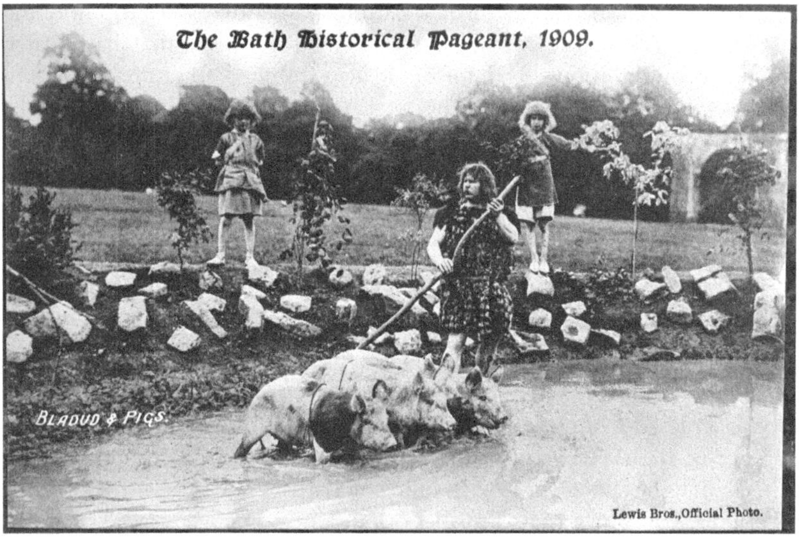

Fig. 1 King Bladud and the Pigs, 'Bath Historical Pageant', postcard, 1909

Bierce wrote a short story in 1874 of the entire King Bladud/pig tale, ending 'he thought to outdo Daedalus and Icarus. [...] He outdid them handsomely; he fell a good deal harder than they did, and broke his precious neck' (Bierce 2002, 202); Moyra Caldecott wrote *The Winged Man* (1993), placing Bladud's flight as the apogee of what he did: 'the people down below [...] saw him hurtle to the earth [...] Lear ran forward [...] Too late' (Caldecott 1993, 267). Stephen Jarvis, who wrote a prehistory of *Pickwick Papers*, *Death and Mr Pickwick* (2015), included his own variation of the fall: 'Bladud plummeted down, down, down. At the instant he struck the earth, the crowd, acting as one, drew in their breath, and this covered the sound of his neck snapping' (Jarvis 2015, n.p.); the title of Vera Chapman's *Blaedud The Birdman* (Chapman 1978) speaks for itself, though its blurb enlarges '[e]ducated by Druids, granted wings by a beautiful naked sorceress, banished and rescued from a swine-herd's mud-cursed realm, he risked his kingdom for the secret of flight, a secret that could dash him to pieces—or change the destiny of man'.

King Bladud's tale, then, offers an insight into the fluid life of myth: what stays, what is reformed, what is cut, what is relegated and what becomes a focus. Through it we see how Bath's notional origin changed as perceptions of its waters changed; while Bladud only retained his nobility by altering entirely his nature and relationship to the hot water, from 'maker' to 'discoverer'. Though myth is often treated as an insight into the way the past told its stories, Bladud's changing myth reflects the time(s) in which it is told, and says as much about 'now' as then. Hence this section has gone to some lengths to show how his unfixed mythology—a pseudo-history that is never crystalized by one, striking piece of literature—reveals much about the attitudes to the place it supposedly reflects. The next section shows the reverse: how the changes that Bath underwent affected, as well as borrowed from, the mythology of Bladud.

2 Bath's History and Bladud

This section is on the history of Bath, not per se, but as it shapes, reflects, animates or questions the King Bladud legend. It focuses, then, on pointed moments in the life of Bath: Bath as a Roman city; Bath as a Catholic-to-Protestant city; Bath as an eighteenth-century party city; and, throughout, Bath as a curative city.

Roman Bath had been founded on a Celtic site, where the Romans had tactfully, or tactically, built their main place of worship to Sulis Minerva, a goddess who fused Celtic 'Sulis' the local goddess of the spa, with the Roman goddess of wisdom and warfare, Minerva. It will be traces of that Sulis Minerva temple that inflected the original Bladud legend: Bladud's dedication of 'his' baths to Minerva shows that the temple must have stayed on, at least in oral memory, up until the eleventh century and beyond; quite possibly bits of it remained visible in Medieval Bath.

Other Roman elements of the city seem to have fed the King Bladud myth too, though which, and in what way, are open to question. The story of Bladud's wings has been traced to a particular Bathonian Roman image, for instance. Known as the 'Gorgoneion', but sometimes also called 'Bladud's head', it is a carving of a male head with Gorgon-like hair out of which wings issue on either side. The suggestion is that a similar image—not this one, as it was rediscovered only in 1790—led to the idea of a man who attempted to fly. That, though, is equally likely to be a modern attempt to back-create a myth from Roman remains, given the date of the Gorgoneion's discovery (Fear 1992, 222–224). An alternative Roman background to Bladud's flying story is that it comes from a different statue or image: of 'Sulis Minerva'. Minerva, when depicted as 'Victory', is typically winged—could a depiction of the goddess in that form have been visible in the twelfth century, and morphed into a winged man (Hammond 2000, 59)? Again, though, the danger is that modern readings are imposing interpretations rather than extracting them—no such image is known in Bath, and any there had been would have shown a godhead of the wrong sex. But Bladud's flying may not have a material origin at all, of course. The name 'Sulis', Celtic for eye or vision, sounds so like the Latin 'sol' that it has often been mistaken for a sun reference: indeed, Bladud's fall onto the temple of Apollo, the sun god, is likely to descend from this. And, as 'sun' is crucial to the Bladud story—his first temple is dedicated to (Sulis) Minerva; his death arises from his attempt to fly to the sun; his ultimate descent is onto a temple of Apollo (Sol)—could it be that the name Sulis Minerva suggested aspects of the story, including the attempt to fly? There is certainly a logic, as well as a pleasing irony, in having a king who first worshipped the sun, and then tried to rival it, being brought down by it, and onto a place set up in its honour (built, according to versions of the story that fuse the Apollo with the Minerva temple, by Bladud himself).

The source of King Bladud's founding a university in Stamford, far from Bath, is hard to reconcile with history, though some of its elements can be sourced. Merlin 'foresaw' that Stamford would become a place of learning,[4] but his prophecy did not mention Bladud as some have claimed (Drakard 1822, 6; Caldecott 1993, 280). And, as a set of Oxford rebels from Brasenose Hall and Merton College did, in 1333, attempt to found a rival university in Stamford, Lincolnshire, that place does indeed have a university connection. How and why, though, did it become linked to Bladud at all? Suggestions include the fact that Stamford and Bath are both near a 'Swineford' and thus connect in the pig story ('Bladud and the Founding of Bath', online)—but pigs entered the myth later so cannot be the source. And, though both Stamford and Bath have 'curative' water, Stamford's Iron water Spa was not to be exploited until 1819, and is abandoned now, so that is not likely to be behind the connection either. Perhaps it is simply that the two places are both on Roman roads. Or perhaps it is that as a worshipper of Minerva, Bladud was perceived to be 'wise' like her, and that morphed into his having an academic bent. Whatever is the case, the effect of making Bladud the founder of a British university some fourteen centuries before the establishment of Oxford or Cambridge, extended Bladud's importance over the nation. Bladud, in this version of the tale, is at the heart of—is, indeed, the source of—British higher learning.

Refinements and alterations to the tale of King Bladud in the early modern period seem to reflect the conflict between Catholicism and Protestantism that defined the age. Until the time of Henry VIII, the ownership and running of the once-Roman baths of Bath had been in the hands of monks: the baths were housed within a monastery complex, and all hospital or therapeutic work that included them was, notionally, religious. Pilgrims certainly attended the baths, as names like The Cross Bath (which sported a central cross at various periods in time, and to which visitors seem to have brought crosses of their own) suggest. With the dissolution of the monasteries under King Henry VIII in 1539, however, the baths became the preserve of secular doctors. And, when Protestant Elizabeth I came to the throne, she tried to stop Bath from becoming a hub of Catholic insurrection by encouraging Protestant doctors to use,

[4] The prophecy, 'Doctrinae stadium, quod nunc viguet ad vada Boum/Tempore venture celebrabitur ad vada Saxi', is translated as 'Science that now o'er Oxford sheds her ray/Shall bless fair Stamford at some future day' in *The Mirror* 1831, 18.

but also explain the science behind, the hot water. As a result, Catholics and Protestants interpreted the actual hot waters differently: to Catholics, they were, as described by one Banwell in 1449, 'a heavenly gift of warm and healing waters' (quoted in Jones 2005, 16): a miracle from God. To Protestants they were, as John Jones wrote in *The bathes of Bathes ayde* (1572), curative waters '*confirmed by reason, and dayly tried by experience*'. This difference is reflected in and may explain the varying Bladuds of the time: Bladud the magician, and sometimes Bladud the bad, is a feature of the inexplicable miraculous water—a Catholic version; Bladud the scientist, and, often, Bladud the good, reveals waters that are natural and scientifically explicable—hence, Protestant.

As part of the Protestant takeover of the meaning of the baths, a statue of King Bladud was placed in the King's Bath, though when is open to question (Fig. 2).

Still to be seen in the King's Bath now, the Bladud statue gave, and gives, a royal but non-religious focus to the place. Tokens of successful cures that might otherwise have been placed on religious icons were suspended, instead, over Bladud. One picture, c. 1682, shows 'The Crutches of Recover'd persons hanging over ye statue of Bladud' (Dingley 1867, xlix); and a 1688 account that lists successful Bath cures includes William Headache who, 'giving glory to GOD, and Honour to the *Bath*' attached 'his *Crutches* near the Throne of K[ing] *Bladud*' (Guidott 1725, 360). The new statue had the advantage, too, of promoting Bath's royal connection, while making the actual 'king' of King's Bath, not Henry I, after whom it was originally named, but Bladud himself, Bath's own king.

The engraved table glossing King Bladud's statue from below is both easier and harder to date. It reads:

> Bladud: son of Ludhudibras; eighth king of the Britains from Brute; a great philosopher and mathematician, bred at Athens, and recorded the first discoverer and founder of these baths eight hundred sixty three years before Christ. That is, two thousand five hundred sixty two years to the present year, 1699.

This table (re)confirms Bladud's academic and non-magic credentials; says that Bladud discovered, rather than created, the baths; ignores Bladud's flight and fall; and eschews, for reasons explored above, what may have been in an earlier table: the pig story. It apparently provides restrained highlights of the 'old' Bladud tale at the very time that the new was

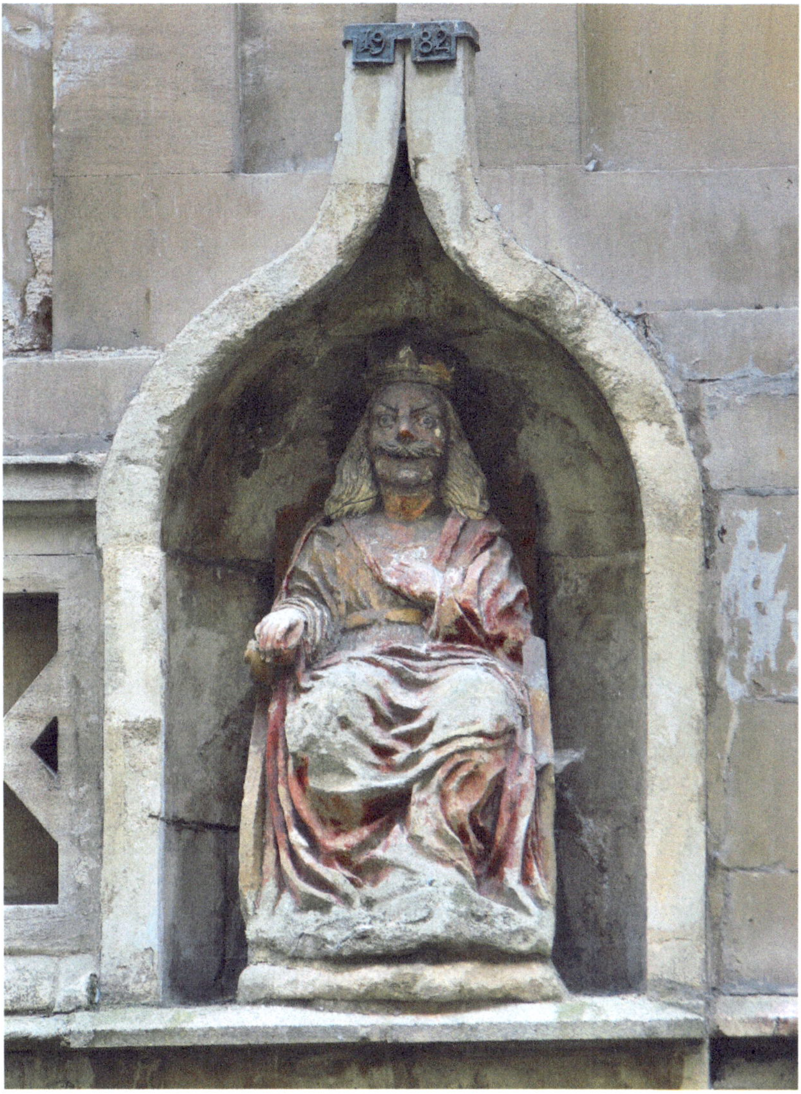

Fig. 2 Statue of King Bladud, date unknown, The King's Bath, Bath

replacing it. But its final sentence, made up of annually changeable information—the year, and Bladud's dates relative to it—suggests all its information is 'updatable'. When that table was painted on wood, it was indeed annually re-inscribed: Thomas Dingley, in *History from Marble*, relates the contents above for its Bladud table, but adjusted to the year 1682 (xlviii); a transcription of the table in Thomas Johnson's drawing The King's Bath and the Queen's Bath, now in the British Museum, has the same contents but, again, with numbers altered for the year 1672. But when the table was fixed in copper in 1699, the story was made permanent in one sense, and wrong in another. It is always out-of-date—and so always hinting that other versions of the tale should be sought for.

The King Bladud statue itself, however, may even have brought about key aspects the new 'pig' story. As it seems, Bath had had an earlier Bladud statue, 'carv'd by some vile bungler's hands' (An. 1753, 11) and affixed on the town's North Gate; on the South Gate had been a statue of Edward III. Both statues have, by different writers, been said to have been moved to become the statue placed in the King's Bath as Bladud (Falconer 1867, 7)—and perhaps both are, for the current statue, according to Laurence Tindall, its 1982 restorer, is a fusion of at least two earlier images, and has a head older than its body. Second-hand and weathered, both of the 'gate' statues will have appeared to have 'skin' that was pitted and worn: in situ, or moved to the King's Bath, 'Bladud' may as a consequence have appeared 'leprous' (Clark 1994, 47). If so, then statues relaying the 'old' Bladud story directly led to the 'new' story. The fact that the Bladud statue in the King's Bath was framed by rejected aids and prosthetics will have helped give substance to the new narrative: he will have seemed utterly symbolic of a man cured.

Local place names, 'Swineford', said to be where Bladud crossed the river Avon with his pigs, and 'Swainswick' ('Swineswick') said to be where he then settled, may be responsible for the pigs in the new Bladud story (Clark 1994, 45), as may Hogs Norton, once the name of the north side of Bath (Wood 1749, 1:75). These 'connections' were also good for the city: they celebrated locality, while extending Bladud's reach into other bits of Somerset. They also, of course, served as 'proofs' of the truth of the Bladud tale: so that what may have contributed key elements to the story were now testament to its genuineness.

It was the new King Bladud tale that had a major effect on the material nature of Bath. As above, the 'new' story encouraged Bladud-pride. Bladud-pride led to Bladud buildings; Bladud buildings shaped the eighteenth-century city, now dedicated to two functions both of which arose from the water: 'cures' (for the old and ailing); parties and amours (for the young who accompanied them). New buildings were needed to house the many elegant families who came to Bath, and the dances they enjoyed while there.

Architect John Wood the Elder, who designed and, together with his son John Wood the Younger, built Bath's iconic circular street of town-houses, The Circus (1754 and 68), was one of the builders responsible for making eighteenth-century Bath. He was also a King Bladud obsessive. According to the crazed books he wrote from a combination of research and wild imagination, Bath had been the centre of Druid activity in Britain, and Bladud had been an Arch Druid—though whenever he was in Greece he moonlighted as a Hyperborean priest of Apollo and was known as Abaris[5] (Figure 3).

Having acquired leprosy in Athens, Bladud/Abaris returned, became a swineherd, learned about the hot waters from his pigs—and then set up a university for Druids in nearby Stanton Drew.[6] As Stonehenge was, Wood went on to claim, an imitation of a Stanton Drew temple, so Bath could be returned to its Bladud glory by acquiring a 'Stone-henge-like' building. Hence The Circus, originally called The King's Circus (the 'King' being Bladud, of course). Its classical shape and design, so often thought to be a peon to Palladianism, was largely constructed from Wood's take on Bladud. The finials on its parapets, stone acorns, are, for instance, Bladud references: they reflect the fact that Druid Bladud was Priest of the Oak—while also suggesting fodder for his pigs. Elegant eighteenth-century Bath was, in significant and surprising ways, shaped by Bladud.

Other Georgian buildings had a Bladud-focus too. A depiction of the king was added to a wall of the Cross Bath when it was redesigned by Thomas Baldwin in 1783. This eighteenth-century Bladud, in opposition to the one in the King's Bath, was shown in his swineherd moment,

[5] See the illustration to his *An Essay Towards a Description of Bath* (1749): William Hoare's 'Bladud, to whom the Grecians gave the Name of Abaris'.

[6] His complicated ideas cover a range of his writings: *An Essay Towards a Description of Bath* (1749); *Choir Gaure, Vulgarly called Stonehenge on Salisbury Plain, Described, Restored and Explained* (1747), *The Origin of Building: or, the Plagiarism of the Heathens Detected* (1741). They are neatly summarised in Harris 1989, 101–107; and their numerological ideas which determined the dimensions of the Circus are explained in Morrison 2011, 43–58; and Mowl 1988.

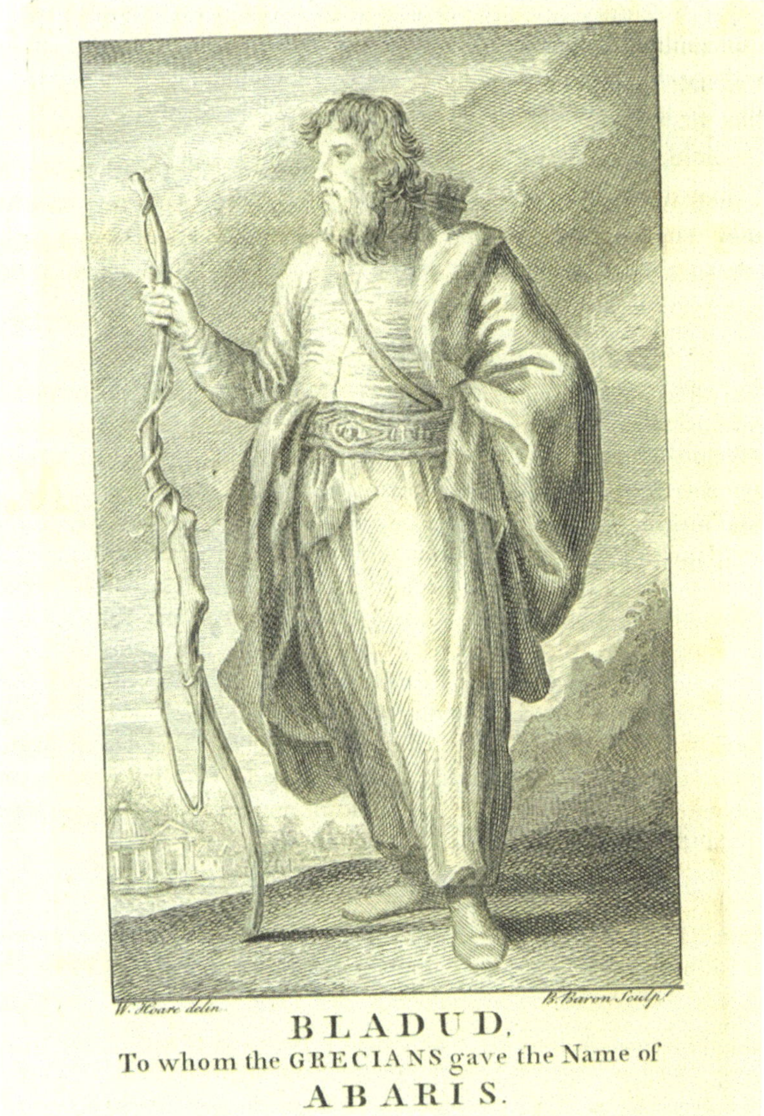

Fig. 3 'King Bladud: to whom the Grecians gave the name Abaris', by William Hoare, engraved by Bernard Baron, in John Wood, *An Essay Towards a Description of Bath*, 1749; reprinted in R. Hippesley, *Bath and its Environs, a descriptive poem, in three cantos, etc.*, 1775

a bow in his hand and a quiver of arrows at his back—so about to be cured by the bath. The image seems to have been partly based on the Bladud/Abaris one from Wood's *Essay* (1749). Other buildings of the period adopted Bladud's name: they include the terrace of 'Bladud Buildings', built 1755–1762; and the 'Bladud Bank' (1790–1841) that they contained, distinguished at the time by the wooden bust of Bladud it had mounted outside. A series of pubs from then and later were given Bladud titles too: The Bladud's Head in Walcot Street; The Bladud's Head in Catsley Place, Larkhall; The Bladud Arms in Lower Swainswick. The cures and flirtations of eighteenth-century Bath, then, had a Bladud background, as cartoons like Thomas Rowlandson's *Comforts of Bath: King Bladud's Bath* (1798)—showing large and ungainly Georgian bathers, wearing cumbersome bathing hats and coats, under the indifferent Bladud Statue in the King's Bath—make clear.

Even Bath souvenirs of the time were distinguished by King Bladud references. In the 1790s, when 'tokens'—local coins that served for small denomination money, or souvenirs—were minted, they generally featured Bladud and his pigs. Of surviving tokens, the most common have, on one side, 'Bladud Founded Bath', containing a picture of Bladud carrying a quiver with arrows—as in the Bladud/Abaris and Cross Bath image—but also incongruously wearing a crown. On the other, the most usual of a range of variants is 'Through his Swine', encasing another picture of Bladud, still with crown and quiver—his shield is on the ground—driving two pigs. The story of the waters' cure of pig and man alike, tellingly part of coinage, now had a literal worth to the city.

But nineteenth-century Bath was less taken with the King Bladud pig story, as Dickens' rewriting suggests. Fewer depictions date from that time, though one painting, *Bladud in Exile* (1807), by Benjamin West, shows a reflective, melancholy Bladud, tending swine and not obviously leprous. The only Bladud statue to be added to the city over that period, by Stephano Pieroni in 1859, was placed on top of a fountain that supplied free mineral water to the people of Bath. It was pig-free: anxiety raised by Darwin's idea that men might descend from 'apes' seems to have put people off stories about the interconnectedness of all biological species. Besides, pigs do not seem to have been to Victorian taste aesthetically. Indeed, Bladud himself came to seem dated. Writes Gibbs of the King's Bath:

> A statue of King Bladud [...] adorns this bath, which it would become the corporation to remove now. Such absurd fables are unworthy of a place here. The substitution of some beautiful Grecian nymph of the fountains, would be more tasteful and ornamental. (Gibbs 1835, 17)

In the twentieth century, however, the 'new' King Bladud tale was sentimentally re-established. The pigs were just too good not to be 'staged' at a time when Herbert Beerbohm Tree's theatrical productions—like the famous *Midsummer Night's Dream* filled with real rabbits—were all the rage. Bladud really came into his own later, however, as the result of two crises. In 1976 the NHS decided it would no longer use the baths for curative bathing treatments 'concluding that plunging patients in the miraculous water was no more effective than turning on a hot tap' (Kennedy 2002, online). Worse, in 1978 a girl died of a meningitis-related illness having bathed in the waters, acquired from the aging pipes that fed Bath's spas. Not only were the baths now said to have no medical healing value; they were also revealed to be injurious to life. Bathing was stopped, visitors were warned not even to touch the untrustworthy water—and the listed buildings in which the baths were housed, quintessential to the look and nature of the city, fell into disrepair. For twenty-five years Bath was a bathing city without baths, while funding was frantically raised for a new, healthy, modern structure—complete with 'wellness suite'—that could re-establish Bath as a major, healthful spa resort.

Enter King Bladud, once more. Damaged Bath, during its dark period, seemed to see itself in Bladud, whose abortive attempt to fly came to renewed prominence. In 1990, under the Victoria Road Bridge in Bitton, the Vizability Community Art Collaboration made a group mosaic, *On the Wings* (Hammond 2012, 101). For the exterior of the Ustinov Studio Theatre, in 1996, Igor Ustinov, son of the actor Peter Ustinov, after whom the building was named, designed a winged figure in bronze and sheet steel with a bird flying towards him: he is called, ironically and defiantly, 'Hopefully'. One other Bladud image, on a frieze for The Podium Shopping Centre and Library, made by artist Barry Baldwin in 1989, shows a different version of a 'fallen' Bladud. Depicted as a soldier (though that has never been part of any of his narratives), he sports a leopard's head for a hat, suggesting, perhaps symbolising, extraordinary strength combined with a clinging spotted skin disease.

And then re-enter King Bladud again. Once the updated 'Thermae Bath Spa' was established (its name vaguely hinting at its Roman heritage), Bladud's 'new' story—the king who was cured by the marvellous water—came back to prominence. Stripped of its mythological status, and treated as fact, Bladud's tale 'showed' how the baths had always been curative (and hid the fact that, recently, they had been the reverse). The website of 'Thermae Bath Spa', opened in 2006, proclaims that 'The natural thermal springs in Bath were first discovered by Prince Bladud around 863BC, who was cured from his skin disease after bathing in the waters' ('Thermae Bath Spa', online). Bladud's cure—not, here, for leprosy, which mineral waters cannot heal, but for a skin complaint, which they can—also enables Thermae Bath Spa to hint at having medical properties it cannot otherwise claim.

With King Bladud's cure comes Bladud's pigs, its source. When a public art event was designed for Bath in 2008, it was organised around, and named for, *King Bladud's Pigs in Art*. A template pig was made by sculptor Alan Dun and 106 copies of it were cast in resin ('Alan Dun: Sculptor', online). The copies were individually decorated by artists and famous people, displayed around Bath for six months, and then sold at auction to raise money for the 'Two Tunnels' cycle path project.[7] So over the last decade, pigs have once more filled the city and raised actual money for it. Bladud himself, however, was relegated. Apart from his name, he barely featured in *King Bladud's Pigs in Art* except in one specific instance. An old Bladud statue—the 1859 one by Stephano Pieroni, which had long been removed from its fountain—was brought out of the gardens of a retirement home where it had been stored. It was repaired and placed in the Parade Gardens in 2009, with one addition: one of Dun's pigs, carved in stone by Nigel Bryant and students from The City of Bath College, was added to it. At least for now, then, Bladud's pigs—ecocritically appealing, and not bound by issues of class and birth as Bladud is—are overtaking the king's narrative.

3 Conclusion: The Bladud Myth Now

Hot water issuing from the earth is odd and requires explanation: is it sinister (does it come from Hell?), or appealing (it is pleasurable to be in). Is it curative or dangerous? This chapter, in telling the story of King Bladud, has shown how attitudes to the water itself over time have altered,

[7] Pictures of the event are gathered in Witty 2008.

and equally been altered by, the myth. Therein lies the interest and inexplicability of Bladud. His pseudo-history, sometimes taken as fact, weaves its way in and out of literary narratives on the one hand; buildings and artefacts on the other; sometimes shaping them and sometimes being shaped by them; always attempting to answer the mystery of what the waters are and mean. Even the two parts of the chapter, narrative and material, have not mapped onto one another in a totally co-ordinated way, because when and whether 'things' inspire or reflect narratives is not always clear; and because the flow of a story, particularly one not always written down, is not in one direction only.

What can be said is that the changing tale of Bladud shows how myths can be made up of embedded historical truths (like the Minerva statue), changed to embrace new truths (like the pig-sounding name Swineswick), and treated as allegories that also are, or come to seem, literal (Bladud's fall; Bladud's cure). That means that the Bladud story is always true and untrue, metaphorical and literal, but in different ways for different periods—not least because the story itself is different in different periods.

Absent from this chapter is what might have governed the narrative shifts further: the oral versions that, perhaps, directed the written and material ones. But King Bladud's permanence, if anything, celebrates their loss, for no telling, or account or building has 'owned' his tale enough to fix it in one form. King Bladud can thus be positively compared with King Lear, his son. Lear was the notional founder of Leicester, but that is largely forgotten, because one writer, Shakespeare, fixed Lear's tale elsewhere: on his troubled old age, his madness, his dreadful relationship with his daughters. Bladud, who has never been chosen as sole focus by a major writer, is not so narratively constrained: he can be focussed on in youth or in age, when wise or foolish, as ill or well. He is thus much better positioned to serve 'his' city where, over time, he has been king, god, magician, academic, sick person, commoner, Druid, star-gazer, overreacher, fallen man, as required, precisely because his wayward myth is so unowned, and so malleable.

It remains to be seen where the Bladud tale will go next. This chapter was started before Covid-19, but finished during the pandemic. Current news is filled with accounts of the way a vicious disease has crossed from bats to people, possibly via another animal. Will Bladud's pigs slope away from his story once more as a result—disease-bearers, no longer charming? Or, will we remember that Bladud was the source of his pig's infection and they of the cure—so that the story can be reinstated as one of redemption, where the animals solve an illness caught from people? Whatever the answer, Bladud's tale will remain like the waters he founded, or discovered, or was cured by—the waters that he symbolises and celebrates—unknowable, compelling, complex, illogical and perhaps a bit magic.

Works Cited

Primary Sources

An. 1711. *Daily Courant* (January 29).

An. 1755. *The Bath and Bristol Guide*. Bath: Printed and sold by Thomas Boddely, in King's-Mead-Street. Sold also by the booksellers of Bath and Bristol.

An. 1831. *The Mirror of Literature, Amusement, and Instruction* (January 8).

Baron, Robert. 1647. *Mirza a tragedie*. London: Printed for Humphrey Moseley… and for T. Dring, and are to be sold at his shop.

Bierce, Ambrose. 2002. The Early History of Bath. In *Cobwebs from an Empty Skull*. London: George Routledge and Sons, 1874. Reprinted Auckland, New Zealand: The Floating Press.

Caldecott, Moyra. 1993. *The Winged Man*. Bath: Bladud Books.

Camden, William. 1695. *Camden's Britannia Newly Translated Into English, With Large Additions and Improvements*. ed. Edmund Gibson. London: Printed by F. Collins, for A. Swalle… and A. & J. Churchil.

Chapman, Henry. 1673. *Thermae Redivivae*. London: Printed for the author, and are to be sold by Jonathan Edwin.

Coryate, Thomas. 1611. *The Odcombian Banquet*. London: Imprinted [by George Eld] for Thomas Thorp.

De Chassanion, Jean. 1597. *The Theatre of Gods Judgements*. London: Printed by Adam Islip.

Dingley, Thomas. 1867. *History from Marble*. ed. Thomas E. Winnington. Westminster: Camden Society.

Falconer, Randle Wilbraham. 1867. *The Baths and Mineral Waters of Bath*. London: Robert Hardwicke.

Gibbs, Samuel. 1835. *Gibb's Bath Visitant*. Bath: Published by Samuel Gibbs.

Guidott, Thomas. 1725. *A Collection of Treatises Relating to the City and Waters of Bath*. London: printed for J. Leake, bookseller at the Bath.

Hardyng, John. 1543. *The Chronicle of Ihon Hardyng in Metre*. London: In officina Richardi Graftoni.

Harington, Sir John. 1653. *A Briefe View of the State of the Church of England as it Stood in Q. Elizabeths and King James his reigne*. London: Printed for Jos. Kirton.

Higgins, John. 1574. *The First Parte of the Mirour for Magistrates*. London: By Thomas Marshe.
Higgins, John. 1619. *The Falles of Unfortunate Princes*. London: Imprinted by F.K. for William Aspley, and are to be sold at his shop in Pauls Churchyard at the signe of the Parrot.
Holinshed, Raphael. 1577. *The Firste [laste] Volume of the Chronicles of England, Scotlande, and Irelande*. London: Imprinted for Iohn Harrison.
I., T. 1595. *A World of Wonders*. London: [By Abel Jeffes] for William Barley, and are to be solde at his shop in Gratiousstreat neere vnto Leadenhall gate.
Jarvis, Stephen. 2015. *Death and Mr Pickwick*. London: Jonathan Cape. Kindle Edition.
Langtoft, Peter of. 1725. A Fool's Bolt soon Shott at Stonage. In *Peter Langtoft's Chronicle*. 2 vols. Oxford: Printed at the Theater.
Marlowe, Christopher. 1604. *The Tragicall History of D. Faustus*. London: Printed by V. S[immes] for Thomas Bushell.
Monmouth, Geoffrey of. 1999. *History of the Kings of Britain* (c. 1136). Trans. Aaron Thompson with revisions by J. A. Giles. Cambridge: Ontario.
Shakespeare, William. 1968. *Mr. William Shakespeares Comedies, Histories, & Tragedies* [*The Norton Facsimile*] (1623). Facsimile by Charlton Hinman. New York: Norton.
Spenser, Edmund. 1590. *The Faerie Queene*. London: Printed for William Ponsobie.
Wood, John. 1741. *The Origin of Building: or, the Plagiarism of the Heathens Detected*. Bath: printed by S. and F. Farley, and sold by J. Leake.
Wood, John. 1747. *Choir Gaure, Vulgarly Called Stonehenge on Salisbury Plain, Described, Restored and Explained*. Oxford: Printed at the Theatre.
Wood, John. 1749. *An Essay Towards a Description of Bath*. n.p.: Printed by James Bettenham and sold by C. Hitch; and J. Leake at Bath.

Secondary Sources

Bartie, Angela, Linda Fleming, Mark Freeman, Tom Hulme, Alex Hutton, and Paul Readman. Bath Historical Pageant. *The Redpress of the Past. Historical Pageants in Britain*. http://www.historicalpageants.ac.uk/pageants/985/. Accessed October 26, 2020.
Borlik, Todd A. 2016. Hellish Falls: Faustus's' Dismemberment, Phaeton's Limbs and Other Renaissance Aviation Disaster–Part 2. *English Studies* 97: 1–11.
Butler, Guy. 1985. King Lear and Ancient Britain. *Theoria: A Journal of Social and Political Theory* 65: 27–33.
Chapman, Vera. 1978. *Blaedud the Birdman*. London: Rex Collins.
Clark, John. 1994. Bladud of Bath: The Archaeology of a Legend. *Folklore* 105: 39–50.

Fear, A.T. 1992. Bladud: The Flying King of Bath. *Folklore* 103: 222–224.
Fisher, Matthew. 2004. *Once Called Albion*. PhD diss.: University of Oxford.
Drakard, John. 1822. *The History of Stamford*. Stamford: Printed by and for John Drakard.
Green, Emanuel. 1902. *Bibliotheca Somersetensis*. 3 vols. Taunton: Barncott and Pearce.
Greer, Germaine. 2000. *John Wilmot, Earl of Rochester*. Horndon, Devon: Northcote House/British Council.
Jones, Nigel R. 2005. *Architecture of England, Scotland and Wales*. Westport, CT: Greenwood Press.
Hammond, Cynthia Imogen. 2012. *Architects, Angels, Activists and the City of Bath 1765–1965. Engaging with Women's Spatial Interventions in Buildings and Landscape*. Oxford: Routledge.
Hammond, Cynthia. 2000. Mending Icarus' Wing: The Poetics of Descent. In *The Poetry of Life in Literature*, ed. Anna-Teresa Tymieniecka, 55–64. London, Kluwer Academic.
Harris, Eileen. 1989. John Wood's System of Architecture. *The Burlington Magazine* 131: 101–107.
Hunt, August. Bladud and the Founding of Bath. *Shadows in the Mist: The Quest for a Historical King Arthur*. http://mistshadows.blogspot.com/2017/01/bladud-and-founding-of-bath.html. Accessed October 26, 2020.
Kennedy, Maev. Bath's Time Comes Again as Spa Reopens (December 31, 2002). *The Guardian*. https://www.theguardian.com/society/2002/dec/31/communities.arts Accessed October 26, 2020.
Levy Jr., H.M., and William Ruff. 1967. The Interpolated Tales in "Pickwick Papers", a Further Note. *Dickens Studies* 3: 122–125.
Morrison, Tessa. 2011. Reinventing the Past: John Wood the Elder. *International Journal of the Humanities* 9: 43–58.
Mowl, Tim. 1988. *John Wood: Architect of Obsession*. Bath: Millstream Books.
Poole, William. 2012. Gloster and Bladud. *Notes and Queries* 59: 536–538.
Strachan, Michael. 1962. *The Life and Adventures of Tom Coryate*. London: Oxford University Press.
Warner, Richard. 1801. *The History of Bath*. London: R. Cruttwell, and sold by G. G. and J. Robinson.
Wiggins, Martin. 2014. *British Drama 1533–1642: A Catalogue: 1598–1602*. Oxford: Oxford University Press.
Witty, Megan. 2008. *King Bladud's Pigs in Bath: A Public Art Project in and Around Bath*. Bath: King Bladud's Pigs. in Bath.

Websites

Bath in Time. Images of Bath Online. https://www.bathintime.co.uk/catalog/product/view/id/10352. Accessed October 26, 2020.

Dun, Alan. Alan Dun: Sculptor. http://www.alandun.co.uk. Accessed October 26, 2020.

Thermae Bath Spa. https://www.thermaebathspa.com. Accessed October 26, 2020.

CHAPTER 7

Creatures of the Bath: Transformations at the Early Modern British Spa

Amanda E. Herbert

In June of 1668, English diarist Samuel Pepys travelled to Bath to visit its hot mineral springs, and marvelled at the women and men who splashed in the city's outdoor pools, describing them as 'strange to see', for '[they] cannot but be parboiled, and look like the creatures of the bath'! (Pepys 1942, 195). For Pepys, frequent bathing made people 'creatures', as if life underwater had turned these swimmers from humans into something else entirely.

Seventeenth- and eighteenth-century Britons believed firmly in the curative powers of mineral spring waters, and at these sites many different kinds of women, men, and children sought relief from disease and injury. By drinking spring water, pumping it over their bodies, and plunging into mineral pools to swim, these health-seekers attempted to make themselves look and feel better, to transform disfigured or sick bodies into ones that were whole and well. But as Pepys' diary entry shows, spas were also feared for their powers of alteration, conversion, and obfuscation. In

A. E. Herbert (✉)
Folger Shakespeare Library, Washington, DC, United States
e-mail: aherbert@folger.edu

S. Chiari and S. Cuisinier-Delorme (eds.), *Spa Culture and Literature in England, 1500–1800*, Early Modern Literature in History,
https://doi.org/10.1007/978-3-030-66568-5_7

the pools, rising steam blurred lines of sight, and shifting sands lining the floors made navigation difficult. The sound of the cities, with bells clanging and crowds of people—both poor and rich—talking, shouting, and singing, felt disorienting and chaotic. The smell of the water was described as off-putting and nauseating. People who drank spa waters thought that they tasted terrible. Use of mineral waters could produce physical side-effects which were recognized as uncomfortable, painful, and unusual. Spas thus were imagined as places of health and healing, but simultaneously as sites of physical danger, sexual ambiguity and intrigue, and even political and social unrest.

This chapter frames its evidence according to the study of the early modern senses: sight, hearing, smell, taste, and touch. In the seventeenth and eighteenth centuries, the senses were recognized as having a hierarchy, with the 'higher' senses offering input to the body that was more refined, encouraging more complex thought and feeling. Scholars of sensory history have worked to recognize this early modern paradigm but also to recover the ways that people who lived in this period themselves reflected upon, experienced, and wrote about their complex sensory worlds (Tullett 2019; Roodenberg 2016; Kambaskovic 2014; Cahill 2009; Cockayne 2007; Harvey 2003; Jenner 2000). Simultaneously, scholars of the body and medicine have recognized that physical sensation was inseparable from emotional and spiritual experience, and that early modern people wrote and enacted lives in which 'feeling' was expressed on the inside just as much as it was on the outside (Walkden 2018; Weisser 2015). This chapter pulls these different strands of scholarship together in order to better understand and interpret the sensory experiences of the spa. For seventeenth- and eighteenth-century people, a visit to the spa was destabilizing, uncertain, and uneasy. Like many early modern medicines, the regime made them feel bad before it made them feel good, but on levels which were so comprehensive that they were described as undoing, unsettling, and even dehumanizing.

Drawing upon travel guides, government documents, private correspondence and diaries, satirical literature, and medical casebooks, this chapter focuses particularly upon the city of Bath in the southwest of England. Bath, a small urban centre in Somerset county, was Britain's largest, most famous, and most popular spa city. But spas flourished around Britain and its early empire: in England, Tunbridge Wells (Kent), Epsom (Surrey), and Scarborough (North Yorkshire); in Scotland, Moffat Wells (Dumfriesshire); in Ireland, Dublin (Leinster); and in territories claimed by Britain in acts of colonization and conquest, such as Jamaica, Nevis, and Virginia. Spas were open to all people, regardless of their race, gender, or socio-economic status. In the baths and pools of mineral water spas, bathers therefore would have rubbed elbows, and other body parts, with many kinds of people, creating an atmosphere bubbling with class tensions, gender troubles, and stage-of-life challenges.

1 Sight

For many early modern bathers, the first destabilizing sensory force of the baths was visual. In hot baths, clouds of rising steam made it nearly impossible to see more than a few feet in any direction. In the sixteenth century, John Leland wrote that the pool in the King's Bath 'rikith [smokes or smoulders] like a seething potte continually' (Smith 1907, 142; *OED*). In the seventeenth century, Thomas Dingley made particular note of the 'steam and vapour' which he believed characterized the pools (Dingley 1867, 50). Spa doctors—especially those who advocated for cold mineral springs—expressed concerns about the steam in hot baths. In his 1711 *Natural History*, Benjamin Allen stated that 'the Steamy, or more purely Spirituous [springs] [...] by reason of the Heat, [are] questionable'. Further denigrating these waters as legitimate medical aids and stressing that they were products of unhealthy industry rather than health-giving medicine, Allen explained that mineral waters that seemed 'steamy [often come] from a Mine, or Quarry' (Allen 1711, 41). Steamy springs were described by another spa practitioner as filled with 'malignant Effluvia or Steams, that are very pernicious where they fall' (An. 1705, 4–5). Medical practitioners weren't the only people who were wary of mineral water steam. For many patrons, the sight of hot steam made bathing downright frightening: in his *Journey Through England*, John Macky explained that watching the steam rise off of the surface of the water of the bathing pools, 'gave me a lively idea of several pictures I had seen [...] of Purgatory with Heads and Hands uplifted in the midst of the smoke just as they are here' (Macky 1722, 130). For Macky and others like him, clouds of steam and lack of clear sight encouraged feelings of confusion and danger, invoking death, the afterlife, and suffering.

Obfuscation led many spa-goers to worry that sexual mores were being overturned and challenged, either just out of sight or far too much in the public eye. As early as the fifteenth century, church officials in Bath had complained that people swimming in the pools occasionally revealed 'their privy parts to the gaze of bystanders'. In the sixteenth century, Dr. John Jones sniffed that male and female bathers would sometimes 'see and embrace each other', which he believed was 'not only undecent, but also […] most uncivil and barbarous' (Wroughton 2004, 110). Seventeenth-century images of bathing show that spa-goers went into the pools both clothed and naked; those who did elect to wear clothing dressed in loose, heavily draped gowns and drooping caps, all of which would have obscured social status and gender identity (Herbert 2004, 120–124). The proximity of bathers both in and out of the spa caused practitioners and patients to worry about uncleanliness, nakedness, lack of privacy, and awkwardness. In Dublin, Peter Belon advocated for the spas but did 'wish there were better Accomodations and Conveniences' located around the springs; any 'natural conveniences […] [like] Shrubs & Bushes' could offer some privacy for changing clothes, urinating, and defecating, but Belon admitted it would be better 'if Rows of Tents were pitched on each side of the Green' (Belon 1684, 70–73). Spa waters were supposed to make bodies whole and well, but being unable to see what happened—or, that too much could be seen—was a consistent cause for worry and unrest.

2 Sound

Early modern people also disliked the sounds of spa cities, which they characterized as discordant, disorderly, and nonsensical; these criticisms were also gendered and reflective of early modern class anxieties. The city of Bath did ring its church bells with frequency: ringing marked moments of political and religious importance, and it marked burials, which were very common in a city filled with sick and injured people. Accounts from one of the parishes in the centre of the city, St. James, show that in 1700 the bells were rung in remembrance of 'when the King landed' (probably a reference to the disembarkation of William of Orange before the so-called Glorious Revolution); on 'the 5 November' (a reference to Guy Fawkes Day); and on 'Coronation day'. St. James' bells were also rung for burials, including the interment of locals, but also burials of lower status people who were not from Bath, such as 'ringing for [a] stranger [who died] at [the] Swalow', a local inn (An. 1654–1780, n.p.). Music and bells were also played for wealthy or notable people to welcome them into spa cities and as part of their treatments. In the summer of 1668, Samuel Pepys noted that after his first swim in the baths, musicians arrived with 'musick to play to me'. Pepys called this 'extraordinary good as ever I heard at London almost, or anywhere' (Pepys 1942, 195), but not all spa visitors were similarly impressed. In his eighteenth-century treatise on Bath, Oliver Goldsmith complained that 'upon a stranger's arrival at Bath he is welcomed by a peal of the Abbey bells, and in the next place, by the voice and music of the city waits [municipal musicians]'. Goldsmith found 'these customs [...] [to be] disagreeable' (Goldsmith 1762, 41–42; *OED*). Satirists made spa city sounds the subject of their works, joking that the 'charming sweet sounds both of fiddles and bells' were actually so loud that they were 'rung so hard that I thought they would pull down the steeple [...] some think it strange they should make such a riot/ In a place where sick folk would be glad to be quiet' (An. 1768, 34–35).

The voices of women and lower status people in spa cities were also condemned and mocked. The anonymous *New Bath Guide* described female swimmers who socialized in Bath's pools as so noisy that they resembled animals like geese or chickens, noting 'how the ladies did giggle and set up their clacks' (An. 1768, 44). Other diatribes were directed against people based on their social status. John Wilmot, Earl of Rochester, wrote in his 1697 poem *Tunbridge Wells* that the rural squires he encountered at the mineral spring produced 'more irksome noise, [with] their silly talk' (Stedman 2013, 222–226; Vieth 1968, 79).[1] Two eighteenth-century anonymous satirical poems followed this theme; in 1717 Bath's practitioners, residents, and patients were accused of making 'noise and Nonsense [...] their Dear delight' (An. 1717, n.p.) and in 1748, the same people were called 'Loit'rers' who made such 'incessant Noise' that 'themselves they stun' (An. 1748, n.p.). For all of these authors, spa cities—where lower and higher status people all used the same facilities and occupied the same spaces simultaneously—were so noisy that they were nonsensical, stupefying, and annoying.

3 Smell

The smell of mineral waters made spa visitors and patients uncomfortable and often induced disgust. Some people were critical of the general cleanliness of the cities in which spas were located. In 1716, the Duchess of Marlborough noted with scorn that she 'never saw any place abroad

[1] In this example Wilmot was writing of 'Sir Nicholas Cully', a recurring literary character who was a buffoon, country squire, and knight.

that had more Stinks and Dirt in it than Bath' (Cowper 1865, 197). Daniel Defoe agreed, calling Bath 'a close city [...] more like a prison than a place of diversion'. Defoe's characterization of Bath as 'close' was no doubt designed to invoke the idea of a close-stool or privy, as he went on to say that the city 'scarce gives the company room to converse out of the smell of their own excrements'. For Defoe, Bath was not a healthy place, but a very unhealthy one, 'where the very city it self may be said to stink like a general common-shore' (Defoe 1927, 168).[2] Even advocates of the spa could not help but recognize that some springs emitted an unpleasant odour, usually because they were sulphurous. Writing about springs in Scotland, Matthew Mackaile noted in 1664 that mineral springs were often denoted by 'the fetide smell, wherewith they are impregnat' (Mackaile 1664, 43). In some instances, revolting mineral water smells, while discomfiting, could simultaneously aid in the identification of mineral springs. Mackaile went on to write that while one of his friends was walking through a mountain valley in Dumfries, 'he smelt a smell like to that of Brampton wells'. Instead of turning away from this unpleasant odour, the man made a point of 'walk[ing] contrary to the wind, following the smell', and eventually, 'upon the top of a little Rock [...] which was covered with mire and clay, he discovered two little Spring-wells' (Mackaile 1664, 43). In this instance, overcoming individual revulsion offered this spa-seeker a significant benefit.

4 Taste

Although patients and practitioners alike believed that drinking mineral waters could be curative, they also recognized that they were hard to swallow. The taste, mouthfeel, and temperature of mineral waters was off-putting to many early modern people, who wondered whether such a substance would cure or kill. In his 1711 *Natural History of the Mineral-Waters of Great Britain*, Benjamin Allen made a point of describing the taste of waters across England. He noted that 'Barnet Water, in Hartfordshire [...] had the Taste of common Pump water, with an Addition of Bitterness' (Allen 1711, 14). In Kent, a spring called 'Shooter-Hill-Water' was described by Allen as 'very bitter, and full of the nauseous Sweet' (Allen 1711, 19). Another spring had only 'a little Bitterness', and

[2] Defoe published these works from 1724–1727.

was praised as 'not so maukish [eg., nauseating] altogether as Epsam', a spring water which Allen deemed nearly impossible to swallow (Allen 1711, 20; *OED*). Patients often described the taste of mineral waters as unusual, strange, or unexpected. At the end of the seventeenth century, Celia Feinnes compared the waters at Bath to boiled eggs (Feinnes 1949, 20).[3] When a Cambridge undergraduate visited a spring at Malton in North Yorkshire, the only praise he could summon when he 'tasted of this water' was that it was 'more steely' than others he had experienced (An. 1725, 40–42). Nauseating and ill-tasting springs were not unique to England; in Scotland, mineral sprngs were described in similar terms. The springs at St. Catharine's Well in Dumfries supposedly had an 'acrimony of their taste, resembling that of the Balsam of Brimstone' (Mackaile 1664, 133–134). That the taste of spa waters resembled or reminded early modern people of brimstone and hellfire was not even the worst thing about them. Taking advantage of the disgust that spa-goers felt when drinking mineral waters, the anonymous eighteenth-century satirist of the *New Bath Guide* joked that 'You cannot conceive what a number of ladies/ Were wash'd in the water the same as our maid is:/ [...] So while little Tabby [the maid] was washing her rump,/ The ladies kept drinking it out of a pump' (An. 1768, 47–49). Here the satirist invoked intersectional, layered fears about uncleanliness and dirt, permeable and unstable social stratification, and extranormative sexuality to make the spa seem distasteful in every sense.

It is clear that repellent flavours—described by early modern writers as bitter, nauseating, and acrid—made drinking mineral waters difficult sensory experiences for many spa-goers. But the mouthfeel of spa waters, the sensations that they created around the lips, palate, tongue, and throat while they were being tasted, swished, and swallowed, was also cause for disgust and unease. The Cambridge undergraduate who visited so many spas in the eighteenth century noted that in Bath, he found 'the water so hot, that tis but just fit to drink'. Although he found this water barely tolerable, the student persisted, writing, 'I drank a Glass of it' (An. 1725, 113–119). Benjamin Allen, who described the taste of mineral springs in his early eighteenth-century natural history, also commented on the texture, temperature, and mouthfeel of spa water. Allen noted that 'Buxton Bath-Water' was neither precisely cold nor hot, but was 'about

[3] Feinnes undertook her travels between 1684 and 1712, and later wrote up her memories of these journeys in manuscript form.

the Warmth of Blood newly exhausted from the body' (Allen 1711, 39). By comparing medical spring waters to freshly shed blood, Allen figured the waters as disturbing, unnatural, and something not typically consumed by early modern Europeans.

5 Touch

Visitors to the spa who chose to bathe in the pools also expressed senses of bodily discomfort and physical and emotional disorientation in response to the texture of the pools, as well as the feeling of floating or swimming. Many spa pools had precarious footing, as they were constructed with a thick layer of sand and gravel on the bottom. The Cambridge student spa-goer noted with surprise that when he swam in the springs at Buxton, he found them 'paved at the bottom with Derbyshire slate'. This made the footing better, but not perfect: 'the water rises from the spring thro' the Cement of the pavement [...] the water in this bath does not stagnate, but is always running', circumstances which must have made it challenging to stay afloat (An. 1725, 56–57). Even when swimmers could keep their footing, the heat of mineral springs made it uncomfortable to stand upright. Samuel Pepys complained during his visit to Bath in June of 1668 that 'the springs [were] so hot as the feet [were] not able to endure' (Pepys 1942, 195). Many bathers did have a hard time staying upright in the water. The strong buoyancy of mineral waters which contained salts made many swimmers feel unbalanced, and they wrote that it was hard to control the movement of their bodies while fully submerged. Eleanor Davies Douglas, known for her apocalyptic and experiential poetry, mentioned in her poem on Bath that swimmers had to be 'by guides supported' (Douglas 1670, n.p.). Even frequent bather and spa-goer Celia Feinnes complained that when she visited Bath, she had trouble staying upright in the water: '[it] is so strong it will quickly tumble you down [...] the spring bubbles up so fast and so strong and so hot against the bottoms of one's feet' (Feinnes 1949, 18–20). For all of these bathers, the pools made them doubt their ability to control the movements of their own bodies.

Feinnes' comments on her uneasiness about swimming at Bath signal that novel and unpredictable buoyancies made even experienced bathers uncomfortable if they knew how to swim, but evidence from city and county records suggests that it was rare for most spa cure-seekers to know how to swim at all. This could only have increased their feelings of insecurity in the water. Although books on swimming for exercise or pleasure did exist, the rarity and novelty of these texts suggests that swimming was not a common practice (Digby 1587; Thévenot 1696; *The Art of Swimming Illustrated by Proper Figures* 1699; *Bathing, and its Effects* 1782).[4] And while some of the larger and well-established spa cities, such as Bath, hired corps of bath guides to support swimmers during their treatments—as alluded to by Eleanor Davies, above—this was not the case in every spa city (Herbert 2014, 123–124). Drowning while bathing in mineral springs was a very real risk; in spa towns, burial records reveal that a large number of people did drown in the pools. Even in the city of Bath, for example, a clerk named John Howell 'drowned in the bathe' in October of 1595. He was joined in this fate by William Prosser (June 14, 1617), John Knowles (August 12, 1623), William Dearing (October 28, 1624), John Burnett (May 8, 1638), and William Brockton (September 12, 1639) all of whom died of drowning in the pools of the city of Bath (An. 1569–1800, n.p.). Feeling uneasy or out of control in mineral waters was not just uncomfortable, it could be dangerous and life-threatening.

After enduring a swimming session, spa patients were told to encourage the waters to move through their bodies by either wrapping themselves in blankets or heavy clothes, or by undertaking exercise, all in order to cause themselves to sweat (Stolberg 2012, 503–522). This component of the cure was widely recognized in treatises about the use of mineral springs. At the very start of the eighteenth century, physician William Oliver required that his Bath patients undertake 'moderate exercise [...] during all the time of drinking', so that harmful discharges from the body could be 'forc'd off by sweat' (Oliver 1704, 221–223). This advice was repeated in ephemera at the end of Robert Boyle's 1684 *Natural Experimental History of Mineral Waters*, where the publisher included an advertisement for what he perceived to be a similar tract: Samuel Haworth's treatise on mineral baths, which promised to show the 'usefulness of Sweating, Rubbing, and Bathing, and the great benefit many here received from them in various Distempers' (Boyle 1684, n.p.). Although sweating was

[4] The first printed book which was substantively about swimming was Everard Digby's *De Arte Natandi* (1587), which was translated and adapted into Melchisédec Thévenot's *L'Art de Nager* (Paris, 1696). The French text was then brought into English three years later as *The Art of Swimming Illustrated by Proper Figures...* (London, 1699). By the late eighteenth century, swimming had become slightly more commonplace, at least enough to warrant lampoons of the activity.

thus understood to be an important and natural process, both patients and practitioners recognized that sudden, unusually rigorous sweating could cause feelings of discomfort and disgust.

Sweat itself was understood to be an off-putting substance. Physician George Cheyne praised mineral springs for their ability to rid the body of 'Foulness [...] and carries it out of the Body, by increas'd Perspiration' (Cheyne 1720, 15–17). The 'foulness' believed to be inherent to sweat was mentioned in explicit detail by a physician named Christopher Meighan, who noted that the 'constant moisture' exuded by his own mineral water patients 'renders their linen remarkably greasy' (Meighan 1764, 53–54). Though sweat was a necessary component of the spa cure which he championed, Meighan's observations also implied that it made his patients 'remarkably' unclean and disgusting (Brown 2011). Some physicians were so wary of sweating as a practice that they told their patients to avoid it; in his manuscript 'Directions for Lady Margaret Grant on How to Take the Waters at Moffatt', in Scotland, an anonymous physician warned that 'after bathing', Grant should 'not go to bed to court sweat as is practiced in some cases'. Avoiding sweating was, according to this physician, 'more safe and innocent than other wise' (An. 1747, n.p.). To keep oneself from becoming sweaty was thus imagined as cleansing to both body and soul.

Patients themselves also expressed reservations about the feel of great quantities of sweat seeping out of and trickling down their bodies. In 1676, Andrea Sall wrote to his friend Jane Gerard that when he bathed in mineral waters, 'in a verie small tyme they make my whole bodie to the top of my head sweat plentifully'. Sall found this sensation to be so unpleasant that it required full-time service and attendance; he explained that he had hired a person 'to stand by me continually wiping the sweat from my face and head while I keep my Legs in the water', in order to complete his cure (Sall 1678, n.p.). William Smith, a minister who lived on Nevis, a Caribbean island claimed by Britain as part of its early empire, described the experience of taking the mineral cure in this tropical environment as painful and frightening because of the volume of sweat he produced. When he bathed in a Nevisian mineral spring, Smith explained that 'in two minutes time the sweat was ready to blind me'. This was so intolerable to Smith that 'in about three minutes more, I was obliged to quit it through faintness of spirit' (Smith 1745, 56–57). For patients like Sall and Smith, sweating provoked feelings of helplessness, vulnerability, and discomfort.

If sweating was considered to be an uncomfortable, albeit unavoidable, consequence of bathing in mineral waters, this was nothing compared to purging. Spa waters were also imagined to provoke the expulsion of faeces, a procedure which—like sweating—was imagined as healthful and important, but which nonetheless made early modern people worry about losing control over or damaging their bodies (Walkden 2018; Wear 2009; Kuriyama 2008, 413–442; Paster 2000, 193–205). Meighan promoted the mineral springs where he worked by offering the praise that 'this water seldom or never purges [...] and this surely adds much to its merit; for purgatives spend their force mostly in scouring the stomach, and bowels' (Meighan 1764, 53–54). Physician George Cheyne criticized spas outside of England for being 'hot, nauseous and purgative' (Cheyne 1720, 50). William Oliver, a physician at Bath, noted that mineral springs could purge, but warned that if the waters 'purge by stool [...] then the use of these waters is lost' (Oliver 1704, 221–223). For Oliver, purging via mineral waters was to be avoided because it meant that the cure was less effective, but he also acknowledged that purging could be dangerous to the body, weakening or damaging it. He admitted that 'purging too much' could be a harmful 'accident' which could occur in patients 'whose digestions are bad, because the fibres of the membranes of their stomach and intestines are weak'. He also gendered this side effect, claiming that women were more vulnerable to mineral water purging than were men, for female spa patients were 'hypochondriack [...] vapours is the common name', and that 'this accident rarely happens to men' (Oliver 1704, 221–223).

Patients at the spa also wrote of purging by stool. Sometimes they framed this bodily function as a positive experience, very often as a negative one, but they always remarked upon it as a notable and unusual circumstance. When Samuel Pepys visited the mineral spring at Epsom in July of 1667, he wrote that he 'did drink four pints, and had some very good stools by it'; as Pepys complained frequently of constipation, and wrote with satisfaction and pleasure when he was able to defecate, it is perhaps unsurprising that he would experience this positively (Pepys 1942, 296). But when Anne Dormer visited Tunbridge Wells in the late seventeenth century, she complained to her sister that her experience of mineral water-induced defecation was 'a tedious time', for she believed that the mineral waters' purgative effects had been harmful: 'I cann scarce say the water did me any good, it pass't so ill, and it purg'd me so much, that I look like a gridiron' (Dormer 1685-1691, n.p.; Weisser 2015, 87-89). By noting that she had lost weight due to excessive purging—so much that she resembled a metal 'gridiron', with her bones showing prominently through her skin—and that the feeling of having the waters in her body had been 'tedious' as they had 'pass't so ill', Dormer demonstrated what she imagined were the debilitative emotional and physical effects of the mineral water purge. Whether they found the mineral purge to be satisfying or painful, almost all spa patients acknowledged that it was inherent to the process of taking the waters. When the spa-going Cambridge student visited Scarborough, he listed his major expense in that city as 'five shillings [...] for the use of the necessary house [e.g. the privy next to the spring]' (An. 1725, 40–42).

6 Humans or Creatures?

Unsettled physical and emotional feelings were thus endemic to the mineral cure. Patients and practitioners alike worried that the spas made it difficult for people to trust their sight, hearing, or senses of smell, taste, or touch, and without these senses—whether 'high' or 'low'—to govern and guide them, spa-goers were left feeling uncomfortable and uneasy. In spaces where the senses could be confused, dulled, or tricked, how would one know how to behave or react? This confusion was made all the worse because spas were open to women and men, young and old, poor and rich. With so many different kinds of people in close proximity, understanding how to behave seemed paramount. Observations about the confusion of the senses at spas were frequently coupled with fears that, without the senses to guide them, bathers might simultaneously be misled, misinformed, or tempted into bending or breaking society's rules, including those governing gender and sexuality, care of the body and best practices of hygiene, and even the socio-economic order.

But it was perhaps the fear that spas broached or disrupted the human–animal divide which made early modern people the most discomfited about the mineral cure (Fudge 2019; Arbel 2017, 201–222; Shannon 2013; Raber 2013; Royster 2005, 113–134). This fear might have been provoked by the fact that some spa cities did actually offer bathing facilities for animals, and some practitioners used mineral springs in order to cure animal diseases and injuries. The mineral spring called 'Dulwich Water', on the border between Kent and Surrey, was known for being 'frequented by Pigeons', and practitioners apparently used the spring to successfully treat a horse suffering from farcy or glanders (today understood as an infection of the bacterium *Burkholderia mallei*) when 'the body of the horse was washed all over with Dulwich water [...] [and] he was by thirst compelled to drink this [...] and was perfectly cured in about three weeks' (Russel 1760, 267–268; Rutty 1757, 171; *OED*). In Bath, a 'horse bath' was drawn onto maps as early as 1610; cartographer John Speed's map of Somersetshire included an inset of the city of Bath, with an image of a pool—with a horse drawn swimming inside of it—labelled 'The horse Bath' on Southgate Street, just south of the city walls (Speed 1610). In October of 1784, another bath for horses was proposed inside of the city walls, 'on the East side of Stall St.' where the pool would be filled with 'the Waste water from the King's Bath in order to make a Hot Bath for horses' (Shickle N.D. Bath Council Books, n.p.). The popularity of Bath's spa for horses was reinforced in two eighteenth-century texts, both of which noted it as a special item of interest in the city. John Wood's 1765 *Essay Towards a Description of Bath* described 'a Bath for Horses, and called the Horse Bath', (Wood 1765, 207) and John Collinson's 1791 *History and Antiquities of the History of Somerset* mentioned 'a bath on the south side of St. James's-church, called the Horse Bath [...] a pool or pond to wash horses in' (Collinson 1791, 41).

While all of this evidence would suggest that mineral spring bathing for animals was a recognized treatment within the period, there are some accounts which attest to the disruptions that animals could cause in the pools. In 1643, the Bath city corporation paid a worker three shillings for the task of 'drawing a dead horse out of the Bath water course' (Shickle N.D. Bath Council Books, n.p.). John Wood also mentioned in his *Essay* that Bath's pools reminded him of 'so many Bear Gardens', where 'Dogs, Cats, Pigs, and even human Creatures were hurl'd over the Rails into the Water, while People were bathing in it' (Wood 1765, 217). Wood's remark that the pools seemed like 'Bear Gardens' was clearly meant to convey that the baths were chaotic, but it was also a pointed one, as, in the early modern period, bear gardens were literal spaces in which animals were baited for sport (*OED*). By comparing a medical practice to a barbarous form of entertainment, Wood demonstrated levelled criticisms against the spa which were both moralistic and social. And Wood's note that many different kinds of animals—pigs, cats, and dogs—appeared in the pools was designed to create senses of unease and worry in among his readers: one could never be sure what kind of creature one might bump up against while swimming or wading in a mineral spring.

That Wood also wrote of the pools as filled with 'human Creatures' brings us back to the quote which opened this chapter, where Pepys called the people who bathed in mineral spas 'Creatures of the Bath'. Wood and Pepys were not the only authors to articulate their belief that what was human and what was animal blurred within the pools. Joseph Browne, an advocate for cold bathing, explained that he had witnessed 'a Poor Man Strip and Leap into this Bath [...] he told me he had Liv'd in the Peak of Darbyshire, and had been a Miner'. Browne described this miner as 'look[ing] more like a Fish than a Land Animal, for his Skin was all Scaby over from Head to Foot'. Browne also called the man a 'Monster, which he look'd more like than a Man', and wrote with disgust and fascination that the man's self-prescribed treatment was to 'was[h] himself [...] four or five times a Day [...] [and] ru[b] off his Scabs as you wou'd Scale a Fish with a Knife' (Browne 1707, 63–64). For Browne, social status, dirt, disease, and the human and the animal were all made uncertain in mineral springs.

Satirists also took advantage of this sense of instability. The anonymous *New Bath Guide* of 1768 described swimmers as 'the strangest fish that e'er were seen', and called these women and men 'stranger wretches', than those humans who did not bathe in springs (An. 1768, 5–6). This satirist went on to poke fun of a medical regimen given to the family's maid, 'Tabby', who has prescribed 'a great many doses [...] [of] *Testic: Equin:* [eg., horse testicles] that she takes ev'ry night'. This was necessitated, the author explained, by Tabby's affliction: greensickness, for 'the poor creature has got the Chlorosis', a disease supposedly suffered by young women who were not sexually active. In addition to inferring that spas were spaces of unauthorized or excessive sexuality, where Tabby was to be cured by swallowing testicles each night, this cure also made her less than human, for, the author remarked 'I never could wonder her face was so green' (An. 1768, 14).

7 Conclusion: Discomfort at the Spa

As this chapter has shown, spas were valued for their ability to make disfigured or sick bodies whole and well. But they were also feared for their powers of obfuscation, alteration, and conversion. By analysing mineral spa cures via the framework of the five human senses, we can see how the women and men who took the waters parsed their interior and exterior feelings about these treatments. This evidence, culled from a wide range of personal papers, government documents, medical casebooks, travelogues, and satirical literature, reveals that drinking or bathing in mineral springs sent mixed physical and emotional messages. Spas were places where intersectional fears about uncleanliness, hypersexuality, class conflict, and the human–animal divide could drive patients and practitioners alike to interpret mineral spring medicine as a dissociative experience rather than a holistic one.

Works Cited

Primary Sources

Allen, Benjamin. 1711. *The Natural History of the Mineral-Waters of Great-Britain. To Which Are Added, Some Observations of the Cicindela, or Glow-Worm.* London: Printed for the author, and sold by William Innys, at the Prince's Arms in St. Paul's Church-Yard.

An. 1569–1800. Register of Burials, Bath Abbey (Sts. Peter and Paul), Bath Guildhall Record Office.

An. 1654–1780. Churchwardens' Accounts and Vestry Minutes for Bath St. James, D/P/ba.ja/4/1/1, Somerset Heritage Centre.

An. 1699. *The Art of Swimming Illustrated by Proper Figures...* London: Printed for Dan Brown, D. Midurnter and T. Leigh, and Robert Knaplock.

An. 1705. *A Letter from a Citizen of Bath, to His Excellency Dr. R.____ [Radcliffe] at Tunbridge.* [Bath?]: [s.n.].

An. 1717. *A Journey to Bath and Bristol: An Heroi-Comic-Historic-, and Geographical Poem.* London: J. Roberts.

An. 1725. *Diary of a Tour Through Several English Counties*, Tour Collection, B10 S3, Bath Central Library.

An. 1747. Directions for Lady Margaret Grant on How to Take the Waters at Moffat, by 'W.P.', Papers of the Family of Grant of Grant selected for, and partly noted in, the 'Chiefs of Grant', GD248/24/2/13, National Records of Scotland.

An. 1748. *Bath: A Poem.* London: Printed for Mess. Longman and Shewell, in Pater-Noster-Row, London; J. Leak, in Bath; and M. Lewis, in Bristol.

An. 1782. *Bathing, And its Effects. A poetical tale. In two parts. In which are interspersed, directions and cautions to those who cannot swim.* London: Printed for W. Goldsmith, No. 24, in Pater-Noster-Row.

Anstey, Christopher. 1768. *The New Bath Guide: Or, Memoirs of the B-r-d Family, in a Series of Poetical Epistles.*

Boyle, Robert. 1684. *Short Memoirs For The Natural Experimental History of Mineral Waters: Addressed By way of Letter to a Friend.* London: Printed for Samual Smith.

Browne, Joseph. 1707. *An Account of the Wonderful Cures Perform'd by the Cold Baths: With Advice to the Water Drinkers at Tunbridge, Hampstead, Astrope, Nasborough...* London: Printed for J. How, in Talbot-Court, in Grace-Church-Street; and R. Borough, and J. Baker, at the Sun and Moon in Cornhill.

Cheyne, George. 1720. *An Essay on the Gout, with an Account of the Nature and Qualities of the Bath Waters*. London and Bath: Printed for G. Strahan, at the Golden Ball, over against the Royal Exchange in Cornhill; W. Mears, at the Lamb without Temple Bar, and H. Hammond, at the Bath.

Cole, G.D.H. (ed.). 1927. *Daniel Defoe A Tour Thro' the Whole Island of Great Britain*, vol. II. London: Peter Davies.

Collinson, John. 1791. *The History and Antiquities of the County of Somerset...* Bath: Printed by R. Cruttwell.

Cowper, Spencer (ed.). 1865. *Dairy of Mary Countess Cowper, Lady of the Bedchamber to the Princess of Wales, 1714–1720*. London: J. Murray.

Digby, Everard. 1587. *De Arte Natandi*. London: Excudebat Thomas Dawson.

Dingley, Thomas. 1867. *History from Marble*. London: Nichols and Sons.

Douglas, Eleanor Touchet Davies. 1670.Bath Daughter of BabyLondon. Hastings Papers, HA Religious Box 1, Folder 28, Huntington Library.

Dormer, Anne. 1685–1691. Letters to her sister Elizabeth Trumbull. Add Ms 72516, F 156–243, British Library.

Goldsmith, Oliver. 1762. *The Life of Richard Nash, of Bath, Esq; Extracted principally from His Original Papers*. London: Printed for J. Newbery, in St. Paul's Church-yard; and W. Frederick, at Bath.

Mackaile, Matthew. 1664. *Moffet-well, or, A topographico-spagyricall description of the minerall wells, at Moffet in Annandale of Scotland...; as also, The oyly-well, or, A topographico-spagyricall description of the oyly-well, at St. Catharines Chappel in the paroch of Libberton...* Edinburgh: Printed for Robert Brown.

Macky, John. 1722. *A Journey Through England...* London: J. Hooke.

Meighan, Christopher. 1764. *A Treatise of the Nature and Powers of the Baths and Waters of Bareges...* London: Printed for A. Millar.

Morris, Christopher (ed.). 1949. *The Journeys of Celia Fiennes*. London: Cresset Press.

Oliver, William. 1704. *A Practical Essay on Fevers, Containing Remarks on the Hot and Cool Methods of their Cure...To which is Annex'd, A Dissertation on the Bath-Waters*. London: Printed for T. Goodwin.

Russel, Richard. 1760. *A Dissertation on the Use of Sea Water...As Also An Account of the Nature, Properties, and Uses of all the Remarkable Mineral Waters in Great Britain*. London.

Rutty, John. 1757. *A Methodical Synopsis of Mineral Waters...* London: William Johnstone.

Sall, Andrea. 1678. Letter to Lady Jane Gerard Baroness Bromley, 24 July 1678, Correspondence of the Dukes of Hamilton, GD406/11525, National Records of Scotland.

Shickle, C.W., tr. N.D. Bath Corporation Accounts, Disbursements, Lands, Water Supply, 17th c., Acc 33:330, B3005, SH1, Local Store, Bath Central Library.

Shickle, C.W., tr. N.D. Bath Council Books Vol. II-IV, 1684–1751, Class B352.0422 BATLocal Store, Bath Central Library.

Smith, Lucy Toulmin (ed.). 1907. *The Itinerary of John Leland in Or about the Years 1535–1543: Parts 1 to 3*. London: George Bell and Sons.

Smith, William. 1745. *A Natural of Nevis, and the Rest of the English Leeward Charibee islands in America*... Cambridge: Printed by J. Bentham.

Speed, John. 1610. Map of Somersetshire and Bath, Bath Central Library.

Thévenot, Melchisédec. 1696. *L'Art de Nager*. Paris: Chez Lamy, Libraire, Quai des Augustins.

Veith, David M. (ed.). 1968. *The Complete Poems of John Wilmot, Earl of Rochester*. New Haven: Yale University Press.

Wheatley, Henry (ed.). 1942. *The Diary of Samuel Pepys*. New York: The Heritage Press.

Wood, John. [1749] 1765. *An Essay Towards a Description of Bath*... London.

Secondary Sources

Arbel, Benjamin. 2017. The Beginnings of Comparative Anatomy and Renaissance Reflections on the Human-Animal Divide. *Renaissance Studies* 31: 201–222.

Brown, Kathleen. 2011. *Foul Bodies: Cleanliness in Early America*. New Haven: Yale University Press.

Cahill, Patricia A. 2009. Take Five: Renaissance Literature and the Study of the Senses. *Literature Compass* 6, no. 5 (September): 1014–1030.

Cockayne, Emily. 2007. *Hubbub: Filth, Noise & Stench in England 1600–1770*. New Haven: Yale University Press.

Fudge, Erica. 2019. *Brutal Reasoning: Animals, Rationality, and Humanity in Early Modern England*. Ithaca: Cornell University Press.

Harvey, Elizabeth D. 2003. *Sensible Flesh: On Touch in Early Modern Culture*. Philadelphia: University of Pennsylvania Press.

Herbert, Amanda E. 2014. *Female Alliances: Gender, Identity, and Friendship in Early Modern Britain*. New Haven: Yale University Press.

Jenner, Mark. 2000. Civilization and Deodorization? Smell in Early Modern English Culture. In *Civil Histories: Essays Presented to Sir Keith Thomas*. eds. Peter Burke, Brian Harrison, and Paul Slack, 127–144 New York, Oxford University Press.

Kambaskovic, Danijela. 2014. "Among the Rest of the Senses...Proved Most Sure": Ethics of the Senses in Pre-Modern Europe. In *Conjunctions of Mind, Soul and Body from Plato to the Enlightenment*. ed. Danijela Kambaskovic, 337–370 London, Springer.

Kuriyama, Shigehisa. 2008. The Forgotten Fear of Excrement. *Journal of Medieval and Early Modern Studies* 38 (3): 413–442.

Paster, Gail Kern. 2000. Purgation as the Allure of Mastery: Early Modern Medicine and the Technology of the Self. *Material London ca. 1600*, 193–205. Lena Cowen Orlin. Philadelphia: University of Pennsylvania Press.

Raber, Karen. 2013. *Animal Bodies, Renaissance Culture*. Philadelphia: University of Pennsylvania Press.

Roodenburg, Herman (ed.). 2016. *A Cultural History of the Senses in the Renaissance*. London: Bloomsbury.

Royster, Francesca. 2005. "Working Like a Dog": African Labour and Racing the Human-Animal Divide in Early Modern England. In *Writing Race Across the Atlantic World: Signs of Race*, ed. P.D. Beidler and G. Taylor, 113–134. New York, Palgrave: Macmillan.

Shannon, Laurie. 2013. *The Accommodated Animal: Cosmopolity in Shakespearean Locales*. Chicago: University of Chicago Press.

Stedman, Gesa. 2013. *Cultural Exchange in Seventeenth-Century France and England*. Burlington: Ashgate.

Stolberg, Michael. 2012. Sweat: Learned Concepts and Popular Perceptions, 1500–1800. In *Blood, Sweat and Tears: The Changing Concepts of Physiology from Antiquity into Early Modern Europe*. eds. Manfred Horstmanshoff, Helen King, and Claus Zittel, 503–522 Leiden, Brill.

Tullett, William. 2019. *Smell in Eighteenth-Century England: A Social Sense*. Oxford: Oxford University Press.

Walkden, Michael. 2018. *The Gut-Mind Connection in Early Modern Medicine and Culture, c.1580–c.1740*. PhD diss.: University of York.

Wear, Andrew. 2009. *Knowledge and Practice in English Medicine, 1550–1680*. Cambridge UK: Cambridge University Press.

Weisser, Olivia. 2015. *Ill Composed: Sickness, Gender, and Belief in Early Modern England*. New Haven: Yale University Press.

Wroughton, John. 2004. *Stuart Bath: Life in the Forgotten City, 1603–1714*. Bath: Lansdown Press.

CHAPTER 8

Bathing in Verse: Christopher Anstey's *The New Bath Guide* and Georgian Resort Satire

Shaun Regan

1766 saw the publication of Christopher Anstey's epistolary verse satire, *The New Bath Guide*. The work quickly became a literary sensation and a commercial success. Four further editions were published during 1766–1767, while a tenth appeared within a decade. Anstey's poem was also something of a game-changer for contemporary depictions of water-based leisure. During the later eighteenth and early nineteenth centuries, *The New Bath Guide* became both a template and a touchstone for poetry focused on British leisure resorts: many writers modelled their texts on the *Guide* and its primary verse form, while a host of imitative and adjunctive verses invoked the poem's central characters and Anstey himself. Satisfying demand for such products that Anstey had created, these watering place verses charted the experiences of fictional invalids and pleasure-seekers at not just Bath but also Bristol, Cheltenham, Tunbridge Wells, Harrogate,

S. Regan (✉)
School of Arts, English and Languages, Queen's University, Belfast, UK
e-mail: s.regan@qub.ac.uk

S. Chiari and S. Cuisinier-Delorme (eds.), *Spa Culture and Literature in England, 1500–1800*, Early Modern Literature in History,
https://doi.org/10.1007/978-3-030-66568-5_8

Brighton, Margate and Ramsgate.[1] Following Anstey, this was a key way in which Georgian leisure was presented to the public: in light anapaestic verse, often extended across lengthy narratives, which detailed behaviours, incidents and opportunities that were characteristic of resorts or specific to individual locations.

A private gentleman of independent means, Christopher Anstey (1724–1805) had himself benefitted from Bath's mineral waters during a visit to the city in the late 1750s. He would go on to purchase a family home in the Crescent around 1770 and become part of Lady Miller's poetic circle at Batheaston. By then, his reputation had been established by *The New Bath Guide*, his first published poem in English and his greatest literary success.[2] Part of the *Guide*'s novelty and appeal lay in its poetic measure. While the work was fêted for its variety of verse forms, the letters of Simkin Blunderhead, whose voice dominates the poem, are mainly written in anapaestic tetrameter: metrical feet of three syllables, with four stresses per line. Anstey's use of this lilting measure, which represented a departure from the iambic metre of much early eighteenth-century satiric poetry, contributed to what Ashley Marshall has described as the simultaneous fragmentation and softening of satiric literature during the third quarter of the century (Marshall 2013, 239–240). Evoking Horatian urbanity rather than Juvenalian disgust, Anstey's anapaests facilitated both pointed ridicule and less judgemental concessions to his poem's leisured targets. To A. B. Granville, in his monumental *Spas of England* (1841), *The New Bath Guide* constituted 'one of the lightest and most amusing satires in the English language'. As Granville attested, Anstey's poem, while satiric, was far from acerbic: less a spur to moral outrage than an invitation to knowing laughter at the 'manners and follies of Bath as a watering-place' during the mid-1760s (Granville 1841, 3:398).

Satiric verse focused on watering holes was by no means a new phenomenon at this time. Harold Love (2008), for instance, has examined an earlier phase of such writing beginning in the later seventeenth century. Yet little attention has been given to the body of resort satires

[1] The coastal spa-town of Scarborough was also addressed in a rare work which, despite not being anapaestic or alluding to Anstey, is relevant to this verse-guide tradition: *The New Scarboro' Guide; or, Memoirs of the Sawney Family, in a Series of Poetical Epistles* (1807).

[2] For further details of Anstey's life and career, see Turner (2005).

written under the influence of Anstey, which continued to appear well into the nineteenth century even as fashions changed and the focus shifted from inland resorts to coastal ones.[3] There are a number of possible reasons for this. The writing itself is of uneven and sometimes dubious quality: 'verse' rather than 'poetry'. In the main, these texts do not gaze either outwards, towards major political events, or inwards, in line with the historical turn towards subjectivity and psychology. There is little sense here of the revolutions in America and France, and their transformative effect on both literature and politics. Instead, in these works, seaside resorts and spas represent places of political repose: where Fox, Burke and Sheridan might take a holiday from parliamentary oratory (West 1788, 15), or where British tourists could indulge a 'smile' at 'Napoleon's threats of invading' (Hofland 1812, 26).[4] At the same time, with their focus on manners and fashions, styles of leisure and behaviour in public places, these verses speak not to the introspection and affectivity that have traditionally defined the ages of Sensibility and Romanticism but to the spaces and networks of 'Romantic sociability', which has emerged as an important focus in literary and cultural criticism of the period (Russell and Tuite 2002; Gilmartin 2017).

The template provided by *The New Bath Guide* was in fact put to a variety of subsequent uses, separately from this focus on British resort culture. During the later eighteenth century, anapaestic poems were published on military and educational themes.[5] In works such as *The Westminster Guide* (1784) and *The New Parliamentary Register* (1791), a number of writers adopted Anstey's model to address parliamentary

[3] Day (1948) discusses anapaestic poems about leisure resorts in a broader section concerning 'Epistolary Satire on Modish Follies'. Seaton (2016) attends briefly to post-Anstey poems about resorts in Britain before focusing on works with Continental settings.

[4] Gary Dyer argues that 'Neo-Horatian works of this time tended to avoid clear political implications, but in effect were comparably conservative' and that 'Horatian satire ultimately is anti-political' (Dyer 1997, 3, 41). While my analysis of resort satires largely accords with this view, Dyer's broad approach tends to efface the particularities of individual works, especially those in the 'neo-Horatian' mould that I am mainly concerned with here.

[5] See for instance *A Sketch of the Campaign of 1793* (London: T. Cadell and W. Davies, 1795); Sappho Search (i.e., John Black), *A Poetical Review of Miss Hannah More's 'Strictures on Female Education': In a Series of Anapestic Epistles* (London: T. Hurst, 1800).

politics specifically.[6] Some Anstey-influenced poems focused on London, while a clutch of anapaestic works ranged beyond Britain, the most significant and best-known being Thomas Moore's Fudge Family verses set in France.[7] Yet both quantitatively and in the popular imagination, this type of verse was most closely associated with resorts in Britain. As Barbara Hofland noted in her own Ansteyan imitation, *A Season at Harrogate* (1812), *The New Bath Guide* was 'the parent of a numerous progeny of watering place bagatelles' (Hofland 1812, [iii]). It is this dominant strain of anapaestic verse that I shall be addressing here. To the writers who followed in his footsteps, I shall suggest, the defining feature of Anstey's poem was its establishment of a new register for evoking the world of provincial leisure: a comparatively tempered satiric mode which, while still *satiric*, was more attuned to the culture of the resorts themselves. While they are by no means uniform in either tone or quality, the 'watering place' verses written in the wake of *The New Bath Guide* likewise maintained a fine balance between popular advertisement and satiric critique. In the process, they extended the mode of amicable resort satire that Anstey had instigated in *The New Bath Guide* itself.

1 Satire and Sociability: *The New Bath Guide*

Structured in the form of 15 verse epistles, *The New Bath Guide* narrates the trip to Bath of the younger members of the Blunderhead family: the country squire, Simkin, his sister, Prudence, and their cousin, Jenny; along with their maid, Tabby Runt. Over the course of its 1600+ lines, the poem surveys the social customs and behavioural codes at Britain's premier resort for medicinal waters and recreation: from the noisy welcome of the Abbey bells and musicians, through early morning bathing (via sedan chair), breakfasts (both public and private), the diversions of gambling and shopping, and the evening balls at the Assembly Rooms. At times, Anstey's poem reads like a satiric-verse analogue to the

[6] The first part of *The Westminster Guide* is addressed to Anstey, while *The New Parliamentary Register* is dedicated to him. Other Ansteyan imitations in the political mould included a number of works published by Ralph Broome in the later 1780s and 1790s, which focused on the trial of Warren Hastings, and subsequent anti-Burkean verse.

[7] [Samuel Hoole], *Modern Manners: In a Series of Familiar Epistles* (London: R. Faulder, 1781); Joseph Moser, *The Adventures of Timothy Twig, Esq.*, 2 vols (London: E. and T. Williams, 1794); Thomas Brown, the Younger (i.e., Thomas Moore), *The Fudge Family in Paris* (London: Longman, Hurst, Rees, Orme, and Brown, 1818).

account given by John Penrose during his own visit to Bath in 1766, with its detailing of daily water-drinking and breakfasting, visiting and promenading.[8] Like Penrose's letters, Anstey's extensive portrayal of this recreational environment testifies to the fact that, in Peter Borsay's words, mid-eighteenth-century Bath possessed 'the most sophisticated complex of leisure facilities to be found in the provinces' (Borsay 1989, 168). More acutely, as Phyllis Hembry observes, within this 'ritualized leisure industry', in which sociability was formalised and pleasure regulated, the assembled tourists were granted 'little time' for 'individual activity' (Hembry 1990, 136).

This is not quite how the poem itself begins. In the opening letter, written by Jenny, Bath is initially apprehended not as a regulated zone of studied sociability but as a pastoral idyll—as 'this fertile Vale' with its 'verdant Meads' and 'genial Springs'. Casting herself as a 'Nymph of Spirit', Jenny's pastoralising is arch, but only partly so (Anstey 2010, 85–86). Soon enough, though, the focus turns to Bath's reputation as a fashionable resort for the improvement of health. In letter 2, having lost both his appetite and his 'Spirits', Simkin calls for the doctor, who does little more than feel his pulse. In this early medical encounter, the rituals of a learned physician, at a fashionable watering place, are contrasted to the country simplicity of Simkin, who quails at the doctor's 'grave' visage and receives a 'Fright' merely from having his pulse taken (Anstey 2010, 89–91).

Notably, Simkin is himself required to translate the doctor's prescription, which is spoken in Latin; once translated, the diagnosis bathetically indicates a case of wind. (Simkin is, as one contemporary joked, the poem's '*flatulent* Hero').[9] The medical profession's implication in the commercial operation at Bath is evoked here as the doctor prescribes medicine for Simkin to take for three weeks, before even venturing to taste the spa's waters. This theme is picked up again in letter 4, titled '*A Consultation of* PHYSICIANS'. Among other things, this letter evokes the proliferation of doctors at Bath, whose waters were being promoted as a cure for 'all Distempers' (Anstey 2010, 100).[10] As Sim observes in

[8] For a summary of his daily routine see Penrose (1983, 73–75).

[9] Letter from 'Aeolus' in *St. James's Chronicle*, issue 905, 18–20 December 1766.

[10] As John Penrose deadpanned in 1766, 'Bath-Waters cure all Disorders, curable or incurable' (1983, 144).

letter 6, moreover, even though they extol the curative benefits of the spa, the physicians at Bath don't appear to partake of the waters themselves:

> Since the Day that King BLADUD first found out the Bogs,
> And thought them so good for himself and his Hogs,
> Not one of the Faculty ever has try'd
> These excellent Waters to cure his own Hide. (Anstey 2010, 112)

At issue here was not just balneology, or balneotherapy, but pharmacology also. The dangers of unregulated medicines are suggested when Tabby becomes ill through 'swallowing Stuff she has read in the Papers', such as 'Water-Dock Essence' (Anstey 2010, 91)—a herbal tincture prepared by Dr John Hill (1714–1775), which also comes in for a satiric swipe in Tobias Smollett's *Humphry Clinker* (1771).[11] Pointedly, the ending of letter 4 sees the doctors' medicines raining down upon their heads, as Jenny throws them out of a window and wonders why so many visitors should head to the spa merely to be 'doctor'd to Death' (Anstey 2010, 100).

In his expansive 1830 edition of *The New Bath Guide*, John Britton contended that Anstey is 'rather too hard on the medical profession, when he represents all the M.D.'s as dolts and dunderheads, practising on the blunderheads' (Anstey 1830, 152). Nonetheless, these encounters with an apparently compromised and ineffectual health industry represent early setbacks to the visitors, who had arrived with an exalted sense of the spa's powers.[12] Disappointed by its promised improvements to health, the visitors turn their attention from doctors and waters to social diversions. A narrative crux arrives in letter 10, in which Simkin '*commences* BEAU GARÇON'. Here, Simkin engages in what Thorstein Veblen theorised as 'conspicuous leisure': a display of recreation that confirmed one's status as a person *of* leisure. As the ambitious protagonist declares: 'I long to do something to make myself known; / For persons of *Taste* and true *Spirit*, I find, / Are fond of attracting the Eyes of Mankind' (Anstey 2010, 133). Such conspicuous displays of leisure, Veblen argued, were supported by the consumption of 'honorific' luxuries, which convey esteem—not least

[11] As Gavin Turner notes in his edition of *The New Bath Guide*, all of the medicines listed by Anstey in these lines were advertised in the *Bath Chronicle* in 1765 and 1766 (Anstey 1994, 109–110).

[12] On the poem's portrayal of illness and its treatment see also Cossic-Pericarpin (2017).

fashionable clothing, the 'insignia' of leisure (Veblen 2007, 53, 113). As he increases his own public appearances, Simkin accordingly decks himself out in the sartorial accessories of male fashion: bag-wig, ruffles, muff, buckles, stockings. Thus accoutred, he regards himself complacently as part of the leading social set: 'I look,' he says, 'like a Man *of the very first World*' (Anstey 2010, 135).

The qualification implied here by 'look' is, though, significant. As his self-fashioning as a 'Beau' suggests, Simkin is at best an effeminised gentleman. Having taken fright at a doctor's touch, he now experiences a feeling of 'Transport' in his 'Bosom' at the Ball, where he finds the assembly of women 'overcoming' (Anstey 2010, 137). Despite his efforts to fashion himself into a modish gentleman, for Simkin at least the distinction between an aspirational squire and a man of true refinement remains intact. Crucially, as the poem's denouement reveals, Simkin is not finally a secure member of the leisure class described by Veblen, lacking as he does sufficient means to support its conspicuous lifestyle. Having frittered away his money in aping the elite, he is thus left lamenting his financial debts, along with the romantic distresses in which this excursion to Bath has embroiled his female companions: Jenny, abandoned by the free-wheeling military impostor, 'Captain' Cormorant; Prudence, a spiritual enthusiast (seduced by the Methodist, Nicodemus [Roger]); and Tabby, impregnated by a Moravian Rabbi.

2 Anapests and Advertisements: Ansteyan Resort Satire

Despite this downbeat outcome, and by contrast to Simkin himself, *The New Bath Guide* was quickly received as a modish triumph. To Thomas Gray, writing in August 1766, for instance, Anstey's poem was 'the most fashionable of books' (Gray 1935, 3:927). A decade later, in 1778, Frances Burney would deem the work sufficiently decorous for the gentleman-suitor, Lord Orville, to read together with the delicate heroine of her novel, *Evelina* (Burney 1994, 328). Except for a few demurrers over the indelicacy of its anti-evangelical satire (in letter 14), this combined reputation for excellence and propriety would continue into the nineteenth century. Reviewing the collected edition of his *Works* that was published by his son, John, in 1808, the *Critical Review* concluded that Anstey 'will delight his countrymen as long as a taste for genuine wit and humour remain among them' and that his poetry had 'added to the innocent stock of irresistible laughter' (An. 1809, 274). The reception of *The New Bath Guide* particularly as *politely* humorous testifies to an important aspect of its success: the extent to which Anstey had deviated from a dominant satiric discourse which presented corruption and disease as metaphors for life at the spa. To Ned Ward in *A Step to the Bath*, Bath was composed of '*Pools of Iniquity*'; it was, he concluded, 'a Valley of Pleasure, yet a sink of Iniquity' (Ward 1700, 3, 16). The 1737 poem *The Diseases of Bath* figured Bath as both sick in itself and sickening to others: its doctors were a 'canibal [sic], man-mangling Brood' while its denizens were the 'scum' of the nation. Evoking images of contamination and bodily pollution, the author of *The Diseases* portrayed the Pump Room as a place of 'sickly, crude, offensive Vapours' that the 'Nostrils snuff up with the tainted Air'; while, in the waters themselves, 'Nameless Diseases join'd pollute the Stream, / And mix their foul Infections with its Steam' (*Diseases* 1737, 5, 4, 13–14). This mode of civic satire would culminate in Matthew Bramble's famously phobic account of the Bath waters, in Smollett's *Humphry Clinker* (1771).

The disgust that these works express at aqueous pleasure-seeking and inter-status sociability offers a stark tonal contrast to Anstey's wry portrayal of Bath. Part of the innovativeness of *The New Bath Guide* was to step outside this discourse; to satirise Bath anew in less scabrous, more accepting terms. This tonal ambivalence, both pointed and generous, would be adopted by writers of resort satire through to the mid-nineteenth century. This period saw the publication of a fascinating mixture of 'Ansteyan' verses, which (in varying combinations) mimicked Anstey's anapaestic rhythm, continued his tale of the Blunderheads, and focused on Bath or on other resorts, both inland and coastal.[13] These works bear witness to what one early nineteenth-century commentator archly termed 'the Hydromania': 'an inordinate and irresistible longing, either for large draughts of certain waters to be found in distant parts of the kingdom [...] or for the entire or partial immersion of the body in

[13] The adjectival form 'Ansteyan' appears in Mangin 1815, 3: 'To relate in our favorite Ansteyan measure, / How matters go on in these regions of pleasure'. According to a footnote in the second edition, also 1815, 'Ansteyan' was the author's own coinage: 'This epithet *(Ansteyan)* is invented' (10).

hot or cold water' (M.M. 1827, 298–299).[14] While the verses themselves were of varying length and form, many were long epistolary narratives, often employing the conceit of visitors writing to family or friends during a recuperative trip to a particular resort. With whatever degree of humility, many also registered their indebtedness to Anstey—indeed, insisted upon the alignment. As this anapaestic 'progeny' attests, the cultural afterlife of *The New Bath Guide* was closely bound up with the literary depiction and popularisation of water-based leisure resorts in the later eighteenth and early nineteenth centuries.[15]

During these decades, a number of resorts gained both prose guide-books and satiric verse-books, often written in the 'splayfoot Measures' popularised by *The New Bath Guide*.[16] While the verse guides offer mixed and sometimes barbed assessments of the fashions and follies, rituals and ridiculous behaviour to be encountered at the resorts, they nevertheless animate the popular images of these arenas in ways that the prose guides—with their histories, descriptive accounts and travel advice—could not. Yet it would be a mistake to view the verse guides as being entirely at odds with their prose counterparts. Repeating Anstey's own trick, guidebooks-in-verse often mimicked the titles of prose guidebooks, and were often published in close succession. The prose *Brighthelmston Directory*, which first appeared in 1769, for instance, was followed in 1770 by *The New Brighthelmstone Directory; or, Sketches in Miniature of the British Shore*: an Anstey-style anapaestic satire. 1770 also saw the publication of both *The Margate Guide*—a prose guidebook—and *Margate in Miniature; or, The New Margate Guide*, a poetic spinoff.[17] A decade later, in 1781, readers interested in the drinking spa at Cheltenham were presented with

[14] As Robin Jarvis notes in a discussion of 'Romantic swimming', the first use of 'hydromania' recorded by the *OED* comes from a letter written by Percy Shelley in 1793 (Jarvis 2015, 251).

[15] Borsay (2000) provides a detailed overview of the resorts and their development during this period. For the movement from inland spas to the sea-side, see also Walvin (1978) and Walton (1983).

[16] The 'Ghost' of the actor, James Quin, describes Simkin's anapaests as 'splayfoot Measures' in the 'Epilogue' to *The New Bath Guide* (Anstey 2010, 175). The phrase was picked up by a number of Anstey's imitators.

[17] *The Margate Guide* repeated material first published in *A Description of the Isle of Thanet, and particularly of the town of Margate* (London: J. Newbery and W. Bristow, 1763). *Margate in Miniature* is not recorded on ESTC; it appears to be no longer extant (Worldcat).

two new works in the forms of *The Cheltenham Guide*—a prose work attributed to Weeden Butler (1742–1823)—and *The Cheltenham Guide; or, Memoirs of the B-n-r-d Family Continued*: Anstey-style epistolary verses attributed to William Fordyce Mavor (1758–1837). Typically, the quality of these verse satires was queried by reviewers, if not outright denied. To the reviewer in the *Monthly*, for instance, *Margate in Miniature* was the 'silliest' of all the imitations of *The New Bath Guide* (An. 1770b, 326). The *Critical* was more cutting; as it concluded, 'What a pack of despicable imitators has the author of the Bath Guide tempted out, to plague the Reviewers, and impose on the public!' (An. 1770a, 232). Reviewing the verse *Cheltenham Guide* a decade later, the *Critical* opined similarly that 'Of all the aukward pretences to the wit, humour, and poetry of the *Bath Guide* that have appeared, this is one of the worst' (An. 1781, 392). Yet the reviewers' commitment to pinpointing and decrying the very worst of the Bath-Guide knock-offs does not encompass their full significance or modern interest. For, even as they engage in satiric mockery, these alternative verse guides also display a countervailing desire to publicise their resort of preference.

The promotional bent of much of the 'resort satire' published during these decades is apparent in some of the verse guides noted above, which appeared hot on the heels of their prose equivalents. Written 'after the model' of *The New Bath Guide*, for instance, *The New Brighthelmstone Directory* (1770) commends Brighton as a place of interpersonal politeness and good humour; extolling the Steyne as 'our great public walk, / Where the ladies assemble to giggle and talk' (*New Brighthelmstone Directory* 1770, vi–vii, 14). Like other Ansteyan imitations, this poem conveys the disconnected conversations of the assembled Company without savaging polite discourse itself, in the manner of Swift's *Polite Conversation* (1738). Indeed, Swiftian allusions serve instead to enliven the scene: the novel and somewhat surreal nature of the enclosed bathing machines is evoked, for example, via a comparison with Gulliver's experience at the end of his Brobdingnagian adventure: 'I could not but think of the wonderful knocks, / Which Gulliver heard on his great wooden box' (*New Brighthelmstone Directory* 1770, 31). At the same time, the curative efficacy of the resort is attributed in this work not to the waters but to the sociability that Brighton facilitates. It is the conversation enjoyed while dining, rather than the benefit of sea-bathing, we are told, that has 'banish'd' the persona's 'spleen' (*New Brighthelmstone Directory* 1770, 62).

The mainly anapaestic *Cheltenham Guide*, one of a number of continuations of Anstey's narrative, likewise lauds its resort of choice; partly, in this instance, through favourable contrasts to its rival spa, Bath. Somewhat implausibly, the work's opening lines see the inspired visitor declaring that 'I feel poetick fire, / When CHELT'NHAM is my theme' (Mavor 1781, v). Nevertheless, the verses that follow present Cheltenham as somewhere that offers health without expense, in a resort marked by '*real* PIETY' (viii). By comparison, as the initial Apostrophe declares, Bath is a place of '*form* and vice; / Where Brother SIM acquir'd the *ton*, / But fell by cards and dice' (vi). The central character here is Tristram, Simkin's brother, who has travelled to Cheltenham (along with Prudence and Jenny) owing to a 'scorbutick taint' in his blood. Refusing to satirise the 'gay vot'ries of Chelt'nham's *sweet* spring', Tristram registers the lack, at Cheltenham, of some of the modish affectations which might seem to taint Bath: as he notes, for instance, the women at Cheltenham wear their own hair (Mavor 1781, 16, 19, 26). More broadly, Tristram relays the visitors' well-bred pastimes: promenading, conversation, tea-drinking. A potential fly in the ointment arrives in the shape of Simon Moreau, Cheltenham's first Master of Ceremonies and the main target in the work of satire directed at Cheltenham itself. This 'Ape, in the shape of a Beau' comes in for criticism for attempting to enforce a rigid '*etiquette*', which leads Tristram to lament 'that forms should efface / The native politeness and ease of this place!' (Mavor 1781, 28–29).[18] Unlike Bath, the poem insinuates, Cheltenham encourages only a *natural* politeness. Pointedly, this rejection of '*etiquette*' is followed by a poem titled 'The Roll of Beauty', in which Flavilla is advised to reject '*politesse*' in favour of her genuine graces (Mavor 1781, 40).

In quite specific ways, *The Cheltenham Guide* also furthered its promotional design by overwriting the less decorous aspects of Anstey's *New Bath Guide* involving its female characters, Jenny and Prudence. The outcome of the trip to Cheltenham resolves some of these issues at the level of plot: Prue here marries a respectable parson, Jerome (as against her earlier, Methodist seduction) while Jenny marries Bevil, 'a man of true virtue, taste, wit, and sound knowledge', by contrast to her earlier liaison with the fortune-hunting Captain Cormorant (Mavor 1781, 106). Intriguingly, Anstey's text is itself cast as the source of Prue's current,

[18] Moreau drew on his experience of Bath and its social regulations (Hembry 1990, 185).

reputational difficulties: 'had she not told her NIGHT VISION *in print*' in *The New Bath Guide*, '[s]he might have pass'd here for a virgin and saint' (Mavor 1781, 24). Letter 7 of *The Cheltenham Guide*, written in the form of a hymn from Prue to Eliza, in effect displaces Anstey's problematic letter 14, which had been the main focus for criticism of *The New Bath Guide*'s indelicacy. The competition between the spas is further evoked as Jenny, despite being the 'queen of the walk' at Cheltenham, rejects her former Bath life in favour of an 'artless' existence that partly involves a reaction against the studied formalities of social decorum (Mavor 1781, 25, 59). Ironically, artlessness is employed here as a commercial selling point; the very quality that Cheltenham sought to capitalise on through its cultivation of easy, non-ritualised sociability. Although technically a mock-Guide, then, *The Cheltenham Guide* does in fact seek to endorse the resort that it describes, as a space of purer and more relaxed recreations than Bath. Indeed, both through direct comparisons and in the happier outcomes granted Jenny and Prudence, the *Guide* intimates that Cheltenham represents a place for restoration *from* the seductions of Bath. In full advertorial mode, the work concludes in the hope that 'all who love health, / Without squand'ring their wealth, / Make *Chelt'nham* their summer retreat!' (Mavor 1781, 110).

Even as they followed Anstey in offering satiric exposés of contemporary resort culture, then, verses written in the wake of *The New Bath Guide* often aimed to sponsor particular resorts. In many cases, they also offered guidebook-style information, either in footnotes or within the verses themselves. Arguing that Brighton 'justly claims a superiority over other watering places', Jane West's *The Humours of Brighthelmstone* (1788) indicated precisely which resorts it outperformed in sociability: "Tis said, that in gaiety Brighton excels / The pleasure at Margate and old Tunbridge Wells' (West 1788, [iii], 9). Like other examples of Ansteyana, West's anapaestic verses covered the daily rituals and available amenities of the resort, while footnotes explained the bathing machines and the particular institutions referenced in the poem itself (such as the tavern ballrooms: Shergold's and Hick's). More expansively, in the late 1790s *The Sea-Side, A Poem* offered a rare anapaestic take on Ramsgate through the lens of Simkin Slenderwit, arrived at the coast for his nerves along with his brother Billy, who is suffering from scrofula.[19] The poem's tone—its relationship to Ramsgate—is suggested from the opening words of letter 1: 'WHO would not, dear Mother, to RAMSGATE repair, / To gain health from the ocean and flirt with the fair?' (*Sea-Side* 1798, 1). Simkin's 'hand-gallop lines' convey back home both the rituals of the resort (such as the timings for bathing) and the pleasures of the seaside. To the upbeat Sim, an Assembly Ball is peopled by 'so many mirth-making elegant creatures,' while his description of Ramsgate pier veers into hyperbole: 'That fabric stupendous! that monument dear!' (*Sea-Side* 1798, 14, 56, 77).

Such uncritical enthusiasm and poetical overreaching are undoubtedly ironised—yet in presenting Simkin's preference for Ramsgate the poem appears to be in earnest. Having surveyed its coastal rivals, the poem gives the touristic laurels to Ramsgate: as Sim declares, 'Both the health to restore and the soul to refine, / O! RAMSGATE! the credit, the glory, be thine!' (*Sea-Side* 1798, 76). Sim's effusions here echoed Simkin's 'Panegyric' on Bath in Anstey's original poem: 'the World to refine, / In Manners, in Dress, in Politeness to shine, / O *Bath*! – let the Art, let the Glory be thine' (Anstey 2010, 115). In many respects, indeed, *The Sea-Side* is paradigmatic of post-Ansteyan verse: epistolary in form, primarily anapaestic in measure, written in self-conscious relationship to *The New Bath Guide*, and focused on a contemporary leisure resort. Importantly, as I have been arguing, the poem's anapaestic epistles are also explanatory and promotional, at the same time that they are allusive and satiric.

3 Blundering Northwards: Versifying Harrogate

A more intricate case is presented by two texts about Harrogate that were both published in 1812. Between them, these works further illuminate the relationship of verse guides to prose guides, the promotion of resorts in verse, the tension between advertisement and satire, and the competition that could exist within, as well as between, resorts. The first of the poems, Barbara Hofland's *A Season at Harrogate*, comprises anapaestic epistles written by Benjamin Blunderhead, the nephew of Anstey's Simkin, to his mother in Derbyshire. Through the letters of Benjamin, who like his uncle

[19] ESTC and Worldcat record only the second edition of *The Sea-Side*, dated 1798. The first edition may have been published in either 1797 or 1798: the six letters that comprise the poem are dated over summer 1797 (July to September).

is bilious, the poem presents a versified survey of the resort at Harrogate, taking in its doctors, beauties, bathing, balls, inns, libraries and shops. Like prose guides of the period, the poem also pays expansive attention to the surrounding area: places such as Plumpton, Harewood, Studley, Ripon, Hackfall and Newby. During outings beyond Harrogate itself, the tourists visit such local attractions as Knaresborough castle, Saint Robert's Chapel, and the famous dropping well. Trips to these sites, which reflect the Romantic-period interest in ruins, antiquities and Britain's past, are here cast as both a novelty and a fashionable desideratum. As Benjamin writes in explanation of these countryside excursions: 'You must know all this summer 't has been much the rage, / For High Harrogate parties new scenes to engage' (Hofland 1812, 78). Being a Blunderhead, Benjamin experiences certain social difficulties in the civilized milieu of the watering place and its fashionable company. Yet for all its hits at the resort and at Benjamin himself, the poem portrays both Harrogate and its vicinity in a primarily positive light. Unusually, for an anapaestic satire, even the doctors at Harrogate are commended: for physicians 'more skilful and kind, / Not a Spa on the Island can promise to find' (Hofland 1812, 89).[20] Indicatively, the ending of the *Season* finds Benjamin still in effusive mode, declaring that he will 'renew' these 'pleasures' the following year at his 'dear Harrogate' (Hofland 1812, 90).

To the reviewer in the *British Critic*, *A Season at Harrogate* had 'copied' the 'style of Anstey' with 'more than common success' (An. 1812, 631). With its extensive notes on the various places visited by Benjamin, which incorporate guidebook-like information, Hofland's poem also evinced an educative, as well as a satiric, impulse. A related, if purposely distinct, take on Harrogate is on show in another anapaestic poem published in 1812, titled *A Week at Harrogate*. To read these works in sequence is a peculiar experience. For substantial sections, *A Week at Harrogate* offers variations on the subject-matter of Hofland's *Season at Harrogate*, to the extent that the earlier work becomes a slightly blurred palimpsest of the later one. *A Week at Harrogate* again features Benjamin Blunderhead as its central protagonist, this time writing from Harrogate to his friend, Simon. As in Hofland's poem, Benjamin here surveys the amenities available to visitors at Harrogate, not least its shops. Barring a few deviations, it also retraces Hofland's itinerary of excursions. Over

[20] A note to these lines, p. 103, contrasts the portrayal of the doctors in 'the memoirs' of Benjamin's 'celebrated uncle' – i.e., Anstey's *New Bath Guide*.

the course of the poem, *A Week at Harrogate* is sometimes acerbic, its Benjamin Blunderhead less decorous than the one in Hofland's *Season*. Early on, for instance, Benjamin observes that the tourists 'spend so much time here, in eating and drinking, / That they've seldom an hour, or a moment, for thinking' (*Week at Harrogate* 1812, 19). Later, when offering his 'gig' to the ladies during a trip to Plumpton, he states that it will hold two women so long as they're 'not over big.' Blithely unaware of the personal insult this implies, he commends himself for his 'polite' action (*Week at Harrogate* 1812, 26). More broadly, though, the poem is interspersed with paeans to Harrogate, which has usurped Bath in Ben's affections and which, he tells Simon, 'hath new charms ev'ry day, / To all so enchanting, so charming, and gay' (*Week at Harrogate* 1812, 42, 60). As a member of the Blunderhead clan, Ben is partly foolish in his aspirations and his enthusiasms. Yet, as in other anapaestic verses of the period, his extolling of his resort of choice is not entirely undercut by either his missteps or his ignorance. Rather, the protagonist here is also the guide *to* the spa, conveying information about its facilities and entertainments even as he records a number of comic mishaps. Like his namesake in Hofland's *Season*, Benjamin departs Harrogate reluctantly, and with a promise, in his case, to return not just the following year but 'each year, whilst on earth I remain, / Those scenes, and those fountains, to visit again' (*Week at Harrogate* 1812, 74).

To a significant degree, *A Week at Harrogate* might be said to have combined the content of *A Season at Harrogate* with the format and diurnal structure of John Cam Hobhouse's *The Wonders of a Week at Bath*, another anapaestic work that was published the previous year.[21] For all their similarities of subject matter, though, there are also some key differences of emphasis between the two Harrogate poems. If Hofland had successfully emulated the style of Anstey, then the author of *A Week at Harrogate* is markedly more beholden to previous literary representations. An early 'Consultation of Physicians', for instance, replays Simkin's experience in *The New Bath Guide*; in both works, the doctors discuss politics rather than their patient's condition (*Week at Harrogate* 1812, 16–17). Later, at Hargrove's library, Benjamin purchases a small pamphlet

[21] Like Hobhouse's poem, and unlike Hofland's, *A Week at Harrogate* covers the journey *to* the resort town and features a running header that summarises the contents of each page.

of poems concerning Harrogate, including one in praise of 'Harrogate-Spaw' which begins 'THY waters, old Bladud, let Ainsty [*sic*] proclaim…' (*Week at Harrogate* 1812, 32). While at the library, he encounters in person not just Anstey's Captain Cormorant but also Micklewimmen, the hypocritical Scotsman from the Harrogate scenes in Smollett's *Humphry Clinker*, which are here reprised in verse. Beyond these literary representations, a more material difference between the works lies in their relationship to their publishers and the genre of tourist guidebooks. While Hofland's *Season* mentions both Wilson's and Hargrove's libraries, in her poem Benjamin's library of choice is that of R. Wilson, bookseller brother to her printer-publisher, G. [George] Wilson. As Hofland's protagonist notes, he goes to Wilson's every morning; it is there that he turns 'to get a new book' (Hofland 1812, 45). By contrast, *A Week at Harrogate*, which was published with Hargrove, fails to mention Wilson's library at all, instead showing Benjamin making repeated visits to Hargrove's own library.

This difference bears especially upon the issue of authorship and the texts' agendas. While both poems have been attributed to Hofland, it seems more likely, as Dennis Butts conjectures, that *A Week at Harrogate* was commissioned by Hargrove and Sons following the publication of Hofland's work by Wilson (Butts 1992, 100–101).[22] This sense of two texts in competition, released by rival booksellers, is borne out not just by Benjamin's numerous visits to Hargrove's but by his engagement with other texts published or sold by Hargrove. Among works mentioned in the poem itself, and advertised at the end of the work, are Thomas Garnett's *A Treatise on the Mineral Waters of Harrogate* and *The Trial of Eugene Aram, late of Knaresborough*.[23] Fittingly, the first item in the appended list of Hargrove's publications is '*The Harrogate Guide*', then into its sixth edition. Within the poem, Benjamin purchases a copy of this prose guidebook from the author, Ely Hargrove himself (*Week at*

[22] Both poems are ascribed to Hofland in Behrendt (2013). Butts suggests the Yorkshire poet, David Lewis, as the possible author of *A Week at Harrogate* (Butts 1992, 101).

[23] The appended list of books printed and sold by Hargrove and Sons, Knaresborough and Harrogate, includes the fifth edition of Garnett's *Treatise*, with an appendix by local physician John Jacques (1810), and the tenth edition of the *Trial* (also 1810).

Harrogate 1812, 20).[24] To Benjamin, the '*Harrogate Guide*' is a thing of wonder. As he describes in a notably bathetic stanza:

> In it, the most ample descriptions abound
> Of the inns, of the waters, and country, around—
> Of the mould'ring remains of those structures, sublime,
> Which are half wash'd away by the current of time:
> Of the past and the present the author relates,
> And has added a map, and a number of plates. (*Week at Harrogate* 1812, 20)

Beyond simply advertising Hargrove's prose guidebook, in this poem published with Hargrove, Benjamin's versified guidebook intermittently refers to its prose model. Rather than including his own notes, as had Hofland, for instance, Benjamin directs his reader to information contained in Hargrove's *Guide*. For his descriptions of the surrounding countryside, moreover, Benjamin not only refers but on occasion defers to the *Guide*. Plumpton, he informs Simon, is 'best describ'd in the *Harrogate Guide*'; Fountains Abbey (a ruin) and Studley are 'Both amply describ'd in the *Harrogate Guide!*'; while 'To have seen the inside' of Ripley castle 'would have been a great treat, / As I learnt, by the Guide, 'tis the *Ingilby*'s seat' (*Week at Harrogate* 1812, 27, 43, 46). A guidebook so authoritative as Hargrove's, it would seem, cannot be rivalled in mere (Blunderheaded) verse. In these promotional anapaests on Harrogate, likely commissioned by Hargrove himself, Benjamin in effect offers a guide to the *Harrogate Guide*, as well as to the place itself.[25]

A Season at Harrogate and *A Week at Harrogate*, then, advertised their publishers while effacing the reading establishments of their main competitor. In their promotional partiality, the poems can easily appear to support critical complaints about the toothless nature of Anstey-style

[24] The work was actually titled *The History of the Castle, Town, and Forest, of Knaresbrough [sic], with Harrogate, and it's [sic] Medicinal Springs*, 6th ed. (Knaresb[o]rough: Hargrove and Sons, 1809). The first edition, not covering Harrogate, had been published in 1769.

[25] Intriguingly, one of the deviations from Hofland's itinerary of outings in *A Week at Harrogate* sees Benjamin failing to reach Bolton. This might possibly be connected to Hofland's plug, in *A Season at Harrogate*, for six prints of views of Bolton by 'T.C. Hofland' (i.e. Thomas Hofland), Barbara's husband since 1810 (Hofland 1812, 103).

satire.[26] Nonetheless, like most anapaestic verses on resorts, the two works also display at least a residual impulse towards satiric critique. Strikingly and perhaps surprisingly, in poems that tend to promote Harrogate, some of their most pointed lines are reserved for the wells themselves, especially the sulphuric well in Low Harrogate. Hofland's poem, for instance, registers the stench and 'nasty' taste of the sulphuric waters and compares taking a bath there—what she terms 'a Harrogate boiling'—to being inside a coffin (Hofland 1812, 14, 23). Describing the 'Manner of Bathing' at the spa, the Benjamin of *A Week at Harrogate* likewise finds the water warm but stinky. Despite his promise to return to Harrogate every year, he thus resolves never to take a bath there again (*Week at Harrogate* 1812, 52–53). Given that the text's frontispiece comprised an illustration of the sulphur well, Benjamin's aversion renders *A Week at Harrogate* somewhat conflicted as a printed, promotional, product.

This uncertainty of design can also be discerned at points in *A Season at Harrogate*. An indicative moment sees Hofland's Benjamin pledging to leave aside his 'moral excursions / And return we again to the list of diversions' (Hofland 1812, 71). As well as anything, this textual segue captures the mixed motivations of many of the anapaestic poems concerning resorts, which to various degrees combined satiric ridicule with representations of sociability, didactic moralising with informational puffery.

4 Conclusion: The Anstey Effect

By no means all anapaestic verses on watering places during this period, certainly, were straightforwardly promotional or *amiably* satiric. The Prince Regent and his entourage were a particular bugbear of Anthony Pasquin (the pseudonymous John Williams [1754–1818]), in works such as *The New Brighton Guide* (1796).[27] The destabilising social effect of inter-status mixing also remained a focus, not least in works about Bath. Gradually, though, this was presented less as *the* central concern, or else began to register in different ways: as in *Eight Letters from Bath* (1830), in which already successful social climbers, here designated the '*Exclusives*,'

[26] See for instance Marshall (2013, 242–243).

[27] Under the same sobriquet, Williams also published *A Postscript to the New Bath Guide* (London: J. Strahan, 1790), an inconsistent anapaestic hodge-podge.

now seek to avoid the '*low mixture*' at the Rooms (*Eight Letters* 1830, 13–14). More broadly during this period, the adoption of 'Ansteyan' measure, continuation of the Blunderheads' tale, and direct allusions to *The New Bath Guide* facilitated promotion of particular leisure resorts—not least Bath's inland rivals and emerging coastal competitors. Above all, perhaps, what Anstey's keywork provided was a pretext, in the full sense of the word: both a model and an impetus, or creative rationale. As later writers asked: why should not Brighton, Margate or Harrogate have a satiric verse Guide, as well as Bath? More specifically, as Richard Scrafton Sharpe noted in his anapaestic *Margate New Guide* (1799), resort culture had not stood still: if Anstey might have viewed Margate as 'unworthy his pen' in the 1760s, 'He cannot, he dare not sure think it so now' (Sharpe 1799, 20).[28]

Increasingly in these verse-guidebooks, satiric critique was tempered with explanation and advertisement. Disputing criticisms of Margate that had been made in George Saville Carey's *Balnea* (1799), along with Anstey's neglect of the resort, Sharpe himself declared 'Shall Margate be slighted? fie! bridle thy tongue' (Sharpe 1799, 21).[29] In a passage which adapts the 'Epilogue' from *The New Bath Guide*, moreover, the author of *The Sea-Side* queried whether satire was even appropriate to coastal pleasures. As the work has Mrs Fussock ask: 'What has SATIRE to do on the shores of the sea? / Where all should be levity, frolic and glee' (*Sea-Side* 1798, 70). The incompatibility between resort leisure and satire that was argued here had clear implications for writers of Ansteyan verse. Thomas Haynes Bayly, the author of a number of imitations of *The New Bath Guide*, wondered whether it was appropriate or even possible to emulate Anstey's anapaestic satire. As an imagined reader asks, iambically and somewhat ironically, in Bayly's *Rough Sketches of Bath* (1817): 'Shall any dare to tread in Anstey's path, / And write satiric verses upon Bath?' (Bayly 1819, 27).[30] Perhaps wishing to bring the *Bath Guide*'s afterlife to a close, even as she added to the progeny, Barbara Hofland cast her

[28] Sharpe's mainly anapaestic poem is structured into ten letters by members of the Bombazeen family and their servant, Fred.

[29] In this defence of Margate, Sharpe's poem differs markedly from contemporaneous works which registered alarm at the heterogenous mixture of classes, both at the resort itself and on the hoy from London. On these more anxious representations see Guest (2017).

[30] I quote from the fourth edition of Bayly's *Rough Sketches of Bath*.

own Benjamin Blunderhead as the 'last of the Blunderhead race' (Hofland 1812, 10). Yet anapaestic satires on resorts would continue to appear, in works such as Bayly's (partly anapaestic) *Epistles from Bath* (1817) and in the form of fictional private letters popularised by Thomas Moore, as in Edward Mangin's *Intercepted Epistle from a Person in Bath, to his Friend in London* (1815) and W.H. Halpin's *The Cheltenham Mail Bag* (1820). Like *The Cheltenham Mail Bag*, some works were now modelled on Moore as much as on Anstey, and tied more specifically to Moore's own characters, as with *Eight Letters from Bath, by the Fidget Family* (1830).[31] Yet Anstey's influence would persist. 1826, for instance, saw the publication of David Huston's *The New Clifton and Bristol Guide. Being a Series of Poetical Epistles written by Simkin B..N..R…D … Now a Visiter at the Hotwells, to his Distant Friends*. Even into the 1840s, in fact, Anstey was still a notable model and touchstone for resort-based verse: the iambic *New Bristol Guide, A Comic Poem* (1847) cited Anstey in its Preface, while the decade would also spawn *The New Torquay Guide* (1843), a verse-guidebook to a coastal resort previously untouched by anapaests.[32]

In a startling comparison, the reviewer of *The Cheltenham Mail Bag* for the *Monthly* averred that 'Anstey, among comic rhymers, is what Homer is among epic bards'. Qualifying this admittedly 'strange' parallel, the reviewer went on to observe that, with the exception of Moore, Anstey's imitators had 'always split on the rock of *individuality*', having little original genius of their own (An. 1821, 216). While they were rarely the finest or most original examples of versification, though, poems modelled on *The New Bath Guide* were prominent among works which imagined the culture and development of contemporary resorts and gave them literary expression. In many cases, I have argued, they adopted from Anstey not just a verse form and family of characters but an involved, not wholly antagonistic satiric viewpoint, which generated opportunities to admire and recommend particular features of a resort even while ridiculing its excesses. As Gary Dyer notes, during this period *The New Bath Guide* and its imitators constituted 'the preeminent example of a non-Juvenalian

[31] By invoking Moore's characters in verses set in Bath, this text (and, to a lesser extent, *The Cheltenham Mail Bag*) returned Ansteyan measure, which Moore had adopted, to the locus of the spa.

[32] *The New Torquay Guide* was reviewed—favourably, and with reference to Anstey—in *The Athenaeum*, no. 827 (2 September 1843), p. 793.

countertradition in verse' (Dyer 1997, 179). Whereas Dyer tends to view such 'neo-Horatian' works as politically (and thus satirically) weak, their comparative lightness, or satiric leniency, can itself be said to have had particular—promotional—purposes, separately from the large-scale political divisions of the day. Importantly, with the upsurge of anapaestic verse came a new attitude to resort tourism—an ameliorative disposition that was more attuned to the 'age of Watering-Places' (An. 1840, 773). The legacy of Anstey's poem lay as much in this accommodating perspective as in the outpouring of anapaests per se. In the terms of the poem's own opening lines, *The New Bath Guide* was itself the 'genial' spring from which flowed this amiable current of versified resort satire.

Works Cited

Primary Sources

An. 1807. *The New Scarboro' Guide; or, Memoirs of the Sawney Family, in a Series of Poetical Epistles.* Scarborough: Hayes and Lacup.

An. 1840. The Monarch of Bath. *Blackwood's Magazine* 48, No. 302 (December): 773–792.

Anstey, Christopher. 1830. *The New Bath Guide; or, Memoirs of the B-n-r-d Family, in a Series of Poetical Epistles*, ed. John Britton. London: Hurst, Chance, & Co.

Anstey, Christopher. 1994. *The New Bath Guide* (1766), ed. Gavin Turner. Bristol: Broadcast Books.

Anstey, Christopher. 2010. *The New Bath Guide* (1766), ed. Annick Cossic. Bern: Peter Lang.

Bayly, Thomas Haynes. 1819. *Rough Sketches of Bath, Epistles, and Other Poems*, 4th ed. London: Baldwin, Cradock & Joy.

Burney, Frances. 1994. *Evelina; or, The History of a Young Lady's Entrance into the World* (1778), ed. Margaret Anne Doody. Harmondsworth: Penguin.

The Diseases of Bath. 1737. London: J. Roberts.

Eight Letters from Bath, by the Fidget Family. 1830. Bath: M. Meyler.

Granville, A.B. 1841. *The Spas of England, and Principal Sea-Bathing Places*, 3 vols. London: Henry Colburn.

Gray, Thomas. 1935. *Correspondence of Thomas Gray*, ed. Paget Toynbee and Leonard Whibley, 3 vols. Oxford: Clarendon Press.

Hofland, Barbara. 1812. *A Season at Harrogate; in a Series of Poetical Epistles, from Benjamin Blunderhead, Esquire, to His Mother, in Derbyshire.* Knaresb[o]rough: G. Wilson.

M.M. 1827. The Hydromania. *Literary Magnet* 4 (July): 297–300.

Mavor, William Fordyce (attrib.). 1781. *The Cheltenham Guide; or, Memoirs of the B-n-r-d Family Continued*. London: Harrison & Co.

The New Brighthelmstone Directory; or, Sketches in Miniature of the British Shore. 1770. London: T. Durham.

Penrose, John. 1983. *Letters from Bath, 1766–1767*, eds. Brigitte Mitchell and Hubert Penrose. Gloucester: Alan Sutton.

The Sea-Side, a Poem, in Familiar Epistles from Mr. Simkin Slenderwit, Summerising at Ramsgate, to his Dear Mother in Town. 1798, 2nd ed. London: T.N. Longman and J. Bell.

Sharpe, Richard Scrafton. 1799. *The Margate New Guide; or, Memoirs of Five Families out of Six; Who in Town Discontent with a Good Situation, Make Margate the Place of Their Summer Migration*. London: R. Dutton.

Ward, Edward. 1700. *A Step to the Bath: With a Character of the Place*. London: J. How.

A Week at Harrogate. 1812. Knaresb[o]rough: Printed for the Author/Hargrove and Sons.

West, Jane. 1788. *The Humours of Brighthelmstone*. London: Printed for the Author.

Secondary Sources

An. 1770a. Review of *Margate in Miniature; or, The New Margate Guide*. *Critical Review* 30, September 1770.

An. 1770b. Review of *Margate in Miniature; or, The New Margate Guide*. *Monthly Review* 43, October 1770.

An. 1781. Review of *The Cheltenham Guide; or, Memoirs of the B-n-r-d Family Continued*, by William Fordyce Mavor (attrib.). *Critical Review* 52, November 1781.

An. 1809. Review of *The Poetical Works of the Late Christopher Anstey, Esq*. *Critical Review* 3rd series, 18, November 1809.

An. 1812. Review of *A Season at Harrogate; in a Series of Poetical Epistles, from Benjamin Blunderhead, Esquire, to His Mother, in Derbyshire*, by Barbara Hofland. *British Critic* 39, June 1812.

An. 1821. Review of *The Cheltenham Mail Bag; or, Letters from Gloucestershire*, by Peter Quince, the Younger [i.e., W.H. Halpin]. *Monthly Review* 2nd series, 94, February 1821.

Behrendt, Stephen C. 2013. Barbara Hofland and Romantic-Era Provincial Poetry by Women. *Women's Writing* 20 (4): 421–440.

Borsay, Peter. 1989. *The English Urban Renaissance: Culture and Society in the Provincial Town, 1660–1770*. Oxford: Clarendon Press.

Borsay, Peter. 2000. Health and Leisure Resorts 1700–1840. In *The Cambridge Urban History of Britain, Volume II: 1540–1840*, ed. Peter Clark, 775–803. Cambridge: Cambridge University Press.

Butts, Dennis. 1992. *Mistress of Our Tears: A Literary and Bibliographical Study of Barbara Hofland*. Aldershot: Scolar Press.

Cossic-Pericarpin, Annick. 2017. Fashionable Diseases in Georgian Bath: Fiction and the Emergence of a British Model of Spa Sociability. *Journal for Eighteenth-Century Studies* 40 (4): 537–553.

Day, Martin S. 1948. Anstey and Anapestic Satire in the Late Eighteenth Century. *ELH* 15 (2): 122–146.

Dyer, Gary. 1997. *British Satire and the Politics of Style, 1789–1832*. Cambridge: Cambridge University Press.

Gilmartin, Kevin, ed. 2017. *Sociable Places: Locating Culture in Romantic-Period Britain*. Cambridge: Cambridge University Press.

Guest, Harriet. 2017. Sociability by the Sea Side: Margate Before 1815. In *Sociable Places: Locating Culture in Romantic-Period Britain*, ed. Kevin Gilmartin, 205–223. Cambridge: Cambridge University Press.

Hembry, Phyllis. 1990. *The English Spa, 1560–1815: A Social History*. London: Athlone Press.

Jarvis, Robin. 2015. Hydromania: Perspectives on Romantic Swimming. *Romanticism* 21 (3): 250–264.

Love, Harold. 2008. Satirical Wells from Bath to Ballyspellan. In *Swift's Travels: Eighteenth-Century British Satire and its Legacy*, eds. Nicholas Hudson and Aaron Santesso, 55–73. Cambridge: Cambridge University Press.

Marshall, Ashley. 2013. *The Practice of Satire in England, 1658–1770*. Baltimore: Johns Hopkins University Press.

Russell, Gillian, and Clara Tuite, eds. 2002. *Romantic Sociability: Social Networks and Literary Culture in Britain, 1770–1840*. Cambridge: Cambridge University Press.

Seaton, A.V. 2016. Getting Socially on the Road: The Short, Happy Life of the Anapaestic Tourism Narrative, 1766–1830. In *Travel Writing, Visual Culture, and Form, 1760–1900*, eds. Mary Henes and Brian H. Murray, 115–138. Basingstoke: Palgrave Macmillan.

Turner, Gavin. 2005. *Christopher Anstey: A Life in Eighteenth-Century Bath*. Bristol: Broadcast Books.

Veblen, Thorstein. 2007. *The Theory of the Leisure Class* (1899), ed. Martha Banta. Oxford: Oxford University Press.

Walton, John K. 1983. *The English Seaside Resort: A Social History, 1750–1914*. Leicester: Leicester University Press.

Walvin, James. 1978. *Beside the Seaside: A Social History of the Popular Seaside Holiday*. London: Allen Lane.

CHAPTER 9

'For Music Is Wholesome the Doctors All Think': The Curative and Restorative Function of Music in Eighteenth-Century English Spas

Pierre Degott

It is probably a truism to say that music, along with other kinds of entertainment, goes together with the universe of spas and bathing. From the very origins of water cures, lack of occupation had to be made up by some kind of entertainment, and we have records, dating back to the early 1640s, of bathers complaining of idleness in Bath (Hembry 1990, 61). It is a well-known fact that English spas, contrary to other resorts in France (Barbeau 2009, 84), were centres of attraction for both the curative function of their waters and the wealth and variety of their social and artistic lives. Alfred Barbeau thus reminds us that as soon as the 1660s Bath began to be 'a centre of pleasure as well as a place of healing' (Barbeau 2009, 19) attended by people who frequented the famous spa not only from necessity but also for amusement: 'Men and women flock hither from all Great Britain, in quest of health but also of pleasure' (quoted

P. Degott (✉)
Département d'anglais, Université de Lorraine, Metz, France
e-mail: pierre.degott@univ-lorraine.fr

S. Chiari and S. Cuisinier-Delorme (eds.), *Spa Culture and Literature in England, 1500–1800*, Early Modern Literature in History,
https://doi.org/10.1007/978-3-030-66568-5_9

in Barbeau 2009, 19), according to Carolus Claromontius [Charles Clermont], the author the *De Aere, Locis et Aquis terrae Angliae*. Some voices even contended that pleasure and leisure-seeking at certain spas ranked far above the mere benefits of the health giving waters, as is the case of the French traveller Henry Misson de Valbourg in his *Mémoires et observations faites par un Voyageur en Angleterre*: 'Mille gens vont passer là quelques semaines, sans se soucier ni des Bains, ni des eaux à boire, mais seulement pour se divertir avec la bonne compagnie. On a Musique, Jeu, Promenade, Bals, & petite Foire perpétuelle' (Misson de Valbourg 1698, 25).

In her analysis of the development of the leisure-industry that took place in early eighteenth-century English spas, Phyllis Hembry also noted that '[…] the emphasis of spa life became more a search for pleasure and entertainment, although still under pretence of taking the waters' (Hembry 1990, 68), acknowledging the fact that by the late century some bathing centres like Scarborough 'had become a pleasure resort rather than a health centre' (Hembry 1990, 214), a statement also confirmed by letter-writers of the period: 'These amusements and the pleasure of seeing company induces many to come who are not really in want of the water' (Drayton Greenwood 1913, 83).

Among notable amusements like shopping, reading, dancing, theatre-going, eating, drinking, flirting, gambling or less innocuous forms of occupation, music would thus rank as one of the many attractions provided by notable English spas. The various aspects of music-making in the early modern period have duly been analysed, and recent scholarship has largely contributed to researching into such areas as repertoire, the choice of ancient or modern compositions, cultural policies, venues, finances, programmes, ticket pricing, rivalries between musicians and performers, rivalries between English and foreign factions, etc. (Rice 2015, 80–82). Studies have been devoted to the musical figures particularly associated to the city of Bath, like the organist Thomas Chilcot (Rishton 1991), the famous Linleys of Bath (Green 1903; Black 1911), the astronomer William Herschel (Brown 1990) or the Italian castrato Venanzio Rauzzini, (Sands 1953) who ran the musical life of the city for several decades (Rice 2015, 173–278). Research has also been done on the Bath careers of such performers as the violinist Franz Lamotte, the flautist Andrew Ashe or the singers John Braham, Gertrud Mara or Elizabeth Billington, who have all left their marks in the history of English music. Recording companies have recently given today's listeners the opportunity of hearing the type of music that would have been played in notable English spas for the sake of entertaining and diverting the public. What needs now to be emphasized is not the dichotomy between the two separate lives offered by the main spas, health-seeking activities on the one hand and the leisure-providing industry on the other, but the interplay and interaction between the two lives, the way both were intimately interconnected in their provision of well-being, medical or otherwise. The purpose of this chapter is thus to show how intimately and intricately music and health-seeking activities were related, the ambivalence with which spas could occasionally be seen having been apparently transferred to the world of music. It is the contention of this essay that music was also used, adroitly and deliberately, for its curative and restorative functions.

1 The Omnipresence of Music

All the various testimonies that have remained to us insist on the part played by music in major English spas, not only in the recreational areas not directly linked to bathing or drinking (play-houses, assembly halls or churches) but also in the places where water-cures, whether the form of drinking or bathing, were actually provided. Samuel Pepys, who spent some time in Bath in 1668, thus wrote in his diaries how the hearing of music would intervene in the course of his cure:

> Carried back, wrapped in a sheet, and in a chair, home; and there one after another thus carried, I staying above two hours in the water, home to bed, sweating for an hour; and by and by comes music to play to me, extraordinary good as ever I heard at London almost, or anywhere. (Pepys 1953, 3: 245 [13 June 1668])

Writing in the mid-eighteenth century, John Wood also reminded his readers of the former habit of serenading ladies of distinction who would go and bathe at the Cross Bath, insisting on the simultaneousness of music-making and taking the waters:

> In the morning [...] the young Lady is brought in a close Chair, dressed in her Bathing Cloaths, to the Cross Bath. There the Musick Plays her into the Water, and the women who tend her present her with a little floating Dish, like a Bason; into which the Lady puts an Handkerchief, and a Nosegay, and of late a Snuff Box is added. She traverses the Bath, if a Novice, with a Guide. (Wood 1749, 2: 437)

In their study of the Pump Room Orchestra at Bath, Robert and Nicola Hyman have also reminded their readers of how music played by such professionals as the City Waits could occasionally be 'amplified by enthusiastic gentlemen bathers joining in song, and thus eventually discouraged' (Hyman 2011, 2). In some extreme cases, singing undertaken by over-enthusiastic patients could be seen as disturbance of the peace and lead to police intervention. John Wood has related occasions when the tumult made by the bathers accompanying the instruments was such that the municipality had to step in and forbid all music thenceforth:

> [...] a Custom that was soon followed with such a Chorus from the Bathers as obliged the Corporation to Meet on the 28th of March 1676 and frame a By-Law to stop the Progress of the Vocal Musick, and put an End to the Gallantries that any ways tended to the Disturbance of the Baths. (Wood 1749, 2:437)
>
> [...]
>
> They assembled together to put an end to a custom which then prevailed of smoaking Tobacco in the bathing Cisterns, singing Songs and making such Disturbances in them as rendering the Baths like so many Bear-Gardens. (Wood 1749, 1: 219–220)

Other commentators like Oliver Goldsmith in his *Life of Richard Nash* have reminded their readers of the habit of greeting visitors not only by the chiming of the city bells, but also by notes of welcome performed by serenading musicians: 'Upon a Stranger's arrival at *Bath*, he is welcome by a peal of the Abbey bells, and in the next place, by the voice and music of the city waits' (Goldsmith 1762, 41). The Bath welcome song seems to have been a local speciality, as can be seen by the following composition by Henry Harington, 'one of the foremost physicians in the city' (James 1987, 659) who also enjoyed a reputation as a glee composer, and who remains as one of those many musicians very much associated today to the musical life of the city of Bath (Fig. 1).

One also knows for sure, as the following quotation by Goldsmith clearly shows, how the life of people taking the waters was punctuated by occasions in which music was ritually attached to the curative process:

> The amusement of bathing is immediately succeeded by a general assembly of people at the pump-house, some for pleasure, and some to drink the hot waters. Three glasses, at three different times, is the usual portion for every drinker; and the intervals between every glass are enlivened by the

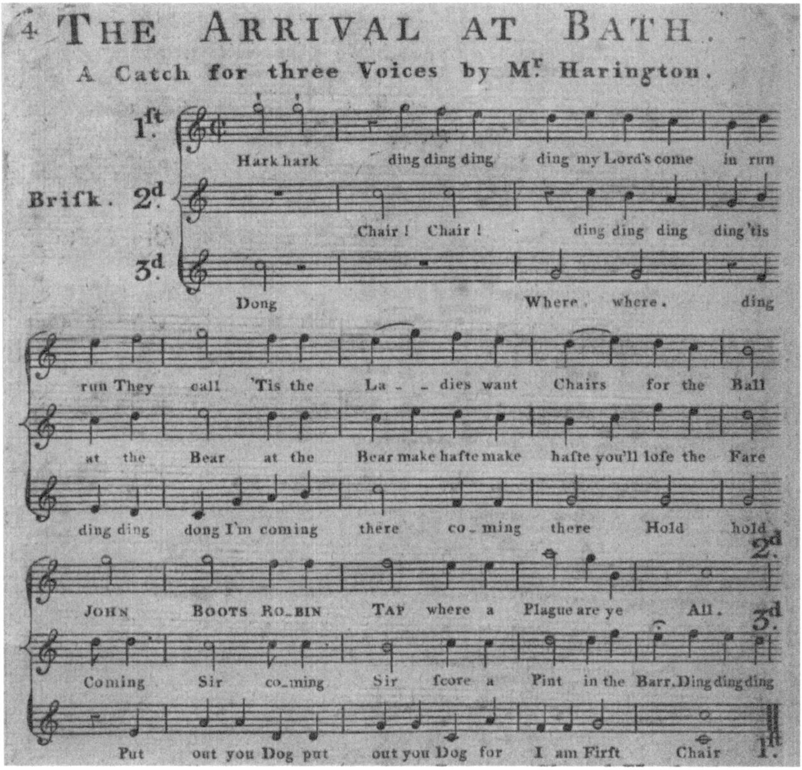

Fig. 1 *Henry Harington, 'The Arrival at Bath',* A Favourite Collection of Songs, Glees, Elegies and Canons, for one, two, three, four and five Voices, as Composed by Mr. Harington of Bath. *London: Longman and Broderip, [c.1780], p. 4. Courtesy of the British Library*

> harmony of a small band of music, as well as by the conversation of the gay, the witty, or the forward. (Goldsmith 1762, 45)

It has also been established, by Wood among others, that many people taking the waters would occasionally perform music *publicly*, as amateurs, in the frame of the entertainment programme offered by the city:

> Concert Breakfasts at the Assembly Houses for some time made another Part of the Morning's Amusement at *Bath*; and the Expenses of these

> were defrayed by a Subscription among Gentlemen; every Subscriber contributing a certain Sum; and for this He had a certain Number of Tickets to present the Ladies with. These Entertainments were esteemed as some of the Politest of the Place; they came to meer Trifles to Individuals; and such People of Rank and Fortune as were well skilled in Musick, took a Pleasure in joining, on these Occasions, with the common Band of Performers. (Wood 1749, 2: 439)

Interference between the valetudinarian and the performing lives of English spas could also come from professional musicians. In that respect, Paul Rice mentions the controversy raised by the interference between the musical and medical activities of the famous singer Sophia Baccheli, known in Britain as Mrs Corri, who had been engaged by Rauzzini on the promise of being given a benefit evening. Some people in the community complained that Mrs Corri, who had actually come to Bath to take the waters for health purposes, had actually intruded herself on the managers of the concerts with the sole purpose of defraying her expenses (Rice 2015, 211). As can be seen, musical life was inextricably enmeshed with circumstances surrounding medical activities.

2 Mixed Attitudes

Another link between music and the waters is the mixed attitude that the two objects generated. It is a well-known fact that hot springs and spa waters, far from being unanimously praised for their beneficial effects on the body and the mind, could also be discarded for their supposedly harmful effects on people's health, but also, and perhaps more importantly, on their morals. Just as the quality of the waters could be questioned, so could the life of dissipation associated to fashionable resorts be called into question. John Wesley's criticism of Bath and the morals of its inhabitants, for instance, has often been mentioned (Hembry 1990, 271), just as one bears in mind what Smollett had to write about the city waters (Smollett 1752). Similarly, music in famous spas could be regarded less as an asset than as a noisy and omnipresent nuisance, criticized for the disruptive tumult it brought about in places where peace and silence would have been expected. Such an attitude is summarized in the following lines from Christopher Anstey's *New Bath Guide*: 'Some think it strange they should make such a riot / In a place where sick folk would be glad to be quiet' (Anstey 1766, 30; see also 31–33, with the story of the gouty Lord Ringbone). The association of music and noise is a constant occurrence in writings devoted to life in spas, as evidenced once again by a certain Mrs. Bradshaw who wrote in 1721 that Bath was 'nothing but noise and nonsense' (Hobart 1824, 76), a point of view that would not have been rejected by the figure of Lady Luxborough (Williams 1945), nor by the fictional Matthew Bramble in *Humphry Clinker*, a character whose frequent headaches are apparently caused by 'the *noise* of the *music* playing in the gallery' (Smollett 1984, 39; emphasis mine). Here, the oxymoronic association of noise and music seems to epitomize the mixed attitude displayed by various people. Smollett's brilliant use of contrasted perspectives in his novel gives an illustrative insight into the way the response to a given object could be at variance (Smollett 1984), just as conflicting points of view can be found in Anstey, where the general attitude towards music is far from being entirely negative:

> Music calls me to the Spring
> That can Health and Spirits bring. (Anstey 1766, 58)

> For Music is wholesome the Doctors all think
> For Ladies that bathe, and ladies that drink. (Anstey 1766, 42)

Here, it is clearly the association between health and music that is brought to the fore.

3 The Healing Power of Music

Whether or not we can take for granted the fact that doctors really thought that music was wholesome is now going to be our final investigation. As a matter of fact, few people would have denied that music could be a comfort for those who sought it. Thomas Rowlandson's famous series of plates *The Comforts of Bath* gives pride of place to music-making, an activity that is apparently which put on a par with drinking, bathing and other restorative activities. But who would have believed that music was actually wholesome, in the sense of health-giving?

Perhaps it is worth reminding at this stage that the often mentioned decision by Richard Nash to introduce music in the Pump Room at Bath early in the eighteenth century, i.e. in the very place where cures were given, had been made in order to counteract the eminent physician John Radcliffe, who had not only questioned in some of his works the beneficial effect of excessive bathing (Radcliffe 1721, 451–452), but had also written a pamphlet specifically intended against the efficacy of the Bath waters, going so far as to threaten to put a toad in the Bath spring so as to poison its waters. As Goldsmith reminds us, Nash's decision, which had actually been taken on the advice of the city physicians (Shaw and Goodwin 2001), was based on the perhaps naïve belief that music could actually 'charm away' poison and therefore be used as a form of cure or remedy:

> In this situation of things it was, that Mr. *Nash* first came into that city, and hearing the threat of this Physician, he humorously assured the people that if they would give him leave, he would charm away the poison of the Doctor's toad, as they usually charmed the venom of the Tarantula, by music. He therefore was immediately empowered to set up the force of a band of music, against the poison of the Doctor's reptile; the company very sensibly increased, *Nash* triumphed, and the sovereignty of the city was decreed to him by every rank of people. (Goldsmith 1762, 25–26)

The case of the tarantula, the spider whose poisonous bite had long believed to be cured by the hearing of music—hence the name of the dance 'tarantella'—is actually mentioned in the scientific works of the time interested in the use of music as a curative agent. Such was the case of the celebrated work by Richard Mead devoted to the treatment of various poisons (Mead 1702) but also, more importantly, of Richard Brocklesby's *Reflections on Antient and Modern Musick, with the Application to the Cure of Diseases* (1749). Some of the ideas expressed in this ground-breaking work, based on solid biblical and classical material but also on the theory of the fluids and how the latter could be affected by sound, were more or less put in application by some of the famous musicians active in Bath in the second half of the eighteenth century. The work by Richard Mead, which also acknowledges the power of music in the cure of the tarantula bite, is thus duly mentioned by the Bath musician Francis Fleming in the third volume of his fictional autobiography (Fleming 1771, 3: 25). Fleming is now mainly remembered for having been the leader of the Pump Orchestra for a few decades, from the 1730s to the 1770s (James 1987, 605–610). The fact that he had read Brocklesby seems to be attested by the fact that he resumes his predecessor's main argumentation:

> The physicians of Bath solicited Mr. Nash to let the Band perform in the Pump-Room, (to which he acquiesced) for the following, among other reasons: 'That the least stroke imaginable upon any musical instrument has such an effect on the human body as to move its component manichulae in all their parts, giving the fibres of the whole body, more or less, according to their degree of tension, corresponding concussions; and consequently the spirits are not only rais'd, or made finer, but the other animal fluids are also briskly agitated, and their preternatural cohesions and viscidities destroyed'.
>
> Music has this advantage above all exercises, that the concussions made upon the fibres by any instrument are short, quick, and easy, whereby the nervous fluid is not only smoothly pushed on in its circulation, but also the natural contextures of all the animal threads are better preserved by their never being overstrained; so that the extraordinary effects of music in many distempers ceases [sic] to be a wonder; and we cannot help expressing our regret that it is not universally practiced, as well for the amusement as benefit of the company where all other medicinal waters are frequented. *Vid^e^ Dr. Mead on the power of music in the poison of the Tarantula*. (Fleming 1771, 3: 23–25)

One can first note that Fleming confirms that it was the physicians who advised Nash to have musicians in the Pump Room. More importantly, he also mentions his regret that music was not *universally* practiced in other spas, a statement that implies not only that there was a genuine medical intent in the use of music, but also that it was a local specificity at Bath. This, again, seems to be confirmed by the book by Philip Thicknesse *The Valetudinarians Bath Guide*, in which music is explicitly mentioned, in the final chapter of the books, as one of 'the Means of Obtaining Long Life and Health' if one is to quote from the book's subtitle:

> [...] there is not a doubt but [music] has a wonderful influence upon the frame of man, and that if it will not cure the bite of the *Tarantula*, yet a fiddle, is nevertheless a good doctor, and it is worth observing, that Music is always encouraged, at places, where company assemble for their health, those who best understand the human body, and the structure of the animal fibre, will most readily allow, that it must operate very powerfully, and that the spirits are not only raised by melody, but that the animal

> fluids are put into brisker motion, and the delicate concussions made upon the fibres by Music being short, quick, and easy, must effect [sic] the whole frame, therefore there is nothing absurd, in attributing extraordinary effects, to the power of Music, and it is rather to be wondered at, why it is not more generally considered in this light. (Thicknesse 1780, 57)

One will note that Thicknesse offers an almost word-for-word paraphrase of Fleming's argument, in a passage that might almost remind us of the genuinely English tradition of debate on music that had been going on since the end of the seventeenth century. It is also to be noted that, later in his developments, Thicknesse suggests an explicit comparison between music and other remedies like those provided by the famous Scottish proponent of electrical cures James Graham, whose works on 'magnetic influences' or what was then called 'electrical aether' are duly mentioned (Thicknesse 1780, 58). Music, like electricity, was thus genuinely and scientifically believed to soothe and heal the 'injured fibers and nerves of the Valetudinarian' (Thicknesse 1780, 58), a fact that reminds us of the scientific approach privileged in Bath by some of the people concerned with the health of their visitors (Turner 1977). Obviously, music was seen as a scientific tool regarded on a par with other forms of therapeutic treatments.

4 Conclusion: Further Investigations

What this examination has shown, so far, is that there was at Bath a deliberate intent to use music with therapeutic purposes in mind. One would of course dream of finding things like traces of medical posology or prescriptions advising on a diet of Purcell or Handel. Until now, no connections between types of pathologies or forms of repertoire have been unearthed, and it is doubtful that such a discovery will ever be made. One does not even know if there were differences, in terms of music programming, between the type of music to be played in the morning, in the course of the cure, or later in the day during the more socially important event of the evening concert. What comes out of the present research is merely the fact that there was in Bath an awareness of the beneficial effect of music and a willingness to put it into practice. Why such experiments were not carried out in other healing-places, or at least in a far less conspicuous way, is another possible subject of investigation. What the present study has mainly brought to the fore is the tendency to treat music as a science, more than as an art form meant to provide emotion, something that seems to be confirmed by the existence in Bath of so many musicians (William Herschel, Henry Harington, Philip Thicknesse...), who also made a name for themselves as scientists. Harington is now remembered for his theories on intervals, as derived from Pythagoras (Harington 1780: 2), and Thicknesse for having devised a kind of harmonic alphabet allowing people to communicate in music (Thicknesse 1772). For many Bath musicians, music was not used emotionally but scientifically, a clue that would incite us to research further in that most intriguing and promising area.

Works Cited

Primary Sources

Anstey, Christopher. 1766. *The New Bath Guide: Memoirs of the B-r-n-s Family. In a Series of Poetical Epistles*. London: Dodsley.

Black, Clementina. 1911. *The Linleys of Bath*. London: Secker.

Brocklesby, Richard. 1749. *Reflections on Antient and Modern Musick, with the Application to the Cure of Diseases. To which is Subjoined, an Essay to Solve the Question*. London: Cooper.

Claromontius, Carolus [Clermont, Charles]. 1672. *De Aere, Locis et Aquis terrae Angliae*. London: Roycroft.

Fleming, Francis. 1771. *The Life and Extraordinary Adventures, the Perils and Critical Escapes, of Timothy Ginnadrake, that Child of Chequer'd Fortune*. 3 vols. Bath: Cruttwell.

Goldsmith, Oliver. 1762. *The Life of Richard Nash of Bath, Esquire. Extracted Principally from His Original Papers*. London: Newbery.

Harington, Henry. [c.1780]. *A Favourite Collection of Songs, Glees, Elegies and Canons, for One, Two, Three, Four and Five Voices, as Composed by Mr. Harington of Bath*. London: Longman and Broderip.

Harington, Henry. [c.1780]. *A Second Selection of Songs, etc. to Which Is Prefixed a Scheme of All the Harmonic Intervals Demonstrated from the Golden Proposition of Pythagoras*. London: Longman and Broderip.

Hobart, Henrietta, Countess of Suffolk. 1824. *Letters to and from Henrietta, Countess of Suffolk, and Her Second Husband, the Hon. George Berkeley, from 1712 to 1767*. London: Murray.

Mangin, Edward. 1815. *An Intercepted Epistle from a Person in Bath, to His Friend in London*. Bath: Gye and Son.

Mead, Richard. 1702. *A Mechanical Account of Poisons in Several Essays*. London: South.
Misson de Valbourg, Henry. 1698. *Mémoires et observations faites par un Voyageur en Angleterre*. La Haye: H. Van Bulderen.
Pepys, Samuel. 1953. *The Diary of Samuel Pepys*, ed. John Warrington, 3 vols. London: Dent.
Radcliffe, John. 1721. *Dr. Radcliffe's Practical Dispensatory. Containing a Complete Body of Prescriptions, Fitted for All Diseases Internal and External, Digested under Proper Heads*. London: Rivington.
Smollett, Tobias. 1752. *An Essay on the External Use of Water*. London: Cooper.
Smollett, Tobias. 1984. *The Expedition of Hymphry Clinker (1771)*. Oxford: Oxford University Press.
Thicknesse, Philip. 1772. *A Treatise on the Art of Decyphering, and of Writing in Cypher. With an Harmonic Alphabet*. London: Brown.
Thicknesse, Philip. 1780. *The Valetudinarian's Bath Guide; Or, the Means of Obtaining Long Life and Health*. London: Dodsley.
Wood, John. 1749. *An Essay Towards a Description of Bath*, 2 vols. London: Bettenham.

Secondary Sources

Barbeau, Alfred. 2009. *Life and Letters at Bath in the Eighteenth-Century*. Stroud: The History Press.
Brown, Frank. 1990. *William Herschel: Musician and Composer*. Bath: William Herschel Society.
Drayton Greenwood, Alice. 1913. *Horace Walpole's World: A Sketch of Whig Society Under George III*. London: Bell.
Green, Emanuel. 1903. *Thomas Linley, Richard Brinsley Sheridan, and Thomas Mathews: Their Connection with Bath*. Bath: n.p.
Hembry, Phyllis. 1990. *The English Spa, 1560–1815: A Social History*. London: Fairleigh Dickinson University Press.
Hyman, Robert and Nicola. 2011. *The Pump Room Orchestra Bath: Three Centuries of Music and Social History*. Salisbury: Hobnob Press.
James, Kenneth E. 1987. Concert Life in Eighteenth-Century Bath. PhD diss., Royal Holloway College, University of London.
Rice, Paul F. 2015. *Venanzio Rauzzini in Britain: Castrato, Composer and Cultural Leader*. Rochester, NY: University of Rochester Press.
Rishton, Tim. 1991. Thomas Chilcot and His Concertos. PhD diss., University College of North Walesm, Bangor University.
Sands, Mollie. 1953. Rauzzini at Bath. *Musical Times* 94 (1321): 108–111.

Shaw, Watkins, and Goodwin, Noël (rev. Frank Brown). 2001. 'Bath'. *Oxford Music Online. Grove Music Online*. https://doi.org/10.1093/gmo/9781561592630.article.41053. Accessed October 26, 2020.

Turner, Anthony J. 1977. *Science and Music in Eighteenth Century Bath. Catalogue of an Exhibition in the Holburne of Menstrie Museum, Bath, 22 September 1977–29 December 1977*. Bath: University of Bath.

Williams, Marjorie. 1945. *Lady Luxborough Goes to Bath*. Oxford: Blackwell.

PART III

Emerging Science: The Therapeutic Uses of Waters

CHAPTER 10

'Water of Paradise': The Role and Function of Balneology in Bacon's *New Atlantis*, *De vijs mortis* and *Historia vitae et mortis*

Mickaël Popelard

In about 1627, an Elizabeth Farrow or Farrer, chanced upon a spring of bubbling water just beneath the cliff to the south of Scarborough. Seeing that the water tasted bitter and that it stained the rocks a red-brownish colour, she decided to share her discovery with her friends and neighbours. The people of Scarborough started to drink the spring water as a local cure for all their ailments. But it was not until after Dr Robert Wittie published his medical treatise about *Scarborough Spa* in 1660[1]—a book in which he promoted the medical virtues of the Scarborough waters and recommended sea-bathing as a medical cure for all ills—that

[1]On Wittie's *Scarbrough-Spaw: or a description of the nature and vertues of the spaw at Scarbrough Yorkshire*, see Lowell Duckert's chapter in the present volume.

M. Popelard (✉)
Département des études anglophones, Université de Caen Normandie, Caen, France
e-mail: mickael.popelard@unicaen.fr

S. Chiari and S. Cuisinier-Delorme (eds.), *Spa Culture and Literature in England, 1500–1800*, Early Modern Literature in History,
https://doi.org/10.1007/978-3-030-66568-5_10

the town's wells became famous, thus making it possible for Scarborough to become a fashionable spa town as well as England's first seaside resort.

This rather well-known story has implications that go beyond the local level of one of Britain's most fashionable spa towns. For the date at which Mrs Farrow (or Farrer) made her discovery happens to roughly coincide with the date at which Bacon's *New Atlantis* was first written and then (posthumously) published. Bacon died in 1626, so there is no way he could have known about the Scarborough wells while writing *New Atlantis*—a work in which baths, springs and wells feature prominently. Robert Wittie, however, was hardly a pioneer in his field. Nor was Scarborough the only watering place in England at the time. Bath, Buxton and a few more local venues like King's Newnham for instance, were already instrumental in spreading the social habit of taking mineral waters. The rise of such spa towns was due in no small measure to the physicians who, from the second half of the sixteenth century onwards, started to publicize and promote the taking of waters in their treatises. Long before Bacon set out to write his scientific utopia, propagandists like William Turner, Walter Baily or Dr. John Jones had already vindicated water-taking as a sovereign cure for many diseases, especially gout. The Cambridge-educated scholar and well-travelled physician William Turner, for instance, deplored that although the baths had been known for a thousand years, 'they were seldom used by the public because of the envy and ignorance of physicians' (quoted in Hembry 1990, 7). This chapter aims at approaching early modern balneology from a theoretical angle by looking at three of Bacon's works on the subject, namely *De vijs mortis*, *Historia vitae et mortis* and *New Atlantis*. It must be made clear from the start that my claim is obviously not that Bacon invented early modern hydrotherapy. Not only were his views on the subject heavily influenced by other writers, both ancient and modern, but he was also part of a culture in which taking the waters had already become a fashionable activity as well as a recognized form of medical treatment. After all, hadn't the Earl of Leicester himself acknowledged, in his famous last letter to the queen, that he '[hoped] to find the perfect cure at the bath'? (Leicester 1588, SP 12/215 f.114).

What I will try to show is that Bacon's defence of water-taking has deeper roots, and indeed philosophical implications, than one might perhaps suspect. In other words, balneology should not be dismissed as a minor, albeit colourful, detail in the grand tapestry of his philosophical system—a system which aims at reconciling not just theory and practice, but also the mind and the senses. On the contrary, it lies at the intersection of several of Bacon's theoretical interests, including his theory of matter and his concern with the prolongation of life. It also foregrounds what I propose to call the sensory quality of his natural philosophy. Far from being an arid, desiccated pursuit, Bacon's writings are bubbling with a strong desire for living life to the full and enjoying all its sensory pleasures. From such a standpoint, the word hydrotherapy, in its technical blandness, sounds perhaps a little too clinical to fully reflect the undercurrent of voluptuousness that can be felt in some of Bacon's philosophical works.

1 Taking the Waters in Bacon's *New Atlantis*

The first point that should be made about balneology in *The New Atlantis* is that it is given pride of place in Bacon's scientific fable. Taking the narrator on a mental tour of the island with a view to showing him their many scientific achievements, the Father of the House of Salomon—the name of the scientific college presiding over the material and spiritual well-being of the island—explains that they

> have also a number of artificial wells and fountains, made in imitation of the natural sources and baths; as tincted upon vitriol, sulphur, steel, brass, lead, nitre, and other minerals. And again we have little wells for infusions of many things, where the waters take the virtue quicker and better, than in vessels or basins. And amongst them we have a water which we call Water of Paradise, being, by that we do to it, made very sovereign for health, and prolongation of life. (Bacon 2002, 481)

A few paragraphs further down, the Father tells his European visitor that they 'have also fair and large baths, of several mixtures, for the cure of diseases, and the restoring of man's body from arefaction [i.e. drying up, withering]: and others for the confirming of it in strength of sinews, vital parts, and the very juice and substance of the body' (Bacon 2002, 482).

As emerges from these two short excerpts, in Bensalem, the taking of waters is a sovereign remedy. There, as in England and the rest of Europe, hydrotherapy is of two kinds: once water has been 'tincted upon', that is to say enriched by adding to it an impressive variety of minerals ranging from vitriol to steel, it can be either taken as a medicinal drink or used for the preparing of 'large and fair baths' (Bacon 2002, 482). It will also be noted that the taking of waters is therapeutic in both the curative and preventive sense of the word. On the one hand, baths are said to help in 'the cure of diseases'. On the other hand, taking a bath of mineral water, or drinking Bensalem's 'Water of Paradise', is also a very efficient way of maintaining health and prolonging life. This does not come as a surprise: in his health-related writings, Bacon ascribes a threefold function to medicine, namely: (i) promoting health; (ii) strengthening and rejuvenating the body and (iii) prolonging life. In *New Atlantis*, Bacon considers the bathing in, and drinking of water within a predominantly scientific and medical context, although he also passes a few remarks of a more social or political nature, suggesting, for example, that baths can be used for pre-nuptial purposes (Bacon 2002, 478).

This is all the more important as the popular addiction to springs and wells had not always been entirely unproblematic from a political and religious perspective. At the height of the Henrician reformation, as well as in the early days of Elizabeth's reign, the taking of waters often carried a politically sulphurous connotation, so to speak. As Phyllis May Hembry explains, Elizabeth feared lest English Catholics might use the taking of waters as an excuse to travel to Spa, in the Spanish Low Countries, where they could easily meet and connive with other Catholic exiles: 'it was this aspect of the question—the English Catholic refugees' search for asylum at Spa near the Catholic university of Louvain in the dominions of Philip of Spain, where they could plot, intrigue and pass intelligence—that concerned Elizabeth I and her ministers' (Hembry 1990, 9). Together with the traditional—and, to Protestants, highly superstitious—view that pilgrimage to wells and springs could bring about miraculous cures, the fear that the taking of waters would be instrumental in furthering Catholic rebellion accounts for it suffering many years of neglect and suspicion during the course of the sixteenth century. Eventually, Elizabeth I's government adopted a more relaxed attitude towards the taking of waters—if only because the existence of baths at home deprived English Catholics of an excuse for travelling abroad. The taking of waters was therefore allowed, provided no miraculous element was claimed to be involved and that the waters could be proven to have genuine mineral and medicinal properties. In the words of Phyllis May Hembry again, the publication of Turner's treatise in 1562

> reflects the clear shift of official policy about the use of healing waters, coinciding with renewed patronage of the baths at Bath and Buxton and the use of certain other springs. The nobility and gentry who responded to his appeal soon found that a sojourn of a week or two at baths or wells was not only a possible cure for disease but a pleasant relaxation from the responsibility of office. (Hembry 1990, 8)

Sir William Cecil himself became a regular visitor of the baths at Bath, a clear indication that the taking of waters had now become a respectable social habit. Such a shift is also clearly reflected in the *New Atlantis* where the baths, springs and wells are in no way conducive to sedition or rebellion. Nor do they involve any miraculous element. The Father of the House of Salomon insists that 'they hate all impostures and lies: insomuch as we have severely forbidden it to all our fellows, under pain of ignominy and fines, that they do not shew any natural work or thing, adorned or swelling; but only pure as it is and without all affectation of strangeness' (Bacon 2002, 486). If the Bensalem waters do retain a sulphurous quality, it is from a strictly medical, not religious or political point of view, being as they are, 'tincted upon sulphur'.

They also perform a political function. Far from undermining the Bensalemite commonwealth, the baths at Bensalem allegedly create a firm foundation for the whole social edifice. They make it possible for husbands and wives to forge stronger marital bonds, or so the Bensalemites argue: 'because of many hidden defects in men and women's bodies, they have a more civil way; for they have near every town a couple of pools, (which they call 'Adam and Eve's pools'), where it is permitted to one of the friends of the man, and another of the friends of the woman, to see them severally bathe naked' (Bacon 2002, 478). For all the Bensalemites' supposed virtue and chastity, it seems that the scopic drive has become institutionalized, as it has been turned into a rite of passage of sorts. Although such a practice strikes us as voyeuristic and morally dubious, it is given moral and political justification on the ground that it helps to combat lechery. According to Joabin, a Jewish islander and one of the narrator's main sources of information about life in Bensalem, they have 'no stews, no dissolute houses, no courtesans, nor any thing of that kind' (Bacon 2002, 477). If the people of Bensalem are the chastest in the world, it is because they place such a high premium on morality. This is not on account of some natural or biological characteristic they happen to have as a people: reverence for morality is primarily a social and cultural construct. The whole point of Bacon's *New Atlantis* is to show how an ideal social organization can channel a nation's intellectual as well as sensual energies towards aims that will benefit not just the nation in question, but mankind as a whole. Thus, if the people of Bensalem were demi-gods naturally inclined to virtue, Bacon's philosophical demonstration would become less, not more convincing. The taking of waters should therefore be conceived of as a cog in a social and scientific wheel whose ultimate function is to make the people of Bensalem not just more virtuous, but also healthier and happier. In the words of the Father of the House of Salomon, 'the end of our foundation is the knowledge of causes, and secret motions of things, and the enlarging of the bounds of human empire, to the effecting of all things possible' (Bacon 2002, 480). At the end of the book is a list of all the wonderful works of nature which are to benefit mankind. Many of these are health-related scientific challenges, including 'the prolongation of life', 'the restitution of youth in some degree', 'the retardation of age', 'the curing of diseases counted incurable', 'the mitigation of pain or the increasing of strength and activity' (Bacon 2002, 488). Among many other useful remedies and 'operations', Bacon insists that baths and wells can also help to restore youth or prolong life. What remains to be understood is precisely how—according to Bacon, at least—the taking of waters can be instrumental in maintaining and strengthening one's health. This can be done by turning to Bacon's *Historia vitae et mortis* (c. 1620) and the earlier *De vijs mortis* (1611–1619), two works in which he lays down the principles of his medical and biological thinking.

2 The Function of Baths in Bacon's Medical Thinking

The key concept in Bacon's medical thinking is that of spirit.[2] In contradistinction to dominant Renaissance medical theories, Bacon believed that ageing and death were attributable to the body's reparable parts being undermined by the gradual failure of the less reparable,

[2] For a more complete discussion of this key Baconian concept, see Rees (1996) and Giglioni (2016).

with the former dying in the embrace of the latter—a predicament he compared to the torture of Mezentius. As Graham Rees explains, 'the root of this failure is the conspiracy between on the one hand the body's internal vital and inanimate spirits and, on the other, the external air' (Rees 1996, xlvii). It must first be reminded that, in Bacon's opinion, the universe consists of two mutually convertible states of matter, namely tangible matter and pneumatic matter. Whereas tangible matter is heavy, gross and inactive, pneumatic matter is weightless, tenuous and highly active. In the sublunar world where men live, bodies are never pneumatic through and through: the middle region, halfway between the Earth's core and the region above the Moon, is where tangible matter meets and interacts with pneumatic matter. Thus, all sublunar bodies, whether they are animate or inanimate, are a mixture of tangible matter and spirit.

To make matters worse, Bacon also believes that there are two types of spirit. Inanimate spirit is present in all tangible bodies at or near the surface of the Earth, no matter whether these bodies are living or non-living. It can be found in stones, rocks and trees as well as in lunatics, lovers and poets—or in lions, goats and foxes, for that matter, as these animal species happen to be regularly mentioned in Bacon's writings.[3] On the other hand, animate (or vital) spirit is the preserve of living bodies only. 'The two kinds differ in that in all varieties of inanimate spirit the airy component predominates whereas in the vital spirits the flamy has the upper hand' (Rees 1996, xlviii). While vital (or animate) spirits are always reluctant to escape the body in which they are enclosed, inanimate spirit, by contrast, is restlessly trying to escape. This is due to the airy nature of the inanimate spirit which longs to conspire with the ambient air because of their common airiness.[4]

[3] See, for example, the following 'facts' from the *Historia vitae et mortis*: 'lions are regarded as long-lived because many are toothless; but this is a deceptive sign, since it could be caused by their rank breath' (Bacon 2007, 179); 'foxes seem very well cut out for long life; they are very well clad, carnivorous, and live in earths; and yet are not noted for longevity. They belong to the canine race, which is short-lived' (Bacon 2007, 179); 'the goat lives about as long as the sheep, and differs little from it in other ways, [...] but it is more highly sexed and that shortens its life' (Bacon 2007, 181).

[4] Escape of the inanimate spirit is one the main causes of decay in inanimate bodies. The other two causes are attenuation (which comes first) and contraction (which comes last). Taken together, the three actions make up what Bacon terms the *actio triplex* of inanimate spirit. First, the spirit attacks the matter enclosing it and converts some of it into itself. This results in the body's weakening, which facilitates the escape of the spirit. Finally come desiccation and decay. To prolong life in animate bodies and increase

Because, as will be remembered, animate bodies contain both inanimate spirit and vital spirits, they are more complex compounds than inanimate bodies. Unlike inanimate spirit, vital spirits do not long for escape since nothing in the outside world is akin to them—theirs being a flamy rather than an airy nature—but they do lead to the consumption of the body enclosing them, which accounts for the need for nourishment. In order to prolong life in living bodies in general, and in human beings in particular, one needs to take into account both the inanimate and the animate spirits. The natural philosopher should therefore operate on two separate, yet interrelated planes: on the one hand, he (or she) must prevent the inanimate spirit from escaping; on the other hand, he (or she) must see to it that the vital spirits do not consume the body by becoming predatory. This is precisely where baths, wells and water-drinking come into play, together with a host of other remedies, some of which are rather fanciful, not to say utterly repellent and outrageous (like bathing in the blood of kittens or infants, for example, a remedy which Bacon cautiously rejects).[5]

According to Bacon, longevity mostly depends on the 'condensing' of animate spirits. These 'are the craftsmen and workers who do everything that happens in the body', they 'should be so worked on and modified that they become dense, not rare, in their substance; persistent, not biting, in their heat' (Bacon 2007, 247). This can be achieved by concentrating them (especially with opiates); cooling them (mainly with nitre); soothing them and finally by curbing their motions (through sleep principally). It would be a mistake, therefore, to assume that baths or water-drinking constitute a sovereign remedy. When it comes to prolonging life, there are much more efficient ways of condensing the spirits. One of them involves the taking of opium, 'which is far and away the most powerful and effective means of condensing the spirits by flight, and next to it opiates, and soporifics in general' (Bacon 2007, 247). Another, which Bacon strongly recommends, is the painting of one's body with woad or other pigments: 'the ancient Britons painted their bodies with woad, and were very long-lived. The Picts did the same; and some think that their

durability in inanimate ones, it is therefore essential to hinder the *actio triplex* of the spirit.

[5] See Bacon (2007, 321): 'it is anciently received that bathing in the blood of infants cures leprosy and restores flesh already rotten. But instances of this brought down popular hatred on the heads of certain kings'.

very name was derived from that. To this day the Brazilians and Virginians paint their bodies, and are (the former particularly) extremely long-lived' (Bacon 2007, 275). Should you run out of woad, rancid salt butter will achieve the desired effect just as well, as the Irish well know:

> [T]he Irish, and particularly the wild ones, are even now very long-lived. In fact they say that within these last few years the Countess of Desmond lived to the age of 140, and cut new teeth three times. Now the Irish habit is to stand in front of the fire without a stitch on, and rub, and so to speak, embalm themselves in rancid salt butter. (Bacon 2007, 277)

Yet, Bacon also insists that the offices and duties of life should always take precedence over longevity, which is why impractical remedies must be rejected in favour of methods compatible with life in society. Living on top on mountains, embalming oneself in rancid butter or painting one's body with woad may be powerful ways of increasing one's longevity, but unfortunately, such remedies also tend to get in the way of one's professional duties. They should therefore be discarded, as Bacon points out: 'I take the view that the duties of life are more important than life pure and simple [...] I put forward remedies and precepts which do not involve abandoning the offices of life or delay or disable them too much' (Bacon 2007, 241). Interestingly, Bacon's list of irrelevant remedies also includes 'constant baths prepared with liquors', thus suggesting that the taking of waters is a sword that cuts both ways. On the one hand, it certainly helps to condense the spirits and prevent their 'flight', to use Bacon's terminology. Examining the effects of baths in the section of the *Historia vitae et mortis* dealing with 'the operations to exclude air' (Bacon 2007, 273), Bacon concludes that special care should be taken to exclude ambient air because it impacts the body in two ways. First, ambient air preys upon the juices of the body and hastens desiccation. Secondly, air also impacts the body in a more indirect way. It is a well-known fact that a body 'closed up and not sweating restrains the enclosed spirit' (Bacon 2007, 273). This leads to its softening the harder parts of the body—which, Bacon believes, is conducive to longevity. According to Bacon, baths can help to prevent communication between the spirits and ambient air by closing skin pores: 'closing of the passages is helped by the coldness of the air itself; by nakedness which hardens up the skin; by cold baths; and by applying astringents, such as mastic oil, myrrh, and myrtle, to the skin' (Bacon 2007, 275). Thus, cold baths, especially when enriched with minerals as in the *New Atlantis*, are listed by Bacon among the most effective ways of achieving longevity in man (and woman): 'but this operation may be better achieved by baths taken infrequently and especially in summertime, baths of those astringent waters which can be safely applied; among these are waters suffused with iron and vitriol, for these firmly contract the skin' (Bacon 2007, 275). What all these remedies have in common is cold, not water. In other words, it is not the baths per se, but rather the cold water they are made of and the minerals they contain that help to close the pores of the skin.

Baths are not inherently beneficial. On the contrary, precautions should be taken to ensure that they do not become dangerous and counterproductive. In particular, hot baths are to be shunned at all costs for they promote the diffusion of the spirits, which, in its turn, leads to their dissolution, thus hastening death, instead of postponing it: 'diffusion is caused by labour too hard, feelings too strong, sweating too much, too much evacuation, warm baths, and sex too much and at the wrong times' (Bacon 2007, 269). As opposed to cold baths, warm baths are therefore detrimental to health. So is excessive bathing. On the other hand, drinking water can help to condense the spirits: 'above all, in youth, and especially in those who have strong stomachs, a good drink of pure, plain water at bedtime is beneficial' (Bacon 2007, 265). All in all, Bacon's preferred diet is quite similar to what he calls

> the austere and almost Pythagorean diet of the kind prescribed by the harsher monastic rules or customs of hermits, whose guiding light was need and poverty. Belonging to this are water drinking, a hard bed, cold air, plain food (i.e. of vegetables, fruits, and meat and fish picked and salted rather than fresh and hot), a hair shirt, frequent fastings, frequent vigils, infrequent sensual pleasures, and the like. For all these things diminish the spirits and reduce them to a quantity sufficient for the offices of life, and this causes them to be less predacious. (Bacon 2007, 261)

Such an austere diet seems hardly compatible with living life to the full. Yet, Bacon adds an important caveat:

> but if the diet were to be a little more pleasurable than severities and mortifications of this kind, and yet always level and steady, the same thing would be achieved. [...] We must also see to it that a body properly nourished, and not starved by the diets just mentioned does not give up timely

> sexual activity, lest the spirits swell up too much and soften and destroy the body. (Bacon 2007, 261–263)

It almost looks as if Bacon was constantly treading a fine line between medical imperatives and the sensuousness of life.

3 'So Shall Nature Be Cherished': Bacon's Voluptuous Philosophy

It would be a mistake, of course, to describe Bacon as a disciple of Epicureanism. But it is perhaps not exaggerated to argue that his interest in balneology also reflects his concern with making life not just longer, but also more varied and more pleasant. Graham Rees contends that 'the aim of prolonging life epitomizes the aims of Bacon's programme as a whole' (Rees 2007, xlvi). While this is no doubt true, it should also be added that prolonging life is not the only goal Bacon sets his sights on. Not every life is worth living. In the (almost) universally shared Christian mindset of early modern Europe, suicide could neither be commended, nor even seriously contemplated. As J. A. Sharpe reminds us, it was not until the late seventeenth century that attitudes towards suicide started to change, leading to what some historians called a (relative) 'secularization of suicide' in the eighteenth century. In the early seventeenth century, by contrast, suicide was still condemned as a felony and 'a flagrant breach of the Christian moral code' (Sharpe 1997, 115). Sharpe quotes one Michael Dalton, the author of a handbook for justices of the peace who argued that suicide was a triple offense: 'against God, against the King and against nature' (Sharpe 1997, 115). As for Bacon, he sometimes seems to turn a blind eye to, and even implicitly condone, the notion that under certain circumstances, taking one's own life is preferable to living in shame or misery. In the classical examples he often quotes and examines, there is little trace of his condemning suicide on religious, political or philosophical grounds (to echo Dalton's ternary accusation). On the contrary, Bacon often seems to realize that life can become so burdensome and so tedious at times that one no longer wants to live, as in the following passage from his essay 'Of death': 'a man would die, though he were neither valiant nor miserable, only upon a weariness to do the same thing so oft over and over' (Bacon 2002, 343). One is therefore tempted to draw the implicit conclusion that the value of life lies less in its length than in its quality. The same precept leads Bacon to conclude, after

Celsus, that 'a man [should] vary and interchange contraries, but with an inclination to the more benign extreme: use fasting and full eating, but rather full eating; watching and sleep, but rather sleep; sitting and exercice, but rather exercice; and the like' (Bacon 2002, 404).[6] In other words, engaging in pleasurable activities becomes a medically prescribed imperative.

As it happens, hydrotherapy serves as an interesting connection between the complementary goals of prolonging life and sweetening it. Certainly, longevity is Bacon's primary goal. As I have already pointed out, Bacon rules out those remedies which are better adapted to pleasure than prolonging life. Among them, he says, are 'baths and ointments (as have been in use)' (Bacon 2007, 231). This should not be taken to mean that Bacon rejects baths and water-drinking altogether for, as has been said, he makes it clear that a distinction should be drawn between hot and cold baths. Cold baths are beneficial because they help to close the pores and, by keeping the spirits enclosed and restrained, to increase longevity. What Bacon rejects is the traditional way of taking the waters, which involves hot or warm baths. The problem with hot baths lies not in the water but in the heat: 'hot baths are as opposite to our operation as anointings are in line with it, for the one opens the passages, while the other blocks them. Therefore a bath without subsequent anointing is very bad; but anointing without the bath is very good' (Bacon 2007, 277). This may sound like a very austere, almost monastic condemnation of a pleasurable activity. Yet, Bacon is also acutely aware that too much austerity is unlikely to increase longevity 'for in flames we see that a rather larger one (provided it is steady and quiet) takes rather less from its kindling than does one which is agitated, and by turns fiercer and calmer' (Bacon 2007, 261). Consequently, it is excess in all things, not pleasure as such, that must be shunned.

So, are we to conclude that Bacon is torn between conflicting objectives? Does it mean that health, longevity and pleasure are all desirable, if also incompatible ends? Does the example of hot baths suggest otherwise? It is my contention that, for all his preoccupation with longevity, Bacon never goes as far as to throw pleasure overboard. On the contrary,

[6] The same piece of advice is to be found in *Historia vitae et mortis*: see Bacon (2007, 231): 'in the meantime we should not despise the advice of Celsus, a physician who was not just learned but practical, who advises variety and alternation of diet, but with a leaning towards the generous'.

it seems to me that his philosophy is suffused with a strong undercurrent of voluptuousness. As a philosopher, Bacon believes that the world is there for our understanding. But science, in Bacon's opinion, is never exclusively conceived of as 'truth seeking' or 'right talking', as would be the case with Aristotle, for example. It is—or should also be—conducive to 'good living' and 'pleasure seeking'. Bacon has an eye for the beauty and diversity of nature. In some passages of the *Historia vitae*, the philosophical inquiry blossoms into an almost poetical, albeit discreet, celebration of the sensory appreciation of life, as is made manifest by the following passage:

> Thus the smell of earth fresh and pure when you are following the plough, or digging, or rooting out weeds, restrains the spirits very well. Leaves falling in woods and hedgerows in late autumn give the spirits good cooling; that is especially true of strawberry plants as they die back. The smell of violets, wallflower, sweet pea, and clary picked as they grow has the same effect. Besides I knew a long-lived aristocrat who, as soon as he woke, had a fresh lump of earth placed under his nose every day, to breathe in its smell. (Bacon 2007, 259)

4 Conclusion: Reconciling Pleasure, Health and Longevity

It is hard to resist the feeling that these lines are not so much about the condensing of spirits as they are about the joy of observing and communing with nature. Not unlike Duke Orsino relishing 'the sweet sound / That breathes upon a bank of violets' (*Twelfth Night*, 1.1.5–6 in Shakespeare 2016, 1829) or Oberon telling Puck about the 'bank where the wild thyme blows' (*A Midsummer Night's Dream*, 2.1.249–250 in Shakespeare 2016, 1098), Bacon is not indifferent to the 'smell of violets'. Paying close attention to the world around us is a source of pleasure. In *New Atlantis*, the Father of the House of Salomon does not say whether the 'large baths, of several mixtures, for the cure of diseases' (Bacon 2002, 482) are hot or cold. But the context in which this piece of information is delivered suggests that the Fellows of the House of Salomon have succeeded in reconciling pleasure, health and longevity. Not only is their science efficient, it also leads to pleasurable results. In Bensalem, life is both easier and more pleasant—or so it seems: 'and in this house we contain also a confiture-house, where we make all sweet-meats, dry and moist, and divers pleasant wines, milks, broths, and sallets, far in greater variety than you have' (Bacon 2002, 485). There is little doubt that the emphasis, here, is on variety. Bacon aims at showing that the Bensalemite scientists are capable of enlarging nature. But they also make it more enjoyable. After all, wine was not listed in *Historia vitae et mortis* as a powerful way of prolonging life, only water was. In Bensalem, however, the tension between pleasure, health and longevity is no longer palpable. Projecting his scientific dreams into Bensalem's utopian space was perhaps Bacon's way of reconciling pleasure and longevity. But a similar undercurrent of sensuality, albeit in a more subdued form, was also detectable in *Historia vitae* or in the *De vijs mortis*. Although, in these two works, the emphasis is clearly on moderation, it is difficult to resist the feeling that Bacon is almost imperceptibly drawn towards what he calls 'the more benign extreme', i.e. the pleasures of life. All in all, if one is to choose between the two extremes, (a certain amount of) pleasure is to be preferred over (too much) austerity: as Bacon himself explained in 'Of the regiment of health', 'so shall nature be cherished, and yet taught masteries' (Bacon 2002, 404). Making life longer is not necessarily incompatible with making it sweeter, too: on the contrary, the two goals are perhaps best understood as going hand in hand. This is particularly obvious in *New Atlantis*, for, in Bensalem at least, it seems that one can take not the 'primrose way to th'everlasting bonfire', as in *Macbeth* (2.3.15, in Shakespeare 2016, 2523) but the warm baths way to longevity.

Works Cited

Primary Sources

Bacon, Francis. 1996. *De vijs mortis*. In *The Oxford Francis Bacon*, vol. 6, ed. Graham Rees, 269–359. Oxford: Clarendon Press.

Bacon, Francis. 2007. *Historia vitae et mortis*. In *The Oxford Francis Bacon*, vol. 12, ed. Graham Rees, 140–377. Oxford: Clarendon Press.

Bacon, Francis. 2002. *New Atlantis* in *The Major Works*, ed. Brian Vickers. Oxford: Oxford World's Classics.

Baily, Walter. 1587. *A Briefe Discours of Certain Bathes or Medicinall Waters in the Countie of Warwicke neere vnto a Village Called Newnam Regis*. London: s.n.

Dudley, Robert, Earl of Leicester. 29th August 1588. *Letter to Elizabeth I*. SP 12/215 f.114, National Archives. https://www.nationalarchives.gov.uk/education/resources/elizabeth-monarchy/earl-of-leicester-to-elizabeth/. Accessed October 26, 2020.

Shakespeare, William. 2016. *The Complete Works. Modern Critical Edition*, eds. Gary Taylor, John Jowett, Terri Bourus, and Gabriel Egan. Oxford: Oxford University Press.

Turner, William. 1557. *A Book of the Nature and Properties as Well of the Baths in England as of Other Baths in Germany and Italy*. Cologne: Arnold Birckman.

Wittie, Robert. 1660. *Scarbrough--Spaw: Or a Description of the Nature and Vertues of the Spaw at Scarbrough Yorkshire. Also a Treatise of the Nature and Use of Sea, Rain, Dew, Snow, Hail, Pond, Lake, Spring, and River-Waters, Where More Largely the Controversie Among Learned Writers, About the Original of Springs is Discussed. To Which Is Added a Short Discourse Concerning Mineral Waters. Corrected and Augmented Throughout the Whole, Together with an Historical Relation of Cures Done by the Waters*. London: Charles Tyus.

Secondary Sources

Giglioni, Guido, James A.T. Lancaster, Sorana Corneanu, and Dana Jalobeanu, eds. 2016. *Francis Bacon on Motion and Power*. Berlin: Springer.

Hembry, Phyllis. 1990. *The English Spa. A Social History, 1560–1815*. London: The Athlone Press.

Rees, Graham. 1996. Introduction to *De vijs mortis*. In *The Oxford Francis Bacon*, vol. 6, ed. Graham Rees, lxv–lxix. Oxford: Clarendon Press.

Rees, Graham. 2007. Introduction to *Historia vitae et mortis*. In *The Oxford Francis Bacon*, vol. 12, ed. Graham Rees, xlvi–lix. Oxford: Clarendon Press.

Sharpe, J.A. 1997. *Early Modern Britain. A Social History 1550–1760*. London: Arnold.

CHAPTER 11

'Minerals in Winter': Robert Wittie's Cold Treatment

Lowell Duckert

According to the Dutch extreme athlete Wim Hof, cold should be everyone's 'warm friend'.[1] The famous 'method' that bears his name—the three 'pillars' of cold therapy, breathing, and commitment—promises a stronger immune system, better sleep, and increased energy. Clothing and temperature control, he claims, leave the human body under-stimulated, thereby 'atrophying the age-old mechanisms related to our survival and basic function'. A steadfast practitioner of 'WHM' learns to unlock their 'inner power [...] the ability of our body to adapt to extreme temperature and survive within our natural environment'. But this glacial guru's well-intentioned advice—'to a happier, healthier, and stronger you'—should give the cryo-curious pause. Could this 'power' be just another attempt at reasserting human resilience and control over inhabitable environments of

[1] For more on the Wim Hof Method, visit: https://www.wimhofmethod.com/practice-the-method (accessed June 2, 2020). Unless specified otherwise, all citations refer to this website.

L. Duckert (✉)
Department of English, University of Delaware, Newark, DE, USA
e-mail: lduckert@udel.edu

S. Chiari and S. Cuisinier-Delorme (eds.), *Spa Culture and Literature in England, 1500–1800*, Early Modern Literature in History,
https://doi.org/10.1007/978-3-030-66568-5_11

'our' own making, an immersive practice meant to harden the permeable body for the sake of self-help? Is this yet another form of hyperborean and masculine forthrightness in the face of frigid adversity, an 'inner' quality that polar explorers prized—and for which they were praised? In *The Way of the Iceman*, Hof speaks rather unkindly of his old 'friend' to boot: 'You can't learn anything from the cold. But you can learn to not do some things' (Hof and de Jong 2016, 17). If we cannot count on cold to set a positive example for living in the climatic 'extreme[s]' of the Anthropocene, what, then, *does* it teach the world's remaining icemen and women, as well as those warm/ed societies set in their anthropogenic ways?

Early modern cryologies, I propose, aid this inquiry. Many medical manuals of the mid- to late seventeenth-century advised against the ingestion of cold water, let alone one's (e.g. Hof's) full on immersion. It was typically believed that an excessive amount of cold plugged the body's pores, trapping its unhealthy elements inside. Humoral theory, the prevalent discourse handed down by the Greek physicians Hippocrates (c. 460–377 BCE) and Galen (129–199), viewed the human body as a combination of four humours (black and yellow bile, choler, and phlegm) suspended in a delicate amalgam. Disease occurred when these fluids lost their equilibrium. Even when remedying outbreaks of burning illness, specialists' cold prescriptions for correcting a patient's humoral imbalances were cautious at best. Treatments tended to question the body's innate integrity rather than uphold it. My analysis complements the study of what Mary Floyd-Wilson calls 'geohumoralism', or, 'regionally framed humoralism' (2003, 2): the palpable impacts that climates made upon one's temperament, complexion, ethnicity, and other identifying features. Scholars have expanded the investigation to include earthquakes (Totaro 2018) as well as the heavens (Chiari 2019). By adding the tangible matter of cold to this conversation, I enlarge the scope of geo/humoral research in order to uncover those 'things' that cryo- and hydrological types of inhuman agency do to corporeal forms.

This chapter draws from a range of literary and natural-philosophical texts invested in the un/healthy effects of cold contact, chiefly the *Scarbrough Spaw* (1660) of Robert Wittie (1613–1684), an English physician who successfully managed to turn his country's exposed eastern coast into a thriving therapeutic resort. While he is persuasive in his defence of a salubrious north and the physiological benefits that come from its coldness, Wittie's most notable accomplishment, I argue, is in situating the

spa-going human subject in wider global–local waters, collapsing hydro-spatial distance by eliminating the separation between embodiment and environment. At his spa/*Spaw*, that is, subcutaneous and subterranean 'veins' intersect. This material-metaphorical mapping of wintry humans and minerals that occurs at the source of a local wellspring recognizes the body's degree of wellness as dependent upon physical degrees of temperature; and yet, it simultaneously checks that same body's capacity to completely compose itself. In conclusion, I ask why we should re-examine past perceptions of cooling in a world that is currently warming. Inuit climate activist Sheila Watt-Cloutier is a passionate advocate for '*the right to be cold*': 'the demand that the global community recognize that the well-being of our environment is in itself a fundamental human right' (Watt-Cloutier 2018, xxii). 'Our home', she points out, 'is a barometer for what is happening to our entire planet' (Watt-Cloutier 2018, xxi). Returning to Wittie's spa-derived macro-microcosmic model can reinsert us in the precarious water cycles of today's cryosphere, calling our attention to (and care for) its porous bodies most at risk.

1 Frost's Impressions, or, Preparing the Palate

It is useful at this early point to situate Wittie's *Spaw* within the period's competing, contrasting, and complementary knowledges about the nature of cold water. Debates at this time centred on what cold—ontologically speaking—actually *was*. Without an understanding of thermodynamics' three laws, some brumal-minded thinkers pondered whether cold might not be a chemically produced *result*, but rather a transmittable *substance* of its own. On a theoretical spectrum extending from the 'privative' (a lack of heat), to the 'positive' (an actual presence), natural philosophers leaning to the latter followed the pre-Socratic thinker Parmenides (c. 450 BCE). A century before Aristotle, he had sought the tangible origin of cold, known more mythically as *primum frigidum*—'first cold' in Latin. Francis Bacon (1561–1626) effectively rejuvenated this (pseudo)scientific pursuit. His *Sylva Sylvarum* is a frost-nipped forest, for it stipulates no less than seven 'Meanes of Producing Cold' (Bacon 1627, 23). Highlighting the creative reciprocity between hot and cold—'nature's two hands, whereby she chiefly worketh' (Bacon 1627, 23)—it is the second cause he identifies—the 'contact of cold bodies, for cold is active and transitive into bodies adjacent' (Bacon 1627, 23)—that etched his name into the millennia-long history of temperature. 'Whosoever will be an Inquirer into Nature, let him resort to a Conservatory of Snow and Ice' (Bacon 1627, 23). But Bacon is less known, perhaps, for a pronouncement he makes later in his monumental tome of natural history: 'whosever will make experiments of cold, let him be provided of [...] a conservatory of snow' (Bacon 1627, 101). Simply put, to find the source of 'frigus'—as he had earlier named it (1608)—one must interact with the stuff of snow.[2]

Let us take his advice, then. The Puritan divine William Fulke's (1538–1589) *A Goodly Gallerye* (1563) is one such laboratory made of snow, and therefore a good place for sussing out its origin. An amalgamation of Aristotle, Pliny, and Seneca, it marks the first time 'meteorology' entered the English language, and it appeared in nine different editions in the span of a century. Fulke's anti-Romanist polemics led to his appointment as master of Pembroke Hall, Cambridge, in 1578. But it was his earlier work of rational investigation into 'Impressiones, named of ther height, Meteora' (Fulke 1979, 25) for which he is best remembered. Fulke found astrological readings and the practice of prognostication antithetical to the truer science of astronomy. Dutifully Aristotelian, he divides meteors into 'vnperfectly' and 'perfectly mixed' (un/resistant to change, respectively), made up of either moist 'vapores' or dry 'exhalations' (Fulke 1979, 26).[3] 'Snowe', he says, 'is a cloude congeled by greate colde, before it be perfectlye resolued from vapors into water' (Fulke 1979, 98). This basic understanding of cold would predominate discussions. Poor Robin, whose *Almanack* first printed in 1664 went through annual publications from 1669–1700, writes in the *Book of Knowledge* (1688) that 'snow is ingendred of Rain, the Cloud congealing through extremity of Cold' (Poor Robin 1688, 92), and John Tulley, observing 'the Natural Causes of Watry Meteors, as Snow, Hail, Rain &c.' (n.p.) from Boston, repeated the same almost verbatim in his *Almanack* (1693) over one hundred years later: 'You must first Understand, that all Watery Meteors, as Rain, Snow, or such like, is but a moist Vapour drawn up by the Vertue of the Sun,

[2] See *Calor et Frigus* (1608); Bacon, ironically, died of pneumonia after stuffing a hen with snow: a reminder that the encounter always retains a lethal edge (a point to which I will return in closing). See Aubrey (1898, 1:75).

[3] The very brief early modern meteorological forecast that follows depends almost entirely on three indispensable studies: Craig Martin's 'Introduction' (2011), the first chapter of Vladimir Janković (2000), and the first two parts of S. K. Heninger (1968), particularly 'Snow'.

and the rest of the Planets into the middle Region of the air, where being congealed or dissolved, upon the earth, as hail or rain' (Tulley 1693, n.p.). Snow seems to be a simple meteor by this summary, the known components of its material composition handed down (or up) through the ages.

Fulke's account proves snow is less easily 'understand[able]', however, when he turns to what snow *does* in addition to what it *is*. If 'hore froste', which is 'nothing els but dewe congeled by ouermuche cold [...] doth often stynke' because it is drawn from fetid places like lakes full of 'stinking' mud (Fulke 1979, 97), the cold cloud gains a sensory quality as much as it collapses spatial differences between lower, middle, and high regions of the atmosphere. Noisome 'matter' (Fulke 1979, 97) that falls to earth might have its formation in the waters at your very feet. Even without a definitive grasp of the water cycle in which melting ice and snow play a major part—a theory that would later be proven by Pierre Perrault (c. 1608–1680)—the hydrological cycle widens to include a number of snowy 'Impressiones' of which we are unfamiliar. For Fulke, fluctuations from 'vnperfectly' to 'perfectly mixed' meant that snow could take on both mineral and vegetable aspects: the stone 'Christal', he maintains, comes from snowmelt freezing again on high hills, and, contrary to its associations with barren landscapes, it 'causeth thinges growing to be fruictfull, and increase, because the cold dryueth heate vnto the rootes, and so cherysheth the plantes' (Fulke 1979, 99). With its vegetative agency—from the Latin *vegetat*, 'enlivening'—snow embraces life forms; its impress fructifies, makes fertile. In its mineralogical makeup, it keeps open the possibilities of metamorphosis; it channels heat, conducts change. Early modern meteorologists described snow in ways that highlighted its 'thing-power', as Jane Bennett deems it,[4] and the influential energy it carried was called 'cold'.

Writers following Fulke grew interested in cold's impressive impacts upon human bodies. How 'cold dryueth' into humans—in more or less 'fruictfull' ways—was a popular subject of conversation in remedial circles. The Spanish physician Nicolás Monardes (c. 1512–1588) champions the 'properties & vertues' of 'the faire Ladie Snow' in *Historia medicinal de las coasas que se traen de nuestras Indias Occidentales* (completed 1574; translated as *Ioyfull Newes out of the Newe Founde Worlde* by John

[4] Defined as 'the curious ability of inanimate things to animate, to act, to produce effects dramatic and subtle' (Bennett 2010, 6).

Frampton in 1577/1580). Chiefly, he defends 'the good that drinking colde doeth' (Monardes 1580, fol. 164r, fol. 172v, fol. 168v). Citing the Latin grammarian Aulus Gellius's (c. 125–180) maxim 'the yeere of Snow, the yeere of Fertility', he, too, contends that snow destroys 'euil hearbes, and doth fructifie and increase them which are good' (Monardes 1580, fol. 166v). Monardes wishes to know how a human body, like a 'good' herb, reacts to the ingestion of cold water and thereby 'increase[s]' their health. Noting that Galen 'doth counsell to drinke colde' (Monardes 1580, fol. 176v), a hot fever would logically abate with a direct dose. (More on allopathic remedies later). Monardes goes on to enumerate four different ways of making cold: air, wells, saltpeter, and snow. Out of the four, 'the colde which dooth proceede of Snowe, dooth not offend as other colde dooth' (Monardes 1580, fol. 168r). Cold water made with snow is, simply put, the healthiest. For testament to this fact, he cites the example of 'many being sicke, and hauing great occassions of sicknes, after that they drinke cold, are whole straight way: and when they have geuen ouer the use of it, they become sicke agayne' (Monardes 1580, fol. 177r). The 'fruictfull' force identified by Fulke that flows through the diagnosed febrile body turns into a treatment.

Like a good doctor, Monardes advises moderation in all things. Too much cold sends one into a steep decline: 'it [will] appeareth', he cautions, 'howe euill the use of the sayde snowe is, and the water which doeth come out of it, if it bee not by the way of medicine onely' (Monardes 1580, fol. 177v). In Robert Barclay's (1582–1621) bestselling romance *Argenis* (1621; translated from Latin by Kingesmill Long in 1625), Arsidas, feted in Mauritania by the governor Iuba, nearly dies after consuming frozen apples in summer. Washed down with beverages served in 'Cups of Ice', the fruits' unseasonable delicacy and aesthetic delight are too rare to pass over: 'But after they were risen from Dinner, and Arsidas was jestingly discommending the use of hot drinkes, he felt all his sinews, by little and little, to faint with extremity of cold; insomuch, as casting up his meat, his life had almost followed' (Barclay 1625, 348). A physician must handle cold with care, lest their patient, like a gluttonous Arsidas, 'too freely' imbibe. Even if 'euill' (but only if misused), the benefits outweigh the risks when taken properly: 'there is no price to bee esteemed too it, nor understanding that can expounde it' (Monardes 1580, fol. 180r). Despite Monardes's acknowledgment that cold's gastrological magic remains a mystery, its inexplicability leads to a ringing endorsement at the end of his short treatise: 'those which are accustomed to drink it herein, let euery man drink cold' (Monardes 1580, fol. 181^{r}). If one is willing to stomach the snow (literally), they will be salubriously rewarded for their cold courage.

2 'Minerals in Winter', or, a Cool Draught

Wittie first took the waters of Scarborough in 1637–1638 after settling in nearby Hull. As one of the dedicatory poems to the *Spaw* insinuates, however, drawing distempered patients to a town on the North Sea coast was not an easy task. His grand therapeutic plan faced an ancient grudge held against the world's northern places: 'All ill from th'North? nay, that's not so, / For here the wholesome waters flow' (Wittie 1660, sig. A4r).[5] The first two-thirds of the *Spaw* lays out an argument worth the poet's ('R.W.') admiration, culling together an erudite collection of Greek, Latin, and biblical authorities who noted the benefits of drinking water—'there is nothing more necessary unto nourishment' (Wittie 1660, 22)—especially when it is cold: 'it is most healthfull being taken inwardly, and is prescribed by Physicians in many cases, both to prevent and cure diseases, and tends much to preserve us in our well being' (Wittie 1660, 40–41).[6] The remaining sections essentially tout the extraordinary virtues of mineral springs. To sell his particular brand of 'wholesome' water, Wittie had to describe both the 'nature' and 'operation' of the substance his potential patrons would ingest. As a physician steeped in the humoral tradition, Wittie believed that bodily imbalances were properly cared for allopathically (as in, by opposites). A cold and moist illness, for instance, required a hot and dry treatment. Scarborough's water could, 'by due and daily use thereof [...] correct cold & moist bodies, and cure such diseases as proceed from the excess of cold and moysture' (Wittie 1660, 192). His prescription appears to have a glaring problem, though, since cold cannot combat cold.[7] Fortunately, the spa's propriety minerals are ushered in

[5] The reference is to the Book of Jeremiah: '*omne malum ab Aquilone.*'

[6] A sentiment often repeated and obviously intended for the reader's edification: 'The principall token of good and wholesome water is, that it be simple or unmixed, and then it loads not the stomach, and easily passes through the Hypochondres, being also soon hot and soon cold' (Wittie 1660, 160).

[7] He does not subscribe, in a word, to the theory of 'counteraction'; see Lemnius (1658) below. See Floyd-Wilson (2003, 23–47) for a history of thought concerning climate effects in the West.

at this critical juncture. The intrinsic heat of salt, iron, and nitre—inorganic compounds he had personally identified in his laboratory—adds the key ingredient of wellness: 'impregnated with the qualities and natures of the said Minerals', the water 'consequently is hot and dry in operation' (Wittie 1660, 192). He persists: 'Nor let any startle at this assertion, that I affirm this *Spaw* water to be cold and moist, and also hot & dry, which are contrary qualities, since it is cold & moist actually in the instantaneous use of it, but doth heat and dry virtually, & in process of time' (Wittie 1660, 192–193). Spa water goes down cold, in other words, but it slowly burns once inside.

Wittie cites plenty of historical anecdotes and paraphrases hosts of (near-) contemporary colleagues like Monardes: for example, melted snow should not 'be drunk alone, because of its exceeding coldnesse' (Wittie 1660, 64–65), even if it 'preserves the earth' (Wittie 1660, 66–67) from putrefaction; and since the spa is 'strongest' in winter, one should beware drinking the water without first exposing it to air, for 'paralytick and convulsive motions' (Wittie 1660, 245) are sure to follow. That being said, his *Spaw* also makes significant contributions to hydrotherapy scholarship. Any generic kind of cold water will drop a body's temperature—'no man need go to Scarbrough for these intentions' (Wittie 1660, 194)—but the minerals' latent heat in his is what causes it to 'peirc[e] into the most narrow and secret passages of the body, & is excellent in opening obstructions, which are the causes of most diseases' (Wittie 1660, 195). As previously mentioned, early modern medical practitioners agreed that an 'exceeding' amount of cold effectively contracted these pores (the narrowing of blood vessels now known as vasoconstriction), either preventing previous sickness from escaping or incubating novel illnesses entirely. Wittie's waters emend this conventional logic: 'Minerals in Winter', the coldest conceivable, actually clear rather than close the body's blocked pathways. He outlines the purgative and diuretic effects in detail—'casting forth plentifully both it selfe and the excrementitious humours' (Wittie 1660, 196)—even conducting a successful experiment on himself.[8] And lest one fears being weakened by this flowing process, with it comes 'a corroberating or strengthening quality, whereby it fortifies the parts, and so arms nature with new strength to the preventing of relapses' (Wittie 1660, 199). The waters both rectify and reinforce.

[8] Three pints in the morning resulted in 'an evacuation both ways' (Wittie 1660, 197).

Visiting his spa even improves the mood. As the beneficiary of a prestigious education—receiving an MD from King's College, Cambridge in 1647—Wittie would have partnered emotional expressions (the passions) with bodily composition (the humors). Where that body was geo- or hydrographically located, moreover, and to what substances it was exposed, influenced the subject's mental and physiological well-being (Floyd-Wilson and Sullivan 2007). In the voluminous *Anatomy of Melancholy* (1621), Robert Burton (1577–1640) attributes 'bad air' as one cause of the affliction, especially in the most drastic degrees: 'Cold air in the other extreme is almost as bad as hot' (Burton 2001, 239). Because melancholy was associated with cold and dry qualities—and produced by an excess of black bile in the spleen—a body made vulnerable to cold air would naturally succumb to the disposition. In Wittie's expert opinion, surprisingly, low temperatures maintain a healthy temperament. Cold and moist waters literally keep the dark materials at bay, in the bowels: 'It is a most Soveraign remedy against Hypochondriack Melancholly and Windiness, suppressing the vapours which fly up to the head, and cheering the heart, as I might instance at large' (Wittie 1660, 205).[9] Come on in to the *Spaw* and get cold, he gestures to his readers; let the water redefine *you*, deep down, on the anatomical and (subsequently) psychological level.

With all four properties swirling around at once, Wittie could advertise a glass of his spa water, ingeniously, as an elemental and alimentary cure-all. For 'hot and sharp humours', he advises an immediate application by 'incession' or 'injection'. In this case, the initial dose of coldness will be 'more cleansing and healing' (Wittie 1660, 208). Those who suffer from intestinal blockages such as 'Colick' should drink it 'a little warm, and the patient should also bathe in it' (Wittie 1660, 206). Here, the traditional cold-water cleanse ('in process of time') is best served tepid, slightly sped up via immersion. Either dunked in or drunk down, delivered lukewarm or straight up from the cool source, hot- or cold-, wet- or

[9] He claims to have cured two ministers this way, pointing out that 'Mr. L.' travels one hundred and fifty miles annually for a drink (Wittie 1660, 205–206). Wittie's most convincing evidence is, again, his own body: 'I have sometimes drunk of it not for necessity but company, or to make some little evacuation from flegmatick humours, being of an athletick constitution, when within three days I found so great an agility and cheerfulness of body and mind then I had before, as I have wondred at it, that if I had stayed a fortnight, I could not have expected more benefit' (Wittie 1660, 230).

dry-induced maladies are guaranteed to disappear. His pitch amounts to an early modern eco-touristic brochure, and is worth reading in full:

> In a word if any intentions be to be performed in a medicinall way, by allaying or mitigating some hot distemper, opening obstructions, evacuating morbifick humours by Urine or Seige, and strengthening the inward parts of the body, it may be fully and compleatly effected by this water, wherein it operates so safely, as I have very rarely observed any ill Symptomes to arise: not have I scarce named any distemper, of which I have not made particular observation, and most of them many times over, or been certainly informed by credible Authors. (Wittie 1660, 209–210)

A potable tonic that can be transported to London and 'found good' (Wittie 1660, 246) or decanted and 'carryed abroad' (Wittie 1660, 247): Wittie managed to package (in words) Scarborough's water as a wondrous elixir, thereby reserving a unique place for cold in the wider history of spa culture.

Still, the popularity of 'the Germane Spaws' (Wittie 1660, 8) and hot(ter)spots like them elsewhere compelled Wittie to contend with, and improve upon, his continental competition. Besides promoting the healthy components of the town's water, Wittie's ancillary aim in the *Spaw* was showcasing his country's balneological virtues in comparison to other regions' famous mineral springs. Essentially valorising the local cold for an international clientele, he penned a series of careful objections set to refute the rumour that 'because of the coldness of our climate, the water is not so well concocted with the heat of the Sun, and so is hard of digestion' (Wittie 1660, 33). The sun's warming rays could not penetrate far enough into the earth's interior—a maximum depth of ten feet, which had recently been mathematically determined—meaning that other factors were responsible for his water's virtuous 'concoction'. He can only conjecture: some unspecified planetary 'influence' (Wittie 1660, 34) upon the minerals within; the earth being warmer in winter than summer, as the natural philosophers say, because of the heat-trapping 'frosts [...] that shut the pores of it' (Wittie 1660, 35); and a belief that God would not unequally distribute healing waters to southern countries alone (Wittie 1660, 35–36). Yet even without an ascertainable cause, England simply 'doth abound more' (Wittie 1660, 36) in medicinal waters which meet the highest standards ('tokens') of sight, taste, and smell set by trusted ancient authorities (Wittie 1660, 37). In short, while 'there is no Country

but it affords wholesome water, even the most frozen Country of Greenland' […] 'the waters of England are good' (Wittie 1660, 32), if not equal, to the rest. To his detractors in 'Spain, France, and the hot Countries', he believes that 'our waters are as wholesome for our bodies, as theirs are for them in those hot climates, and much more then theirs would be for us' (Wittie 1660, 36). It is 'good' enough, that is, to drink at home. One need not binge abroad.

Despite its ostensible subject matter—the 'Nature and Vertues of the Spaw at Scarbrough' (Wittie 1660, sig. A1^{r})—Wittie's study also engages one of the most contentious hydrographical debates of his era: 'the Original of Springs' (Wittie 1660, sig. A1^{r}). Springs originate, he opines, from rain and snow entering secret passages in the earth, 'which are like unto small fibres of veins, not discernible by the eye, terminating in the skin in all the parts of our bodies' (Wittie 1660, 127). By referring to a popular metaphor of the human body as a geological system—here, a subterranean tangle of mineral and sanguine 'veins', soily and cutaneous 'skin'—Wittie locates the spa-goer in a micro- and macrocosmic overlay presciently known as the water cycle, while carefully distinguishing the site-specific efficacy of Scarborough's water from similar springs around the world. A willing body materially taking in the waters of Scarborough does just that: waters infiltrate via ingestion or immersion and reach to the nerve endings ('terminat[ions]') with their restorative strength. Although 'wholesome' waters exist globally, *England*'s (not *Greenland*'s) are 'good' precisely because of the local terroir. The mineralogical image allows him to expand upon his ecumenical and cosmopolitan argument made earlier—'whether it runs East, West, North, or South, they [are] all indifferently good and wholesome' (Wittie 1660, 162)—but in a slightly more nationalistic 'vei[n]'. By coldly equating his countrymen's vascular makeup with the countryside's vaunted mineral networks, Wittie's spa and *Spaw* are conversant with the aforementioned notion of 'geohumoralism'. Following the logic of humoral theory, a cold, windy, and wet island like England should render its citizens prone to melancholic and phlegmatic characteristics. Some northern authors attempted to reframe this dynamic in their favour, drawing upon Aristotle instead of Hippocrates to argue that cool climates in fact *removed* these dullish humours instead of compounding them, leaving one hot, moist, and primed for colonialist action. Wittie, to be fair, did not have this kind of 'strengthening' in mind for Scarborough—'cheerfulness' appears to be his private goal—yet the *Spaw*'s nationalistic undertone intimates, nevertheless, the far from 'good' racial and ethnic repurposing of cold. His wintery minerals, for now, may steel the body's constitution in healthful, less harmful, ways.

Our tasting would probably end here. But while musing upon river water, one of the several 'sorts' (Wittie 1660, 46) he eruditely describes, Wittie worries that he has 'wade[d] too far into this stream, least I lose my self and my Subject' (Wittie 1660, 169). Contrary to his talk of ends, their progress would not terminate in an overheated body, at least, but perspire back out through the 'secret passages' (Wittie 1660, 195), or, pores, as he once revealed. (A self-regulating, evaporative cooling process more commonly known as sweating.) Wittie in the water, remarkably, starts to 'lose [his] self'. A corollary of geohumoralism was the dissolution of a unified, place-based identity. 'The environment', Floyd-Wilson continues, 'necessarily produced and destabilized early modern English selves' (Floyd-Wilson 2003, 4). In Wittie's case, the cryo- and hydro-components of his spa's seaside environment loosened the borders of somatic integrity as well. His overlay of 'veins' regulated via that body's specific environment advances upon Monardes's blue-blooded prescription, for it helps us to see the body's temperance, its 'wholesome'-ness, as reliant on regimens of minute temperature adjustments. At the same time, his template strains that same body's ability to stabilize itself, since it displays the ecological pressures of cold airs and waters constantly exerting themselves upon fleshly boundaries, checking that idea of 'wholeness' that a holistic spa, especially, would guarantee its soundest, most cryophilic customers. Confining mineral waters within any perimeter is an impossible task. With either a sip or a soak, in sum, the self (the 'Subject') becomes outspread. Inadvertently or not, the *Spaw's* regional advocacy offers a bracing lesson in ecological attachment, the 'trans-corporeal' (Alaimo 2016) and -national currents of cold. We depart along similar 'stream[s]' of thought, wondering about (and thereby enlarging) rather than resolving (and thereby constraining) the incompletion of interconnectivity, dwelling on parts not wholes, drinking to new possibilities rather than 'corroberating' what came before.

3 Feeling 'Exquisete' in the 'Extream'

Any imaginative possibilities nevertheless met sizable intellectual resistance from medical experts well-versed in cryo-genesis: both the creation of cold and the engendering of its ills. Cold's fruitive nature, I have suggested, existed on a physiological spectrum somewhere between 'good' and 'euill', sickness and health, internal and external, regional and universal. A modicum of cold could be prescribed every now and then, yet contact with snow and ice was to be avoided for the most part, leaving meteors' 'Impressiones' unwelcome and unwanted. Wittie's methods, simply put, were unorthodox; as such, his cryo-therapeutic insights, rendered dubious, could be roundly ignored. Surveying early modern climate history, it is not hard to see why the *Spaw*'s instructions proved difficult to swallow. When it was published in 1660, England had been enduring one of the harshest intervals of the Little Ice Age known as the 'Maunder Minimum' (1645–1715).[10] A year after Wittie's death, John Peter, a physician, penned *A Philosophical Account of This Hard Frost*, one of the most graphic descriptions of overexposure available at the time. Airborne 'Particles of Cold', 'Corpuscles of Cold' (Peter 1684, 3), and 'Atomes of Cold' (Peter 1684, 6), being 'conceived in the Frozen Womb of the Earth', coagulate into ice and snow after colliding with 'Liquid Watery Bodies' (Peter 1684, 3). Like Fulke, his foremost concern is the 'Impressions' (Peter 1684, 6) these 'Atomes' make upon himself and his fellow Londoners. Severe temperature swings from freezing to thawing are unhealthy because these fluctuations weaken the body's fortifications:

> [W]hat quarter then can we expect should be given to the various Juices of our Bodies? Can any Extream be Friendly to Nature? Can such sudden Alteration of the Weather prove otherwise, than mightily prejudicial to our Healths? Those Passages of our Bodies which were so long so closely lock'd up, will now be laid open, and become laxe and penetrable, liable to receive such Exotick putrefactive Ferments. (Peter 1684, 9)

The aftershock of cold, to put it another way, is profoundly dangerous. 'Exotick' (meaning exogenous) invaders can more easily seize someone whose pores *were* so strongly 'lock'd up'. Once inside these widened routes, and 'having undoubtedly imprinted on our Bodies such Morbisick predispositions (like seeds of various Diseases)' (Peter 1684, 6), the returning frost effectively shuts in the attacker. Peter's logic, then, helps explain why seemingly sealed-off bodies can still become unwell in the depths of an unrelentingly 'Hard' season like his own. '[I]n Cold,

[10]See Fagan (2000) for an accessible study of this approximately two-degree drop in Celsius.

Raw, Thawing Weather', particles 'insinuat[e] themselves into our gaping Pores', where 'they there stagnate' (Peter 1684, 9). Without adequate evaporation, in sum, the sickness ferments. It should be said that all parts of his prognosis—exposure to 'Extream' shifts in weather; unrestrained fermentation and unreplenished 'Juices'; the cultivation of previously-deposited spores—are in addition to the detriments that cold 'Particles' already pose on their own. The only remedy, in the end, is to see what sort of disease sprouts. There is no 'quarter', indeed, in Peter's estimation; one does not come in from the cold, the cold comes into you. The vulnerable body in and out (again) of winter awaits an inescapable fate: becoming a parasitical 'Womb' of ferment- and fomentation, a breeding ground for alien things eager to break forth upon first thaw and attach upon others. Catching a cold has never sounded so 'putrefactive', nor so terrifying.

As Peter's hostile and horrific imagery demonstrates, cold's animus became more acute in the seventeenth century, all but securing its irredeemable association with 'Extream' affliction. Wittie's *Spaw* had to contend, rightly, with this eco-catastrophic feeling, and professional allies were hard to find. Chapters on 'cold, an enemy to the Nerves and bones' in studies of natural philosophy, like *The Secret Miracles of Nature* divulged by the Dutch doctor Levinus Lemnius (1505–1568), remained commonplace (Lemnius 1658, 288). Cryo-phobic proclamations like his and Peter's insist that the 'enemy' eventually gets in. 'It hapneth sometimes' (Lemnius 1658, 289), so one should be ready for it. To 'help lims oppressed with cold' (Lemnius 1658, 290), for example, Lemnius advises (poorly) that one should soak and scrub the member with cold water, believing that 'snow and cold water raise up heat' (Lemnius 1658, 290). He, like many others, adhered to the classical idea of antiperistasis, ἀντιπερίστασις—Greek for 'against a standing round, circumstance'. This doctrine held that one circumstance (such as an increase in cold) sharpened its contrast (an increase in body heat). Combating cold with cold thereby makes sound medicinal sense, 'for by *antiperistasis* or *contrarietie*, the heat comes in the cold being driven away: which every man may make proof of, by handling Snow or Ice, for his hands will presently grow hot, and look very red' (Lemnius 1658, 290).[11] Lemnius could count on the benumbing experience being ubiquitous enough to state:

> I think there is no man but hath sometimes proved in himself, what bitter pains the joynts endure by reason of the nerves, that have a most exquisete feeling, when they grow stiffe with a more intense and peircing cold, the blood being either extinguished, or running inward into the inmost parts; so that at the first coming of cold, the hands will wax red, and by and by, as the blood grows cold, they will grow wan and dead, being deprived of the vitall blood and Spirits. (Lemnius 1658, 289)

It seems unlikely that Lemnius would describe the painful 'peircing' of cold as 'exquisete' with the connotations of beautiful and delicate. Instead, the 'exquisete' notes a heightened period of sensitivity, which he accurately ascribes to a decrease in circulation ('running inward') or a complete evacuation ('extinguished').[12] Lemnius's word choice introduces two physio-phenomenological aspects at once: it proves that to be 'benummed with cold', is, on the contrary, *to feel*, perhaps to feel an intensification of feeling itself. Un/comfortably numbed like so, what is marginal (the extremities) moves to the centre (the core) and vice versa, the body bravely adapting to the onslaught of cold stabs. Cold, that is, does not just reveal the body to be porous, but makes it more so. Lemnius agrees with Peter and Wittie on this somatic point, but his message, importantly, is a little less antagonistic. His outlook aligns, unexpectedly, with the latter. By using the literal meaning of the word, 'sought out', from the Latin *ex-* ('out') and *quaerere* ('seek'), he insinuates a different route for others—Wittie (1660), and now us—to take: those who proactively, not just defensively, 'sought' the cause of cold, who had

[11] Such redness is due to skin irritation, also known as 'ice burn,' rather than heated blood flow. Although it seems dangerously outmoded, the suggestion to rub frostbitten limbs with snow persists to this day.

[12] William Harvey's (1578–1657) discovery of circulation was but a quarter-century old. The numbness of hypothermia hurts because it triggers the pain receptors of nerves close to the surface of the skin; a similar hardship, hyperemia, is also unpleasant because the second-'coming' blood rush causes vessels to dilate too much, hitting these same nerves. Persons with Raynaud's disease have vessels that overreact to the cold, narrowing suddenly in a bout of vasospasm, and are thereby susceptible to both discomforts.

the nerve to find its origin after feeling its 'exquisete' touch. One reaction to this secretive, shivery, and sometimes-vicious realm of open/ing 'passages' and snarled 'veins' is, crucially, to stay in it.

4 Conclusion: Soaking with the Trouble[13]

Wittie's *Spaw*, far from an outlier, sits squarely therefore within the seventeenth century's heated debates over the nature of cold, dialogues that took place, no less, during the chilliest period of the Little Ice Age in the Northern Hemisphere. When explaining how an object's temperature stays the same and yet feels more or less cold to bodies' 'sensitive parts', Robert Boyle (1627–1691) referred to bathers in his seminal *New Experiments and Observations Touching Cold* (1665).[14] *Spaw*-seeking, or, seeking *through* spas; this, ultimately, is why Wittie's mineral winters matter still: not only was he conversant with the contentious cohorts of cryo-logists who took part in a larger climatological dialogue about their changing world, but he does so by locating the subject in inter/national waters, in 'peircing'-coldness that collapses hydro-spatial distance and human-nonhuman distinctions at the place of the skin. What an 'exquisete' feeling that was—*and that could be*. In *Biogea*, the late French polymath Michel Serres remembers the advice his mountain guide once gave him about the cold: 'If you curl up into a ball', he said, 'if you defend yourself and get dressed, the enemy will penetrate down to your liver: cold is more invasive than you. No. Present yourself, uncover yourself, go toward it, make it your friend; it'll respect you. Turn the *against* into a *for*'. Yet without going beyond the lethal limit' (Serres 2012, 175). This advice might seem useless to someone stuck in the ice,

[13] An homage to Donna Haraway's (2016) insightful phrase for engaging the ecological tensions of the present.

[14] 'This may be exemplified by what has been observ'd by those that frequent Baths, where the milder degrees of heat, that are us'd to prepare those that come in for the higher, seem very great to them that coming / out of the cold Air dispose themselves to go into the Hot Baths, but are thought cold and chilling to the same persons when they return thither out of much warmer places; which need not be wondred at, since those, that come out of the cold Air, find that of the moderately warm Room more agitated, then the cold Ambient would suffer the External Parts of their Bodies to be, whereas the same warm Air, having yet a less agitation then that in which the hotter parts of the Bath had put the sensitive parts of the Bathers Bodies, must seem cold and chilling to Them' (Boyle 1999, 4:230).

alone, waiting to die. Glaciers crumble, of course, and crises do happen. But Serres's point is that the cold keeps producing more. It births a sense of belonging: not how to live in a harsh world in which humans do not belong, and certainly not that the world belongs to us, but a belonging that means cohabiting the world with mineralogical beings that we cannot control, nor possess, nor objectify. Try *feel*; or, better yet, *drink*, *bathe*. Serres's 'lethal limit'—the 'edge'—is in dialogue with these early modern philosophers. While more alpine than aquatic, his epiphany is due to an immersive experience—one of Wittean proportions—within a cold atmosphere. To spa in this spot is to observe the union of life with death, the curls and furls of pain and pleasure. The question becomes how to 'make [cold] your friend', how to take the 'Extream' along with the 'exquisete', how to make 'good'. Here are chancy, accident-prone waters: what is left to test remains up for meditation. The experiment, the promise, of non-division is ours to try.

There is something to be learned by dipping into a cold *Spaw* (pace Hof), both in terms of what to do and what to resist. One parting 'Impression[e]' with which to leave you is this: the point ('limit') of lethality is important to consider, especially the question of *who* is more susceptible (penetrable) than others. Arctic communities, whose diets depend upon marine mammals like whale and seal, are, astonishingly, the most contaminated bodies on the planet at the moment. PCBs (polychlorinated biphenyls), pesticides, mercury, and other pollutants travel from south to north, where they sink and stay within food chains and flesh. The 'Arctic Paradox' appears permanent (Cone 2005). And while cold kills, so does the loss of it. 'If we allow the Arctic to melt', argues Watt-Cloutier, 'we lose more than the planet that has nurtured us for all of human history. We lose the wisdom that is required for us to sustain it' (Watt-Cloutier 2018, xx). Feeling cold in a seventeenth-century *Spaw* might not be the most relaxing experience, admittedly, because Wittie's wide-ranging 'veins' urge us to 'go toward' our warming waters, and their lethal tang, today. Emersion, in short, is not an option. There has never been an exit. As the historian of medicine, Roy Porter, puts it: 'the histories of the spa and of its surrounding balneological disciplines can serve as illuminating epitomes of medicine itself in the world we have lost' (Porter 1990, xii). But a cold world is one which primarily Indigenous communities are *losing* at present, which is precisely why a return, to feeling *with* wet, wintry others of the recent past offers a valuable lesson right now: it is in these brisk waters where we might learn how to brace ourselves for balmier futures, to build company better than before, and to soak in the uncertain 'beyond'.

Works Cited

Primary Sources

Aubrey, John. 1898. *Brief Lives*, ed. Andrew Clark. Oxford: Clarendon Press.

Bacon, Francis. 1627. *Sylva Sylvarum: Or a Naturall Historie in Ten Centuries*. London: John Haviland and Augustine Mathewes.

Barclay, Robert. 1625. *Argenis*, trans. Kingesmill Long. London: G. Purslowe.

Boyle, Robert. 1999. *The Works of Robert Boyle*, eds. Michael Hunter and Edward B. Davis. London: Pickering & Chatto.

Burton, Robert. 2001. *The Anatomy of Melancholy*, ed. Holbrook Jackson. New York: New York Review of Books.

Fulke, William. 1979. *A Goodly Gallerye*, ed. Theodore Hornberger. Philadelphia: American Philosophical Society.

Lemnius, Levinus. 1658. *The Secret Miracles of Nature in Four Books*. London: Jo. Streater.

Martin, Craig. 2011. *Renaissance Meteorology: Pomponazzi to Descartes*. Baltimore: Johns Hopkins University Press.

Monardes, Nicolás. 1580. *Historia medicinal de las coasas que se traen de nuestras Indias Occidentales*, trans. John Frampton. London: William Norton.

Peter, John. 1684. *A Philosophical Account of This Hard Frost from Whence Is Rationally Concluded What Effects It May Probably Have upon Humane Bodies, as to Health and Sickness*. London: Printed for Sam. Smith at the Prince's Arms in St. Pauls Church Yard.

Poor Robin. 1688. *Poor Robin's Book of Knowledge Shewing the Effects of the Planets, and Other Astronomical Constellations*. London: R. Wild.

Tulley, John. 1693. *An Almanack for the Year of Our Lord, MDCXCIII*. Boston: Benjamin Harris.

Wittie, Robert. 1660. *Scarbrough Spaw, or, a Description of the Nature and Vertues of the Spaw at Scarbrough in Yorkshire*. London: Printed for, and are to be sold by Charles Tyus, at the three Bibles on London Bridge, and by Richard Lambert in York, neer the Minster.

Secondary Sources

Alaimo, Stacy. 2016. *Exposed: Environmental Politics and Pleasures in Posthuman Times*. Minneapolis: University of Minnesota Press.

Bennett, Jane. 2010. *Vibrant Matter: A Political Ecology of Things*. Durham: Duke University Press.

Chiari, Sophie. 2019. *Shakespeare's Representation of Weather, Climate and Environment: The Early Modern 'Fated Sky'*. Edinburgh: Edinburgh University Press.

Cone, Marla. 2005. *Silent Snow: The Slow Poisoning of the Arctic*. New York: Grove Press.

Fagan, Brian. 2000. *The Little Ice Age: How Climate Made History 1300–1850*. New York: Basic Books.

Floyd-Wilson, Mary. 2003. *English Ethnicity and Race in Early Modern Drama*. Cambridge: Cambridge University Press.

Floyd-Wilson, Mary, and Garrett A. Sullivan Jr., eds. 2007. *Environment and Embodiment in Early Modern England*. New York: Palgrave Macmillan.

Haraway, Donna. 2016. *Staying with the Trouble: Making Kin in the Chthulucene*. Durham: Duke University Press.

Heninger, S.K., Jr. 1968. *A Handbook of Renaissance Meteorology*. New York: Greenwood Press.

Hof, Wim, and Koen de Jong. 2016. *The Way of the Iceman: How the Wim Hof Method Creates Radiant, Longterm Health—Using the Science and Secrets of Breath Control, Cold-Training and Commitment*. Little Canada: Dragon Door Publications.

Janković, Vladimir. 2000. *Reading the Skies: A Cultural History of English Weather, 1650–1820*. Chicago: University of Chicago Press.

Porter, Roy, ed. 1990. *The Medical History of Waters and Spas*. London: Wellcome Institute for the History of Medicine.

Serres, Michel. 2012. *Biogea*, trans. Randolph Burks. Minneapolis: Univocal.

Totaro, Rebecca. 2018. *Meteorology and Physiology in Early Modern Culture: Earthquakes, Human Identity, and Textual Representation*. New York: Routledge.

Watt-Cloutier, Sheila. 2018. *The Right to Be Cold: One Woman's Fight to Protect the Arctic and Save the Planet from Climate Change*. Minneapolis: University of Minnesota Press.

CHAPTER 12

Mineral Waters as a Treatment for Barrenness in Eighteenth-Century Britain

Sophie Vasset

In eighteenth-century England, barrenness is understood on a continuum: unlike our contemporary perception of infertility as the inability to conceive a child, a great variety of situations could be at the origin of a woman's (as the problem relied mostly on women) inquiry into fertility treatments (Oren-Magidor 2017). A common reason for barrenness given by doctors was the 'mechanical obstruction' of reproductive organs, that is to say, some malformation, protuberance or excrescence in the reproductive parts that could hinder either sexual penetration or the entrance of the sperm. Such a condition was often called 'impotence' in women, by contrast with barrenness in which no obvious sign of mechanical obstruction could be detected by the midwife or surgeon who would examine their patients (Vasset 2017). Female impotence, therefore, was a situation in which no conception was thought to occur.

By contrast, miscarriages were considered as signs of barrenness—they represented a constant worry for eighteenth-century women, as shown by

S. Vasset (✉)
UFR Études Anglophones, Université de Paris, Paris, France
e-mail: sophie.vasset@u-paris.fr

S. Chiari and S. Cuisinier-Delorme (eds.), *Spa Culture and Literature in England, 1500–1800*, Early Modern Literature in History,
https://doi.org/10.1007/978-3-030-66568-5_12

their writings, and remedies can be found in more than a few eighteenth-century midwife recipe collections.[1] Even stillbirths or the death of very young children, when repeated and in the absence of healthy, living children, led to being perceived as barren—Queen Anne's numerous pregnancies and unrelenting attempts at various treatments for barrenness is one of the most blatant examples of barrenness being understood as more than simply the inability to conceive (Oren-Magidor 2017). Secondary infertility, the twentieth-century term referring to the want of a second child, also broadens the concept of infertility and in times of high infant mortality, and reflects, among other, the pressure for a male heir: a lack of additional income for poorer families whose grown children would later support them, or the uncertainty of proper inheritance channels in wealthier families, caused women to look for treatment against barrenness.

In popular medical culture, barrenness was the object of overlapping medical theoretical frameworks that could be invoked within the same text to explain various forms of infertility. Firstly, as seen above, barrenness was made distinct from female impotence, which was presented as a physical obstruction preventing conception. Secondly, in mechanical medicine, a major theoretical trend of the early modern era, barrenness was thought to possibly result from the internal obstruction of the fluids. This idea was also commonly accepted in popular medical culture: for example, *The Ladies Physical Directory*, a popular health manual and collection of recipes from the middle of the century, states that 'Preparatory to the Cure of Infertility in either Sex; it is proper to use evacuation', and describes the ways in which this may be practised, with no connection to the reproductive system: 'Bleeding, lenient Purgatives such as the Solutive Electuary and a gentle Vomit of Ipecacuanha, especially if the Person be plethoric, or cacohymic, cannot but be of great Service' (An. 1727, xx). Thirdly, the humoral framework posited that excess and want regulated the body. The humoral qualities of the organs, whether cold, hot, moist or dry were summoned to account for their dysfunctions. For example, an excessively cold and moist womb was often presented as a cause of barrenness (Evans 2014, 69), as well as other symptoms. A recurrent subject in medical treatises on women's diseases is 'fluor albus' (or *the whites*) as a potential sign of infertility. 'Barrenness mostly proceeds from

[1] See Evans and Read (2015, 3–23).

the Fluor Albus, or too great a Quantity of the Whites (for few Women are without some)', writes the Lancaster surgeon man-midwife Henry Bracken in *The Midwife's Companion*, 'and that the Womb is thereby so continually moistened with slippery Matter, that the Semen or Seed (tho' of a viscours or slimy Nature) cannot be retained by it, but, either sooner or later, slips back again' (Bracken 1737, 20). Finally, excess and want could also affect the whole body, and Sarah Toulalan noted the recurrent trope of the meagre women and overweight men and women whose body frames were seen as barren by early modern medical authors (Toulalan 2017). The frontier between moral, religious and medical discourse was particularly blurred in these cases: excess in all its forms was to blame, as it often took the form of sin in the shape of gluttony, venery or idleness. At the opposite end of the moral and religious spectrum, want of desire and lack of orgasm or pleasure were recurrently invoked throughout the eighteenth century as reasons for barrenness, as Jennifer Evans has shown, and were fought by the use of aphrodisiacs.[2] Barrenness also lurked in the medical discourse against masturbation, prostitution or excessive venery, and was sometimes considered a consequence of venereal diseases, or of an intense mercury treatment which was prescribed for syphilis (Gallagher 2019).

No matter how desperate their cases were, patients were systematically encouraged to keep hope. Barrenness, it was argued in popular and official medical treatises alike, was not incurable. Treatments existed, ranging from the binary cures of humoral medicines based on diet and evacuation, to cure-alls such as the prolifick elixir. Maubray, whose writings on midwifery are a mix of social concern, common sense and quasi-magical remedies, encourages his reader to hope for a cure: 'I can scarce, because of either of *these*, call a *Woman* really BARREN; since I have known some of the most difficult of *these Cases* to have been duly *cur'd*, and diverse *Women* to have conceived, after many Years' (Maubray 1724, 385).

What were, in this context, the effects expected from mineral waters on barrenness? In this chapter, I will attempt some answers by looking at how popular medical cultures accounted for the fertilising powers of mineral waters. Next, I will look at how the cases of royal women, and especially of Queen Anne, had an impact on the popularisation of certain treatments.

[2] Evans's analysis goes against Laqueur's claim in *Making Sex* that the notion of orgasm as necessary for conception disappeared in the eighteenth century (Laqueur 1990; Evans 2014; Fissell 2004).

I will turn then to Scarborough, a smaller spa town than Bath or Royal Tunbridge Wells, and examine how literature and medicine interacted in the promotion of the use of the waters for barrenness.

1 The Mineral Water Cure in Popular Medical Treatises

Treatments for infertility were numerous. They were designed, sold and bought under a great variety of circumstances. They could be procured by doctor's prescription or through the apothecary's counsel, but they were also the result of family advice and might be prepared at home, following the guidelines of health manuals and recipe books. Recent scholarship has shown that a thorough study of treatment could not indeed be restricted to evidence of a doctor's prescription or official medical discourse. Lay medical knowledge, mostly held by women, was transmitted through medical recipes, published and unpublished, as the scholarly part of the 'recipe project' have shown.[3] Elaine Leong's work on the circulation of recipe books inside and outside of the domestic sphere, as well as Jennifer Evans's book on the role of aphrodisiacs have shown how treatment was co-designed by healthcare professionals and users, and transmitted across classes and generations (Leong 2018; Evans 2014). Mineral waters were thus part of this large pharmacopeia, and the waters were often taken in parallel with other types of treatment. Some mineral waters were more specifically identified as a fertility treatment such as the sulphurous waters of Bath or Buxton, and the chalybeate waters of Tunbridge Wells. The relation between specific indications for barrenness and the chemical composition of these waters—sulphurous (sulfur-based), chalybeate (iron-based), saline (sodium or magnesium based) or further mixes of the three—is unclear and hard to trace, even though chemical analysis was part of the due process of establishing the medical virtues of spas (Hamlin 1990; Coley 1990).

To understand how the waters could be prescribed for the cure of barrenness, it is best to start from the medical framework presented above. The effects of waters were accounted for by three major medical

[3] The scholars of this collaborative long-term online project gather, transcribe and make material on early modern receipts available to all, providing historical context and innovative analyses of the meaning and practices around early modern recipes (See 'The Recipes Project', online).

principles. First, impregnation could work internally (by drinking) and externally (by baths, showers and local application). According to this principle, the micro-elements of the water were thought to fortify the juices of the body, or conversely, attack the sick parts like a solvent. In the case of barrenness, it could help nourish the 'juices' if the organs were considered too weak, or dissolve an obstructing tumour. Motion was the second principle, as waters were thought to increase motion of the internal fluids: drinking the waters helped moving the fluids between the organs, whether it meant the digesting fluids or the humours, or the less material animal spirits, which could also clear inner blockages (Courvoisier and Kleiman-Lafon 2018). The third principle was hot and cold: the temperature of the waters would be seen as an active agent on the fibres of the body (muscles, nerves and skin), either too lax or too tense, and much was published in the eighteenth century on the effects of cold or warm baths, which were also prescribed as a domestic remedy.

The lists of ailments that waters could cure was long, as shown in the title page of a treatise on 'Berry's Shadwell Spaw', one of the spas of London which was not as famous as Islington or Hampstead, but was popular enough in mid-eighteenth-century London to have its salts extracted from the water, and sold for dying purposes:

> Directions for [the Use] of That Extraordinary Mineral-Water, Commonly Called, Berry's Shadwell-Spaw: In Sun- Tavern-Fields, Shadwell, near London. More Especially, in the Several Distempers Wherein It Has Proved / by Experience, of the Greatest Efficacy and Success; Such as Colds, Lax, or Weak Fibres, and Affected Nerves; the Palsy, Rheumatism, and Gout; the Yaws, Venereal Distempers, Gleets, and Fluor Albus; the Leprosy, King's-Evil, Scurvy, and Consumption; the Dropsy, Jaundice, Fistulas, and Ulcers; Fluxes, and Inward-Bleedings; Broken Constitutions by Intemperance, or Otherwise; the Diabetes, Sore-Eyes, Catarrhs, and Other Defluxions of Humours, &c. By Diederick-Wessel Linden, M. D.

The great variety of diseases which water treatment is supposed to alleviate might seem reminiscent of quack medicine and its recourse to some of the same rhetoric. As I have argued elsewhere, such retrospective statements do not help us understand either the cultural background in which those treatments were perceived or the potential relief they could procure patients. The author of the treatise on Shadwell Spa, Diederick-Wessel Linden, was no quack doctor: his work on mineral waters was extensive and much discussed in other medical treatises, and his methods included comparison with other mineral waters, especially with those of his native country, Westphalia. He analysed the chemical elements of the water, and presented several case histories, which were the common methods of the official medicine of the time. The long list of diseases, therefore, was both promotional—emphasising the successful cures—and pedagogical. Readers would not necessarily consider the use of waters for themselves if they did not identify, in the title page, the ailment they suffered from. This cloud of medical terms is meant to attract people with a variety of ailments, and even includes variations of the same. Markedly, the indications for barrenness is twice mentioned, as the waters cure the 'fluor albus' and 'Broken constitutions by *Intemperance*', which everyone would have understood at the time to be the consequences of venereal disease and mercury intake, well-known to cause barrenness.

2 Royal Visits

From 1680 to 1720, Tunbridge Wells and Bath were regularly visited by royal women who were struggling to have a child. The political, social and personal pressure exerted on these royal bodies to beget a male heir was, of course, extremely high. Their medical history is relevant for the history of barrenness as these women explored every possible treatment. In 1664, Catherine of Braganza and Charles II visited Tunbridge in hopes of future conception, to no effect. According to Evans, this did not hinder the growing reputation of water treatment (Denbigh 1981, 18) and after the visit of Catherine of Braganza to Tunbridge, 'water cures gained a reputation for treating reproductive disorders that extended to popular culture as well as to medicine' (Evans 2014, 147). Such visits were indeed documented and commented upon in periodicals and journals; they were celebrated by public festivities. As Bath and Tunbridge became centres of public interest for a few weeks' time, the royal visits greatly strengthened their reputation regarding barrenness. They also 'tied with wider ideas about sexuality' as Jennifer Evans explains, 'as fears were often expressed that the aristocracy were less fertile than the lower classes. Writers contrasted the vigorous and virile sexuality of the agricultural, rural classes and the "impotent nobility, whose sexuality was debilitated by urban luxury"' (Evans 2014, 25; Ganev 2007).

Thirty years later, Catherine of Braganza's niece, Anne, Princess of Denmark, later Queen Anne of England, endured eighteen pregnancies with no surviving heir at the end of the Stuart line. She was treated while she was still Princess of Denmark, a period during which she visited the Bath and Tunbridge Wells regularly. She made regular donations to the town of Tunbridge Wells until a request 'for the Upper Walk to be paved' she had made was not accomplished in due time (Denbigh 1981, 19). Her reliance on the waters to fight barrenness was encouraged by her numerous pregnancies. What's more, watering places were a convenient spot outside of the main political centre where political tensions would lead to the Glorious Revolution. Anne was at Bath when James abdicated, and she returned to find William of Orange on the throne (Green 1970, 42). Anne's persistence in finding a treatment for her barrenness, on top of what she understood at the time to be a form of internal gout, leaves very few first-hand accounts in spite of a prolific correspondence. A few allusions to her general medical condition or sympathies expressed to female relations who have just lost a child tell us of the permanent treatment she was receiving. In 1688, as she writes to her sister, she presents such cures as an escape from the Papist atmosphere at court:

> I intend, next week, and it please God, to go to Tunbridge, which the doctors tell me is the best thing I can do to hinder me from miscarrying when I am with child again. I confess I am very glad I am advised to go thither, for it is very uneasy to me to be with people that every moment of one's life one must be dissembling with, and put on a face of joy when one's heart has more cause to ache. (Gregg 2014, 59; BM, Loan 29/10/9)

Although at that time in her life, she had already miscarried four times and had lost her two baby daughters to the smallpox, she hoped for 'being with child again' and feared 'miscarrying again', turning to Tunbridge for a healthy pregnancy. She will show similar confidence early in the first year of her reign:

> I intend tomorrow (and it please God) to take physick in order to drink the spaw waters, which my doctors have adviced me to and I have a great inclination for them myself, hoping they may make my Lady Charlotte for unless I can compass that, it is feard my vaypours will rather grow upon me then decrease. (quoted in Gregg 2014, 106)

Anne perceived her barrenness and miscarriages to be connected to 'vapours', which could also be used to talk about a false pregnancy. She often invoked other physical reasons: most often her internal gout but also, earlier in her marriage, a brisk dance or a fall. She remained confined for several pregnancies, avoiding too much movement. Her getting ready to taking the waters by a preliminary treatment was characteristic of the prescriptions of the time: water treatment was thought to be potentially harmful if the body was underprepared. Anne's conclusion to her letter is yet another proof of the persistence of her hopes, and the political pressure that materialised in her sick body—she had to be carried to the throne for coronation because she was disabled at the time, and remained so until the end of her reign—to procure an heir to the Stuart line: 'I can never have any manner of hopes of the inexpressible blessing of another child, for though I do not flatter myself with the thought of it, I would leave no reasonable think undon that might be a means towards it' (Marlborough and Godolphin 1975, 186, n. 7). This poignant testimony of the resilience of barren women gives us a glimpse of the level of expectations that barren women could have from water cures, which were not in any way the pleasurable, relaxing experience advertised by twenty-first-century cultures of well-being, but a rather uncomfortable, perhaps painful experience of sweating and purging, at best.

Just before the Glorious Revolution, there was a triangular dynamic of barren royal women at court, as Mary of Modena, the Queen, struggled to conceive at the same time as her husband's daughters, Mary and Anne, from his first marriage with Anne Hyde. Anne's recurrent miscarriages and the loss of her two baby daughters was made even more ominous by the birth of Mary of Modena's son, whose legitimacy was questioned by the 'warming-pan scandal': the new-born was said to have been brought in a warming-pan while the whole birth was a fake. The powerful effect of Bath waters on barrenness is related in the hearings that followed the warming-pan scandal. Margaret Dawson, Mary's lady-in-waiting 'noted that previously the queen had been unable to conceive, but that following her visit to Bath, there was an alteration in her temperament that allowed her to bring a pregnancy to full term' (Oren-Magidor 2017, 29). The event left a permanent mark in Bath, with the gift of a cross by the royal couple as an acknowledgement for the effects of the water. It was an obvious sign of Jacobite sympathy, and the cross was taken down in 1783 when Thomas Baldwin, who had just been made architect of the City, redesigned the 'Cross Bath'.

The historiography of spas has been very much influenced by Royal visits and travel narratives, a form of writing which regularly mentioned spas and helped fashion the very identity of the town. Phyllis Hembry's book on English Spas traces the genealogy of such visits as the necessary components of economic success and a growing reputation as spa towns, which was certainly true. Although it is logical to assume such cures were limited to the elite who could afford travel and time off, the history of mineral waters, as Jérôme Penez or Anne Borsay have shown, should not be restricted to an aristocratic practice. First, because major spas like Bath, Harrogate, Cheltenham and Tunbridge had systems in place to subsidize for the poor (Borsay 1999), secondly because the number of spas available reached far beyond Tunbridge, Bath and Harrogate. In fact, there were numerous spas and wells of mineral waters all over the country: Phyllis Hembry's seminal study lists 152 towns with spas between 1515 and 1815. Local spas were used in smaller towns, as it was regularly recorded by water doctors, who often complained of the excessive drinking of potentially dangerous mineral waters by common people who used them with no prescription. Should the waters acquire the reputation to cure infertility, they would become part of the numerous cures that women from a great variety of social classes would attempt, sometimes prompted by their friends and families, sometimes by doctors, and which can still be read about in promotional material, broadside sheets and ephemera.

3 The Example of Scarborough in Literary Miscellanies

I would like to look beyond the main referential texts for spas, and beyond the two major spas of eighteenth-century England, Bath and Tunbridge Wells, to explore how the fertilising virtues of spas could be represented in smaller towns. Austen, Smollett and Burney's novels are regularly quoted in eighteenth-century studies of spa towns, for their protagonists visit Bath for health and leisure, making unexpected encounters that spice up the plot. Spas, however, were mentioned in many other genres, and more specifically in a form of literature quite Spopular at the time, the *Miscellanies*. Miscellanies were collection of the best poems, letters, epigrams and satirical pieces that were collected for a particular year. Their origins varied: some pieces came from periodicals, others (songs, particularly) from broadside sheets, some were published for the first time in the collection (Batt 2012). Title pages often targeted the visitors of one or several spas, as it was the case for The Bath, Bristol, Tunbridge and Epsom Miscellany. Containing, Poems, Tales, Songs, Epigrams, Lampoons, Satires, Panegyricks, Amours, Intrigues,

&c., published in 1735. Not all verse was satirical and many lyrical poems were praising the pastoral surroundings of the spas; their authors became known as the 'water poets' (Denbigh 1981; Vasset, 2022). 'Scarborough: a poem', published in *The Scarborough Miscellany for the Year 1733*, starts in a similar lyrical tone, as the narrator describes the towns and landscapes he travels through until he faces the prospect of the spa town on the sea:

> Thy Scenes, O *Scarborough!* tempt the vagrant Muse
> To roam thy Shades, and sip they healing Dews,
> To climb at early Down thy craggy Steep,
> And view bright *Sol* emerging from the Deep. (An. 1732, 10)

The poem then describes the beauties of the surroundings, and of the town itself, and proceeds to describe the socials scenes 'from Morn to Ev'ning view', starting with drinking the waters early in the morning:

> First at the Well they take the brackish Glass,
> And oft repeat, (for quick the Water pass)
> This purifies the Blood from Vicious Taints,
> And the Wan Cheek with blooming Beauty paints. (An. 1732, 10)

The tone remains lyrical even if the subject is medicinal: the allusion to the bloom of the cheek, often considered to be part of the British identity in eighteenth-century portraits, is the visible version of the invisible work of the waters on the blood. The narrator continues to praise the effects on the waters, and turns to its fertilising virtues, telling the story of Thomas St Quintin and his Wife:

> When languid Nature's genial Pow'rs decay,
> These Springs new Vigour to the Nerves convey,
> This Truth *St Quintin* knew, sev'n Years ally'd
> By *Hymen*'s Ties to a young beauteous Bride,
> Their anxious Breasts no Hope of Issue cheers,
> The Husband droops, the Wise dissolves the Tears,
> At Length advis'd to *Scarb'rough* Spring they flew,
> And e'er ten Moons their waingin Orbs renvew,
> The Pleasing Birth of an auspicious Boy,
> Dispels their Fears, and seals their mutual Joy. (An. 1732, 15)

Such a representation of a sterile couple striving together to take the waters is rare enough to be noted: in the vast majority of literary representations of infertility, as we will see in the next section, women are represented without their husbands. The poem stages a sentimental portrait of a couple expressing their shared sadness at the barrenness of their relationship. The level of anxiety, sadness and hopelessness expressed in the poem are also rare pieces of lyrical expressions of barrenness, more often dealt comically in other poems. Finally, the poem continues on a case of secondary infertility:

> But again for four successive Years,
> The matron's Womb no second Burthen bears,
> Again they droop, again the Spring repeat,
> And with a Female Birth their Joys compleat.
> *Ye barren Fair from ev'ry Climate come,*
> *Drink but these Waters and Mothers go home.* (An. 1732, 15)

Although blatantly promotional, the end of the poem becomes more critical of spas as cure for barrenness, dwelling on the abuses, the rumours and fashionable sociabilities, including the adulterous woman trope to be studied in the next section. Printed on the same page as the poem, a note gives a medical reference for this narrative development. It presents a case taken from a medical book, which, interestingly, is a local visit to the spa from a neighbouring Yorkshire town by a couple who was not part of the elite:

> Mr *Thomas St Quintin* of *Flamborough*, Yorkshire, and his wife, were seven Years and half married, during which time she had never conceived, upon Report of the Efficacy and Virtue of the Water, he brought her to *Scarborough*, where she drank fourteen Days; within a Month after she conceiv'd, which prov'd a Son: Then having a Interruption for four Years, he brought her to the Waters again; after a Fortnight or three Weeks, that she had left the Waters, she conceiv'd again; This prov'd a Daughter. (Wittie 1667, 191)

The medical reference plays several roles in such a context: it brings authenticity to the narrative, gives the poet the status of a learned writer, participates in the promotion of the spa and displaces the trope of the 'miracle cure' that was commonly associated with spas to that of a 'medical cure', referenced and studied. Of course, the limit between miracle cases and medical ones is unclear, especially in the case of barrenness, which according to Daphna Oren-Magidor was often lived as a deeply religious experience (Oren-Magidor 2017). Yet the choice of Wittie is quite relevant in the context of medical writings on spas at the time: Wittie's *Scarbrough--Spaw: Or a Description of the Nature and Vertues of the Spaw at Scarbrough Yorkshire* was not the only treatise written about Scarborough. Wittie, a Yorkshire physician himself, got involved in a controversy with William Simpson of York on the nature and virtues of the waters. According to J. A. R. Bickford and M. E. Bickford, the quarrel increased so much that it 'descended to the coffee houses of York' (Bickford and Bickford 2004). Until the mid-eighteenth century, the two authors were the main medical references on Scarborough Spa and their chemical analysis of the waters, although the very object of their disputes, gave the spa a medical history that pervaded the culture around it.

4 The Adulterous Woman Trope

One common belief about infertility in the eighteenth century, or more generally 'in the past', is that it was always, and often incorrectly, blamed on the woman. In fact, all medical treatises dealing with barrenness point out that either sex could be barren in a married couple, as common events would show. Indeed, many widows remarried and had children with their second husband. The debates on reproduction also gave much fertilising power to the male sex, which implied that infertility could rely on the man. And yet, a clear gender bias emerges as most treatments for barrenness targeted women, from medical recipes to mineral waters. The representation of barrenness in eighteenth-century literature confirms the gender bias, as it deals with the 'adulterous barren woman' trope, a term coined by Daphne Oren-Magidor in her book *Infertility in Early Modern England* (Oren-Magidor 2017, 108). She gives the example of John Eliot's 1658 poem about a barren women cured 'by the pipe, rather the water cock' and comments on the recurrence of comic stories of adultery in the context of barrenness: 'descriptions of the baths by the Earl of Rochester, Thomas Hobbes, Jonathan Swift and others all suggested that it was not the waters of the bath that were curing barren women who went there, but rather the sexual freedom associated with being away from their husbands and in the company of young women' (Oren-Magidor 2017, 109). She concludes that '[t]he trope of the adulterous barren woman was used to great humorous and satirical effect because it allowed a mockery of impotent or emasculated men while also strengthening the popular misogynist few of women as lustful and uncontrollable' (Oren-Magidor 2017, 109). I have shown elsewhere how such misogynist comments were particularly associated with travel narratives that abounded in anecdotes exoticizing religious rituals and treatments for infertility (Vasset 2019, 23–33).

The representation of mineral treatment for barrenness in early modern satire relies on the same narrative device: barren women are sent by their doctors to visit the waters, and end up sleeping with 'beaux', or the Doctors themselves. Many poems staged the licentious spirit of watering places, most famously by the Earl of Rochester on *Tunbridge Wells*, first published anonymously in 1675. Towards the end of the poem, a couple looking for 'means to increase their family' turns to the waters on the advice of a midwife:

> Thy silly head! For here walk Cuff and Kick,
> With brawny back and legs and potent prick,
> Who more substantially will cure thy wife,
> And on her half-dead womb bestow new life.
> From these the waters got the reputation
> Of good assistants unto generation. (Rochester 1968, 143–148)

The 'potent prick', presented as the key to cure infertility, objectifies the two men, restricting their masculinity to hair and erection. In parallel, the woman is reduced to her reproductive organs: her 'half-dead womb' is cured by penetration, as the joke implies this womb has lost life because of the impotence of the husband.

Other satirical pieces I have come across are more indirect: for example, the scurrilous satirical piece entitled *An Exclamation from Tunbridge and Epsom against the Newfound Wells at Islington*, as the title suggests, stages a bitter diatribe against one of the London Spas. It became very popular in the early eighteenth century and was even called 'The New Tunbridge Wells':

> Here [in Tunbridge and Epsom] disappointed wives met with seasonable Refreshments; the barren by virtue of our *Metalsome* Waters, and the application of and *able Doctor* behind a bush, found Nature relieved, grew fruitful and blest with their rejoicing husbands with many a hopeful *Heir*. (An. 1684, 2)

Rochester's rakes, 'Cuff and Kick', are here replaced by an 'able', potent doctor who will replace the impotent and absent husband, confirming once more the double standard of misogyny and mockery of impotence evidenced by Daphne Oren-Magidor.

Along a very similar line, *A Letter from* Tunbridge *to a Friend in* London *being a character of the Wells, and Company there*, published in the 1714 *The Tunbrige and Bath Miscellany*, and adapted from a 1713 issue of Steele's periodical, *The Guardian*, describe the spas' merits as such: 'The chief Virtue ascrib'd to these Waters are the following two: they very often cure the Greensickness in Maids, and cause Fruitfulness in Marry'd Women, provided they are but properly administered by a young physician' (An. 1714, 7). Greensickness in maids is a disease that was ascribed to young virgins, who had a variety of symptoms such as melancholy, winds or *pica* (eating dirt), coming from their unsatisfied desires. Barrenness becomes the married woman's pendant for greensickness, and pleasurable sex is the therapy.

In another miscellany the comic piece 'BATH, A Song – On the Multiplying Virtues of the Bath Waters, Humbly inscrib'd to the Citizen's Wives' was to be sung to the lively and gay 'Tune of, *How long, egregeous* Moore, &c'.[4] The original song compares 'human race and worms' to the advantage of the worm and starts as a pastoral, evoking nature and healing in four verses:

> What might(y) Wonders have been done
> By *Bath*'s alluring Streams
> Shou'd I thro' all their Courses run,
> Some wou'd appear like Dreams. (An. 1735, 13)

After the fifth stanza, the tone changes as the poet mentions the ambiguity of the effects of the water cure. Water can corrupt bodies and manners; they can kill, or even worse, bring shame to respectable families:

> VI
> These Waters, by Experience found,
> From Death do Thousands save;
> With many Vertues they abound,

[4] The tune of 'How Long, Egregious More' was found in *The Convivial Songster* (1784, 225).

Yet send some to the Grave.

VII.
Three Brace of Does, plump, fat, and sleek
Each had a Jet-black Scut,[5]
From *London* came in *Passion-Week*,
And soon began to Rut.

VIII.
The stimulating Salts began
To put their Blood in Mo(tion);
They tired each Doctor to a Man,
Who were at their Devo(tion).

IX.
In *London* long they had been deem'd
Barren as desert Ground,
But now they fruitful are esteem'd,
For they are Pregnant found

X.
Their Pregnancy, as some Folks say,
Was caus'd by *Change of Diet*;
They jaunt, they dance, or sing all Day;
At Night they are not quiet.

XI.
Their Husbands Heads may ack for this;
Their Wives must bear the Blame;
And what they call the *Bliss of Bliss*,
Will terminate in Shame. (An. 1735, 13)

The song playfully revisits the medical theories on mineral waters: motion (as one would expect in a song) is at the heart of early eighteenth-century medicine, as presented earlier. The waters 'put the blood in motion', their potential danger ('send some to the grave') is either an implication that they can be toxic or that they have a real medicinal effect, and as any *pharmakon*, kill or cure. As for the 'stimulating salts', other than the lovely assonance, the expression recalls aphrodisiacs while referring to the minerals (salts were often sold in spa towns like Cheltenham or Epsom).

[5] The mark of venereal disease.

5 Conclusion: The Persistence of Hope

One of the common traits that medical treatises, letters from royal women, lyrical poems and comic jokes have in common is that they all present barren people, most of them women, in a long course of treatment. If the case of Queen Anne is certainly the most extreme and her persistence in taking the waters certainly heightened by political pressure, it mirrors the degree of trust that women or couples could have in the mineral waters, as shown by the example of St Quintin and his wife in Scarborough. In a culture that had become suspicious of miracles, especially those associated with waters that might have been praised as holy waters in the past, the recurrent joke on the 'real nature' of the cure and its adulterous origins was a counterpoint to the high expectations created by medical and popular literature on spas.

Works Cited

Primary Sources

An. 1684. *An Exclamation from Tunbridge and Epsom Against the Newfound Wells at Islington*. London: J. How.

An. 1714. *The Tunbridge and Bath Miscellany for the Year 1714: Giving an Exact Description of Those Places, with Characters of the Company. To Which Is Added, the Lampoon, and Some Other Pieces Written There Last Summer*. London: printed for E. Curll at the Dial and Bible against St. Dunstan's Church in Fleet-Street.

An. 1727. *The Ladies Physical Directory: Or, a Treatise of All the Weaknesses, Indispositions and Diseases Peculiar to the Female Sex from Eleven Years of Age, to Fifty or Upwards. By Which Woman and Maids of the Meanest Capacity May Perfectly Understand the Symptoms, Nature, and True Cause of Their Own Illnesses, and Readily Know How to Manage Themselves under All Their Infirmities*. London: Two Blue Posts.

An. 1732. *The Scarborough Miscellany: An Original Collection of Poems, Odes, Tales, Songs, Epigrams*. London: J. Roberts.

An. 1735. *The Bath, Bristol, Tunbridge and Epsom Miscellany. Containing, Poems, Tales, Songs, Epigrams, Lampoons, Satires, Panegyricks, Amours, Intrigues, &c.* London: T. Dormer.

Bracken, Henry. 1737. *The Midwife's Companion; Or, a Treatise of Midwifery*. London: J. Clarke.

Ibbetson, J.C. 1793. *A Picturesque Guide to Bath, Bristol Hot-Wells, the River Avon, and the Adjacent Country: Illustrated with a Set of Views*. London: Hookham and Carpenter, Bond-Street.

Linden, Diederick Wessel. 1749. *Directions for [the Use] of That Extraordinary Mineral- Water, Commonly Called, Berry's Shadwell-Spaw: In Sun- Tavern-Fields, Shadwell, Near London. More Especially, in the Several Distempers Wherein It Has Proved by Experience, of the Greatest Efficacy and Success; Such as Colds, Lax, or Weak Fibres, and Affected Nerves; the Palsy, Rheumatism, and Gout; the Yaws, Venereal Distempers, Gleets, and Fluor Albus; the Leprosy, King's-Evil, Scurvy, and Consumption; the Dropsy, Jaundice, Fistulas, and Ulcers; Fluxes, and Inward-Bleedings; Broken Constitutions by Intemperance, or Otherwise; the Diabetes, Sore-Eyes, Catarrhs, and Other Defluxions of Humours, &c*. London: Printed for the proprietor; and to be had at the Shadwell-Spaw, in Sun-Tavern-Fields, Shadwell; and F. Jones, Mineral Water Purveyor to His Royal Highness the Duke of Cumberland.

Marlborough, John Churchill, and Sidney Godolphin. 1975. *The Marlborough-Godolphin Correspondence [1707–1710]*, vol. 1, ed. Henry L. Snyder. Oxford: Clarendon Press.

Maubray, John. 1724. *The Female Physician: Containing All the Diseases Incident to That Sex, in Virgins, Wives, and Widows; Together with Their Causes and Symptoms, Their Degrees of Danger, and Respective Methods of Prevention and Cure*. London: James Holland.

Rochester, John Wilmot. 1968. *The Complete Poems of John Wilmot, Earl of Rochester*, ed. David M. Vieth. New Haven, CT: Yale University Press.

Wittie, Robert. 1667. *Scarbrough--Spaw: Or a Description of the Nature and Vertues of the Spaw at Scarbrough Yorkshire Also a Treatise of the Nature and Use of Sea, Rain, Dew, Snow, Hail, Pond, Lake, Spring, and River-Waters, Where More Largely the Controversie Among Learned Writers, About the Original of Springs Is Discussed*. York: A. Broad.

Secondary Sources

Batt, Jennifer. 2012. Eighteenth-Century Verse Miscellanies. *Literature Compass* 9 (6): 394–405.

Bickford, J.A.R., and M.E. Bickford. 2004. Wittie [Witty], Robert. *Oxford Dictionary of National Biography*. https://doi.org/10.1093/ref:odnb/53735 (accessed October 26, 2020).

Borsay, Anne. 1999. *Medicine and Charity in Georgian Bath: A Social History of the General Infirmary, c. 1739–1830*. Aldershot: Ashgate.

Coley, N.G. 1990. Physicians, Chemists, and the Analysis of Mineral Waters: "The Most Difficult Part of Chemistry". *Medical History. Supplement* (10): 56–66.

Courvoisier, Micheline, and Sylvie Kleiman-Lafon. 2018. Actes du colloque 'Les Esprits Animaux. *Épistémocritique*. https://epistemocritique.org/actes-du-colloque-les-esprits-animaux/ (accessed October 26, 2020).

Denbigh, Kathleen. 1981. *A Hundred British Spas: A Pictorial History: With 42 Maps and 81 Illustrations Based on Old Prints and Photographs*. London: Spa Publications.

Evans, Jennifer. 2014. *Aphrodisiacs, Fertility and Medicine in Early Modern England*. Woodbridge: The Boydell Press.

Evans, Jennifer. 2015. The One-Sex Body on Trial: The Classical and Early Modern Evidence. *Journal of the History of Medicine and Allied Sciences* 70 (3) (July 1): 464–466.

Evans, Jennifer, and Sara Read. 2015. 'Before Midnight She Had Miscarried': Women, Men, and Miscarriage in Early Modern England. *Journal of Family History* 40 (1) (Winter): 3–23.

Fissell, Mary E. 2004. *Vernacular Bodies: The Politics of Reproduction in Early Modern England*. Oxford University Press.

Gallagher, Noelle. 2019. *Itch, Clap, Pox: Venereal Disease in the Eighteenth-Century Imagination*. New Haven: Yale University Press.

Ganev, Robin. 2007. *Milkmaids*, Ploughmen, and Sex in Eighteenth-century Britain. *Journal of the History of Sexuality* 16 (1): 40–67.

Green, David Brontë. 1970. *Queen Anne*. London: Collins.

Gregg, Edward. 2014. *Queen Anne*. New Haven: Yale University Press.

Hamlin, C. 1990. Chemistry, Medicine, and the Legitimization of English Spas, 1740–1840. *Medical History. Supplement* (10): 67–81.

Laqueur, Thomas Walter. 1990. *Making Sex: Body and Gender from the Greeks to Freud*. Cambridge, MA: Harvard University Press.

Leong, Elaine Yuen Tien. 2018. *Recipes and Everyday Knowledge: Medicine, Science, and the Household in Early Modern England*. Chicago: Chicago University Press.

Leong, Elaine, and Lisa Smith. The Recipes Project. https://recipes.hypotheses.org (accessed October 26, 2020).

Oren-Magidor, Daphna. 2017. *Infertility in Early Modern England*. Basingstoke: Palgrave Macmillan.

Toulalan, Sarah. 2017. "If Slendernesse Be the Cause of Unfruitfulnesse; You Must Nourish and Fatten the Body": Thin Bodies and Infertility in Early Modern England. In *The Palgrave Handbook of Infertility in History*, ed. Gayle Davis and Tracey Loughran, 171–197. London: Palgrave Macmillan.

Vasset, Sophie. 2017. Female Impotence or Obstruction of the Womb? French Doctors Picturing Female Sterility in the 1820s. In *The Palgrave Handbook of Infertility in History*, ed. Gayle Davis and Tracey Loughran, 311–333. Palgrave Macmillan, London.

Vasset, Sophie. 2019. The Circulation of Anecdotes on Female Barrenness in the Eighteenth Century. In *Intermediality and the Circulation of Knowledge in the Eighteenth Century*, ed. Peter Wagner, 23–33. LAPASEC n°6. Wissenschaftlicher Verlag Trier.

Vasset, Sophie. 2022. *Murky Waters: Spas in British Medicine and Literature in the Long Eighteenth Century*. Manchester: Manchester University Press.

CHAPTER 13

Drowning in Health: Murky Perceptions of Mineral Water and Alcohol in Eighteenth-Century Medical Literature and Social Mores

Vaughn Scribner

In 1768, Diederick Wessel Linden—a German physician-turned-English-mineral spring water-expert—related an odd anecdote involving mineral water and ale. Apparently, 'a gouty, gummy, bloated habit of body' drove one London coachman into the country tavern trade. Hoping to brew his own beer, the coachman dug a well in his new tavern. At forty feet, he discovered mineral water infused with 'coarse salt' and 'marle [calcium-rich] earth, which made the water soft'. The tavern keeper's first batch of mineral water-brewed ale came out 'uncommonly fine', which delighted him. And the more he drank, the more he realized that 'the quality of the ale was so greatly cathartic, that a quart of it was a strong dose'. The mineral water had turned his ale into a purging physic, infused with

V. Scribner (✉)
Department of History, University of Central Arkansas, Conway, AR, USA
e-mail: vscribner@uca.edu

S. Chiari and S. Cuisinier-Delorme (eds.), *Spa Culture and Literature in England, 1500–1800*, Early Modern Literature in History,
https://doi.org/10.1007/978-3-030-66568-5_13

salt and minerals but without 'any other taste uncommon to malt liquor [that] could be perceived!' Soon thereafter, the tavern keeper invited his friends for a house-warming party where 'the fine ale was not spared'. But when the guests began to vomit (i.e. 'purge') their mineral water ale, they accused their host—'remarkable [...] for playing tricks to cause mirth'—of spiking the ale with Jalap (a purgative drug), and left the house in a huff. Linden explained that the tavern keeper continued to drink the medicinal ale by himself, and 'tho' it daily purged him briskly, yet it never weakened, but on the contrary invigorated him [...] And he had the satisfaction of being cured from his gout'. The mineral water ale's healing reputation soon gained steam after a clergyman touted its benefits, 'as several others have done since' (Linden 1768, 55–58).

Linden's recollection demonstrated the murky, but inherent, overlap between mineral water and alcohol in eighteenth-century medical literature and social mores, as well as ongoing arguments over the health of both consumables. In this case, the supposed medicinal qualities of mineral water coalesced with the salubrity of ale to create the ultimate elixir. Yet, mineral water and alcohol were not always so curative, nor were their consumers and observers so sure of their propriety for the health of the human body, or civil society, for that matter.

Although historians often link the eighteenth century with 'enlightened' progress, especially relating to medicine and nature, contemporary opinion regarding the 'health' of ingesting mineral water and alcohol remained confusing at best, and contradictory—even dangerous—at worst. Modern science generally equates consuming water with health and alcohol with illness, but eighteenth-century Britons hardly relied upon such dyads. Rather, these two consumables were inverse, reciprocal, and competitive, often all at the same time. This chapter argues that perceptions of mineral-infused water and alcohol—and coinciding public spaces around these consumables—especially reveal the murkiness of health, science, and social order in the eighteenth-century Atlantic World.

Eighteenth-century physicians and leaders found themselves at an impasse. Just as mineral water might heal the sick and indigent, so too might its overconsumption or mishandling lead to illness or even death. Alcohol, similarly, was often touted as a medicine and social lubricant by those very men who damned it as a poison to human and societal health. Many of the same arguments raged over mineral spas and taverns: how were citizens to govern these popular public spaces according to the most current notions of health and civility? There was no easy answer.

Modern historians have echoed their eighteenth-century predecessors' lack of consensus regarding the consumption of mineral water and alcohol. A litany of scholarship exists on eighteenth-century consumption of, and attitudes towards, alcohol and mineral water, respectively, but a comparative study of these two beverages and their coinciding public spaces proves elusive (Porter 1990; Hembry 1990; Borsay 2012, 155–169; Hardy 1984, 250–282; Scribner 2016, 409–449; Clark 1983; Cowan 2005; Jennings 2016; Nicholls 2009; Salinger 2002; Curl 2010). As historian Phil Withington recently remarked, 'while the historiographical interest in intoxication is clearly extensive [...] it also makes for a somewhat fractured and disparate field of enquiry'. Withington continued by lamenting the absence of alcohol 'treated together' with other consumables (Withington 2014, 16–17). A handful of scholars have 'treated' mineral water and alcohol together, but have almost always considered them as opposing forces to demonstrate the rise of addiction studies and the temperance movement (Porter 1985, 385–396; Clark 1988, 63–84). Similarly, various volumes consider taverns and spas in the same chapter on 'public pleasures' or the 'topography of pleasure', but do not critically compare these two spaces, their consumables, or their place in the 'health' of British and transatlantic societies (White 2012, 293–344; Porter 1994, 169). As this chapter demonstrates, alcohol, mineral water, taverns, and spas must be understood as homogenous rather than heterogenous; inverse, reciprocal, and competitive consumables and consumer spaces which necessarily defined eighteenth-century Westerners' ever-evolving, ever-contradictory, notions of bodily and societal health.

'Health' and 'medicine' remained developing-but-mercurial concepts in the eighteenth-century. Defined by the Englishman, Samuel Johnson, in 1755 as 'freedom from bodily pain or sickness [...] welfare of mind; purity; goodness; principle of salvation', health became a catch-all for citizens, well and ill alike. Medicine ('any remedy administered by a physician', according to Johnson), meanwhile, became the vehicle for a band of physicians more than happy to claim they were able to cure the litany of ailments which seemed to multiply by the day (Johnson 1785, n.p.). Because notions of health and medicine were still (and still are) developing around simultaneous ideologies of nature, science, and humanity, so too were those men and women who professed to have the cures.

While vernacular healing retained its ties to magic and religion, a new sort of healer—the professional physician—appeared in the eighteenth century. Yet he did not bring clear answers. As historian Roy Porter noted, 'the eighteenth century has been dubbed the golden age of quackery [...] hardly any eighteenth-century scientific advance helped heal the sick directly [...] the net contribution of physicians to the relief and cure of the sick remained marginal' (Porter 1997, 266, 284). Armed with a paltry education (a brief stint at a hospital or a few lectures on anatomy) and a need for funds, physicians generally did more harm than good in their supposed healing regimes. As the English poet, Matthew Prior, barbed in 1714, 'Cur'd yesterday of my Disease, I died last night of my Physician' (Prior 1835, 208).

Eighteenth-century medicine often dissolved into outright dissension among its squabbling ranks (Harley 1990, 138–164; Coley 1990, 67–81). Should Herman Boerhaave's theories of the human body as a network of pipes and vessels which controlled the body fluids be trusted as the basis of health, or should new research into the body and soul, anatomy, or more complicated mechanical theories of the body overturn Boerhaave's seemingly reductionist assertions? Physicians became symbols of all that was good and bad in the supposed advancement of health and medicine: they agreed on everything and nothing, hammering out tracts in an attempt to demonstrate their supremacy in physic and healing and, hopefully, gain a coterie of wealthy clients determined to bask in all the modern luxuries of health, science, and sociability.

1 Intoxicating Brews

This is where mineral water and alcohol came in. As critical beverages in the eighteenth-century British Atlantic World, mineral water and alcohol served as key representations of larger confusions surrounding bodily health. Mineral water—a mysterious tonic infused with strange ingredients from the innards of the earth—sprang forth as a mystical representation of nature's wonders. Popular vernacular had long attributed magical qualities to mineral springs, with lore of holy intervention and healing marking these bubbling, stinking spigots. Britons accordingly flocked to various springs throughout England, Wales, Scotland, Ireland, North America, and the Caribbean in search of divine intervention at best, and perhaps a luxurious, relaxing experience at worst (Hembry 1990, 1–3). Yet even with the supposed modernity of the

Enlightenment, eighteenth-century physicians remained just as confused as laypeople regarding mineral waters' medicinal properties. These self-appointed medical maestros used a carefully constructed toolbox of scientific methods to 'explore the *Secrets* Earth contains' (Linden 1752, xii–xiii) and hopefully harness these 'fountains of health' (Smythson 1785, 597). In doing so, they defined mineral water as a 'liquor' which might heal or harm the human body, according to consumption patterns and guidance.

Alcohol, meanwhile, remained a staple of British society. Most Britons trusted alcohol far more than water (pure or mineral) and relied upon it as their main beverage: babies slurped nips of spiced wine, while adults engaged in a seemingly endless flow of alcoholic beverages, ranging from 'small beer' to fuel labourers' calorie-depleting days to night-time bowls of inebriating rum punch. Yet, as with mineral water, physicians began to view alcohol as a beverage that might do as much harm as good if not consumed correctly. They weren't necessarily wrong. After all, the 'gin craze' of the 1730s crippled London, and white, male North American colonists consumed an average of seven shots of hard alcohol a day, in addition to beer, cider, and wine (Clark 1988, 63–84; Rorabaugh 1991, 17). As the eighteenth century progressed, physicians approached alcohol and mineral water with equal measures of hope and caution. They could both cause death, not to mention the disintegration of Western society.

Eighteenth-century British physicians considered mineral water, like alcohol, an intoxicant; a substance which they believed might engender an 'altered state' of human consciousness and bodily control (Humphrey 2001, 585). Taking this into account, physicians often used the same terms to describe alcohol and mineral water: e.g. 'brew', 'distill', 'ferment', 'liquor', and 'spirits' (Monro 1770, 9; Linden 1752, 3–4, 45–49, 70, 143, 165–166; Linden 1768, 15–17; Sutherland 1764, 26, 66, 149; Hales 1739, xxviii, 60). In 1793, furthermore, the English physician, Thomas Beddoes, argued that 'dizziness with a degree of intoxication, is a very common effect of liquors containing carbonic acid'. He continued to explain Pyrmont (Germany) mineral water 'occasions a glow, exhilaration, and confusion of ideas similar to that which follows the use or abuse of spirituous liquors', finally adding that Siberia had a mineral spring which locals called 'the well of drunkenness' (Beddoes 1793, 8–9).

Linden, similarly, repeatedly compared the production of mineral water to that of alcohol. In one case, Linden wondered how fellow physicians could label mineral waters according to only one of their many compounds, exclaiming, 'Would not the Brewer be laughed at if he called Water Beer, though Water is the Chief Ingredient? But it cannot be called Beer, unless the whole Mixture is compleat: I think the same of Vitriol'. Later in the same work, Linden clarified the use of 'fermentation' regarding mineral waters, referred to the chalybeate waters of Tunbridge Wells, England as 'liquor', and compared the mineral water of Shadwell Spa (right outside London) to multiple alcoholic beverages: not only was the Shadwell water 'of a light *Yellow*, nearest the Colour of the *French Brandy*', but it also 'sparkles when poured into a Glass, like a fermented vegetable Juice, such as *Cyder*' (Linden 1752, 3–4, 46–49, 70, 143). Some physicians followed the lead of ale brewers by trying to 'brew' their own 'artificial chalybeates' (see Fig. 1), while others bottled mineral waters for exportation (Lewis 1784, 89; Priestley 1772; Linden 1752, 53; McIntyre 1973, 1–19). Another English physician, finally, worried about the accuracy of mineral water analysis, since every nation utilized alcoholic measurements (wine gallons, ale gallons, pints), which differed according to country (Monro 1770, xi). Though modern consumers are more likely to understand one as artifice and the other as coming from the natural world, contemporary imbibers thought mineral water and alcohol were two sides of the same coin; mysterious liquors brewed, distilled, and fermented by the hand of nature for man's careful consumption.

Physicians also applied near-identical categorization to mineral water and alcohol in their quest to order the natural world. In 1770, the English physician to His Majesty's Army and St. George's Hospital, Donald Monro, published *A Treatise on Mineral Waters*. Effectively a compendium of scholarship on mineral waters over the past two centuries, the book was organized by 'dividing each kind [of water] into such classes as appeared most likely to give a clear and distinct idea of their nature, and properties'. He provided the 'general characteristics' and 'virtues' of each water before adding other scholars' reflections on each water (Monro 1770, xiii–ix). Order and classification proved paramount to the effectiveness of Monro's organization, with temperature and clarity defining the extremes of the scale (cold pure water at one end, and hot mineral water at the other).

As demonstrated by Fig. 2, Monro believed that pure water, which he termed a 'liquor', was most 'proper [...] for the common uses of life', and could thus be consumed more regularly with fewer dangers. Yet pure water also contained fewer benefits compared to mineral water, which rested on the other extreme of the scale. Monro asserted that hot mineral

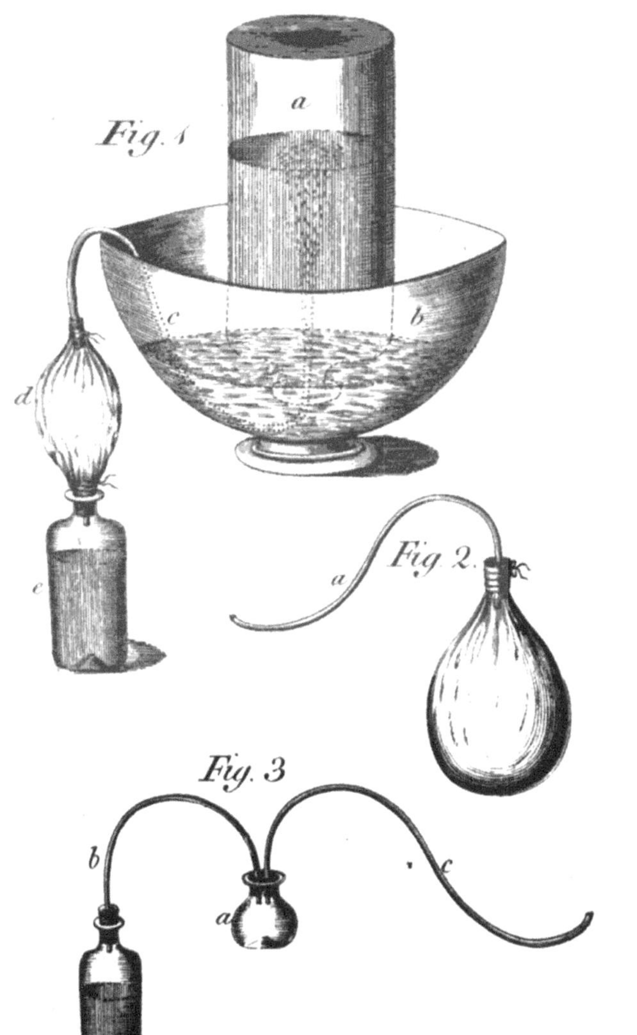

Fig. 1 'Priestley's Illustration of Creating Artificial Chalybeate Water', in Joseph Priestley, *Directions for Impregnating Water with Fixed Air; In Order to Communicate to It the Peculiar Spirit and Virtues of Pyrmont Water, and Other Mineral Waters of a Similar Nature* (London: J. Johnson, 1772)

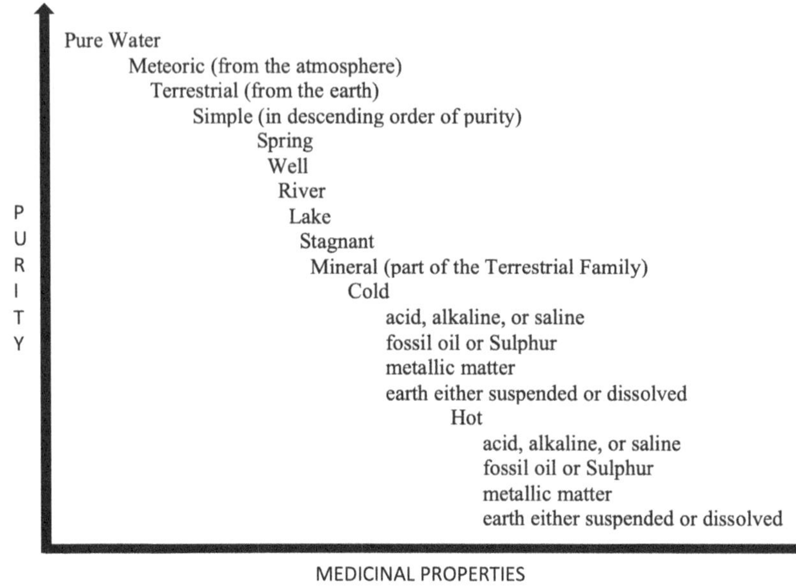

Fig. 2 'Monro's Water Chart', created by Vaughn Scribner from Donald Monro, *A Treatise on Mineral Waters*, vol. 1 (London: D. Wilson and G. Nicol, 1770)

water promised the greatest possibilities to cure 'many disorders incident to the human body', yet also might do more harm than pure water because of its heat and un-checked mineral content (i.e. lack of purity). Ordering the natural world proved problematic. The renowned physician had to admit that 'a great difficulty arises in classifying [mineral waters] properly; for we seldom meet with any which are impregnated with one matter only; but generally with several'. He subsequently grouped each mineral water according to the most prevalent substance, but with the qualification, 'tho' at the same time the water may be impregnated with other matters, which might seem to entitle it to be put in another class' (Monro 1770, v, 3–4, 9, 14–15).

Only fourteen years later, the American physician, Benjamin Rush, and the English physician, John Lettsom (whom Rush had met while studying in England), co-produced a 'moral and physical thermometer' which echoed Monro's ordering of waters. Published in Rush's 1784 *an Inquiry into the Effects of Spirituous Liquors in the Human Body* and Lettsom's *History of Some of the Effects of Hard Drinking* (1786), the 'thermometer' (Fig. 3) charted the healthiness (physical and mental) of consumables ranging from drinking water on one end to consuming 'drams of Gin, Brandy and Rum' throughout the day and night on the extreme end of intemperance and ill-health:

Here was a 'modern' assessment of alcohol and water consumption, replete with the dangers of intoxication according to standards of mental and physical health. Rush and Lettsom also, importantly, both imitated and built upon Monro's organization of water's gradations of salubrity in their chart, thereby further demonstrating the overlap of mineral water and alcohol in the eighteenth-century. But would people listen? Did they even care?

2 Mineral Water: A Medicine (in Moderation)

Arguing that Great Britain had 'a greater number and variety of waters than in any part of Europe' (Ruddy 1757, v), British physicians studied mineral waters in gulps. Yet, they seemed to spit out as much as they swallowed. Practically, physicians approached mineral waters according to contemporary notions of medicine, which led them to organize their studies of mineral waters into three stages. First, they hoped to understand the physical characteristics of mineral waters (colour, smell, and temperature, especially). Second, they applied a variety of chemical tests, both to liquid water and its evaporated residue, to determine the composition of the waters. Third, they surveyed—through personal and anecdotal observations—certain medicinal effects of the waters. Since modern germ theory did not yet exist, physicians did not study the 'quality' of the water. Rather, laypeople and physicians alike judged water according to its clarity, taste, and smell. Unfortunately, they agreed on little else (Hardy 1984, 254; Tomory 2014, 290).

Most physicians approached their studies with the contention that 'observations are, in no branch of medicine, so necessary as in that of mineral waters [...] experience is the touchstone' (Sutherland 1764, introduction, n.p.). Yet 'experience' yielded more confusion than direct 'observation'. The Swedish professor, Torbern Bergman, complained in the late eighteenth century, 'an accurate analysis of waters is justly considered as one of the most difficult problems in chymistry' (Bergman 1784, 109). Bergman was right—though tract after tract analyzing mineral

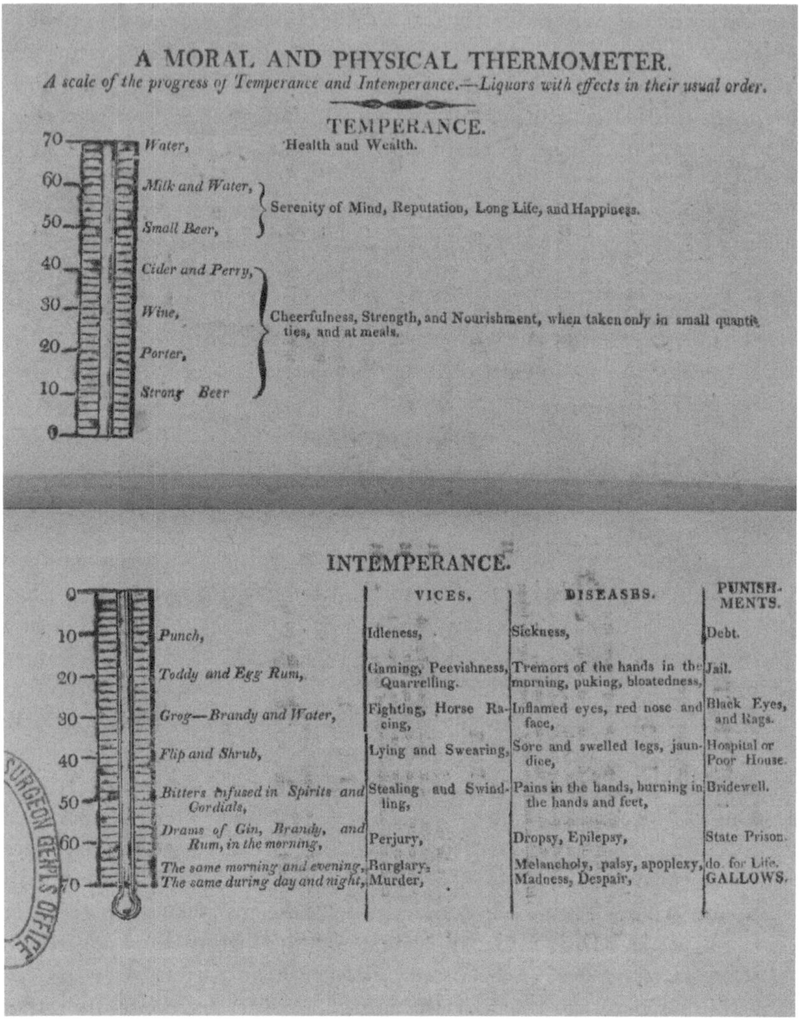

Fig. 3 'A Moral and Physical Thermometer: A Scale of Temperance and Intemperance—Liquors with Effects in Their Usual Order', in Benjamin Rush, *An Inquiry into the Ardent Spirits Upon the Body and Mind*, 6th ed. (New York: Cornelius Davis, 1811; originally printed in 1784) (Courtesy of U.S. National Library of Medicine, Bethesda, MD)

waters appeared in Europe and Britain during the eighteenth century, no one could come to a consensus. The first in-depth, wide-ranging, systematic effort at investigating Britain's mineral waters was Thomas Short's *The Natural Experimental and Medicinal History of the Mineral Waters...* (1734). Short established some baseline tests, but was ultimately stymied by mineral waters' volatile components, which he found 'lost to our senses...either an acid, alkali, iron, sulphur or the inflammable matter'. By 1766, Short doubled down on his despair, exclaiming that the methods of studying mineral waters remained 'confused, inconclusive and wide of the Purpose, in so much that it would be surprising if the Examiners should have made any beneficial or instructive Discoveries' (Short 1734, 14; Coley 1982, 125).

The inconclusiveness and sporadic nature of tests, combined with physicians' egos (not to mention their need for funds), often resulted in confused, contradictory, and sometimes dangerous prescriptions of mineral waters (Brodie 2014, 20). Monro's 1770 *Treatise on Mineral Waters* serves as an excellent summary of these squabbles, going so far as to list every known mineral spring in Great Britain, America, and Western Europe, along with the most current analysis of each water. However, a reader comes away with a muddled understanding of the waters, as most of the entries followed along his description of the 'Dog and Duck' Tavern's mineral spring (situated in St. George's Fields, Lambeth, in the County of Surrey): 'authors differ much with respect to the quantity of solid contents they have obtained, by evaporation, from this water'. Furthermore, Monro noted that Dr. Fothergill argued that 'young strong people' could drink the waters freely, while 'persons advanced in years' might be harmed by consumption (Monro 1770, 136–137).

So, were mineral waters healthy or dangerous? It depended upon who you asked, which spring you referred to, how much water you consumed, under whose guidance you did so, and for what purpose. Such ambiguity both helped and harmed physicians' efforts at convincing citizens to imbibe mineral waters. In 1768, Linden opened his *A Medicinal and Experimental Analysis of Hanlys-Spa* by asserting 'the salubrious Properties of Medicinal-mineral-water Fountains (when judiciously administered) have long been found to be of the greatest service to the human body'. In one sentence, Linden succinctly described the benefits and dangers of mineral waters: healthy, but only 'when judiciously administered'. Watching on as quack physicians prescribed mineral waters with little-to-no understanding of their effects, Linden (along with plenty other physicians) worried that rogue doctors might lead patients to 'make too free with, or to handle this two-edged sword, in an ignorant, and unskilled manner'. Linden continued to explain that, although 'we have a most excellent natural medicine in [mineral] water [...] it is with this, as with all other most powerful Medicines [...] that they are as powerful to hurt the human constitution, if injudiciously used, as they are able to do good, when properly taken'. The German physician believed, furthermore, that it was 'impossible to expect an honest confession of the blunders, the Doctor has jointly committed with his Friend Mr. *Comprehensive*' by not realizing that 'these waters, like other remedies, greatly differ from each other in their qualities' (Linden 1768, 49–50, 88–90).

Others joined Linden in his mistrust of certain mineral water purveyors. The English physician Alex Sutherland warned drinkers against following 'the unreasonable suggestions of designing meddlers; for the saving of paltry fees, they too often throw away the expences of long journeys, and their lives sometimes to the bargain' (Sutherland 1764, introduction, n.p.). After a visit to Bath in 1713, similarly, the English 'spectator', Richard Steele, exclaimed, 'the Physicians here are very numerous, they had almost killed me with their humanity' (Steele 1829, 257).

The dangers of 'taking the waters' extended beyond Britain and Western Europe. Three thousand miles across the Atlantic Ocean, the Philadelphia Humane Society counselled citizens in 1787 to 'avoid drinking [cold water] while you are warm, or, drink only a small quantity at once, and let it remain a short time in your mouth before you swallow it' (*Pennsylvania Gazette*, July 4, 1787). Physicians from Linden to Edward Baynard warned citizens of the danger of being 'so hot, as to sweat or to be ready to sweat' when consuming cold mineral water (Linden 1752, 89; Baynard 1715, 299; Meacham 2009, 13; Thomson 1812, 141). Ultimately, the Philadelphia Humane Society's announcement demonstrated the widespread effect of physicians' findings, no matter their (lack of) efficacy.

Besides admonitions, thinkers engaged in a variety of low-brow tussles over mineral waters. For instance, a select group of doctors nastily debated whether Bath, England's famed mineral springs contained sulfur in the second half of the eighteenth century, which resulted in accusations of bribery, lies, conspiracy, and outright ignorance (Coley 1982, 130–132). With so much money being made among physicians, surgeons, and apothecaries, this debate held real weight (and never really resolved itself).

Yet the prolonged argument over Bath also revealed various medical practitioners' underlying anxieties, for many of them were making their trade up as they went, hoping to collect a quick pound without too many questions.

It should come as no surprise that, upon analyzing England's Glastonbury waters (which were bottled and sold throughout London as a medicinal mineral water), Linden found that the water had a horrible smell 'such as is generally occasioned by animal Substances, in a putrefying state'. When the physician poured oil of Vitriol (sulfuric acid) on the noxious substance, 'there appeared on the Top a slimy Matter, very much resembling animal Substance; and it seemed natural to conclude, that this foetid Smell was contained in the slimy matter only' (Linden 1752, 338–339). The purveyors of Glastonbury water were adding some sort of animal byproduct to their water to mimic the often-disarming smell of sulfuric mineral water. But this shocking revelation did not stop Dr. Linden from including a full advertisement of other bottled mineral waters at the end of his tract, replete with branding and celebratory descriptions (Fig. 4). He had bills to pay, after all. Medicinal morals only went so far.

3 Alcohol's Adversaries... and Adherents

As demonstrated by the opening anecdote about the tavernkeeper's mineral water ale, alcohol and mineral water were not understood as mutually exclusive.[1] Physicians well realized the public's insatiable appetite for alcohol. Linden had to concede in 1752 that 'persuading the Bulk of Mankind to give them strong Liquors with their Food, and to drink good common Water with it [...] is an Attack upon a Luxury, too powerfully established to be shaken by the Physician's Remonstrances' (Linden 1752, 85). As such, extolling the virtues of mineral water did not necessarily coincide with damnation of alcohol. The British physician, John Pringle, argued that soldiers who consumed a diet of water and alcohol were 'preserved by taking these liquors in moderation' (Pringle 1752, 88), while Linden admitted that, though he had 'formerly recommended [...] to drink Mineral–water at meals, instead of small beer',

[1] They still are not. The Superior Bathhouse Brewery in Hot Springs, Arkansas, claims to be the first brewery to utilize thermal spring water as their main ingredient (see 'Superior Bathhouse Brewery Website', online).

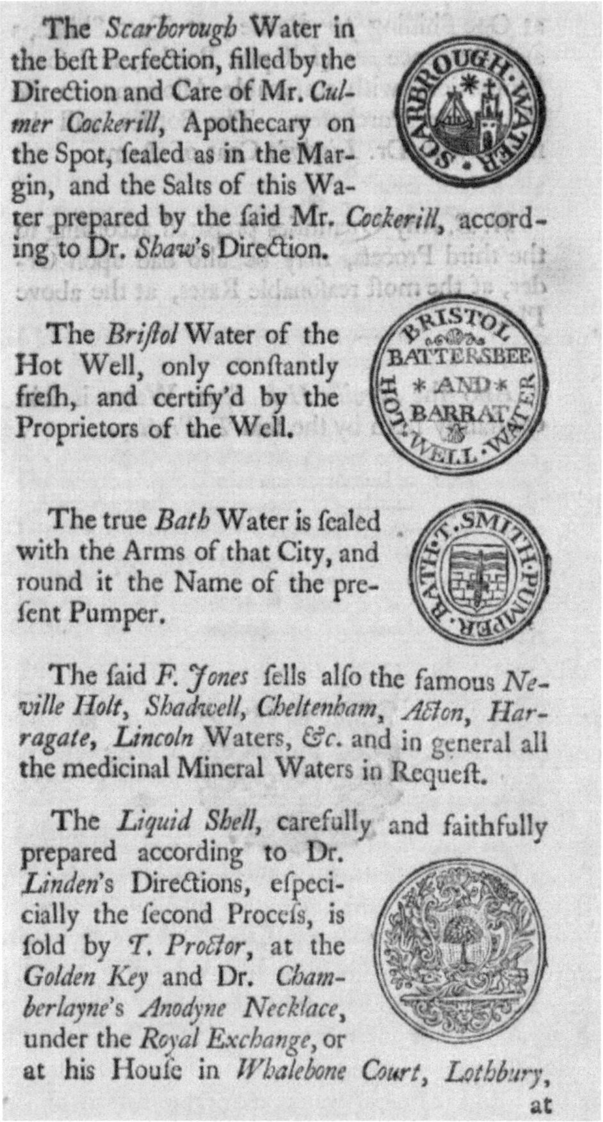

The *Scarborough* Water in the beſt Perfection, filled by the Direction and Care of Mr. *Culmer Cockerill*, Apothecary on the Spot, ſealed as in the Margin, and the Salts of this Water prepared by the ſaid Mr. *Cockerill*, according to Dr. *Shaw*'s Direction.

The *Briſtol* Water of the Hot Well, only conſtantly freſh, and certify'd by the Proprietors of the Well.

The true *Bath* Water is ſealed with the Arms of that City, and round it the Name of the preſent Pumper.

The ſaid *F. Jones* ſells alſo the famous *Neville Holt*, *Shadwell*, *Cheltenham*, *Acton*, *Harragate*, *Lincoln* Waters, *&c.* and in general all the medicinal Mineral Waters in Requeſt.

The *Liquid Shell*, carefully and faithfully prepared according to Dr. *Linden*'s Directions, eſpecially the ſecond Proceſs, is ſold by *T. Proctor*, at the *Golden Key* and Dr. *Chamberlayne*'s *Anodyne Necklace*, under the *Royal Exchange*, or at his Houſe in *Whalebone Court*, *Lothbury*, at

Fig. 4 'Bottle Water Advertisements', in Diederick Wessel Linden, MD, *A Treatise on the Origin, Nature and Virtues of Chalybeate Waters, and Natural Hot Baths* (London: T. Osborne, 1752), n.p.

experience taught him 'that this is a very wrong proceeding'. Linden explained that 'because mineral-waters have elastic spirits' they would 'disturb the food they are mixed with' and cause indigestion (Linden 1768, 123). Thus, for this physician it was low-alcohol beer at dinner and mineral water at least four hours thereafter.

Pringle and Linden were hardly alone in their water/alcohol regimen. In an especially in-depth example, the renowned Scottish physician, George Cheyne, recommended in 1720 drinking mineral waters along with 'generous, un-mix'd Wines, both of them in small and constantly equal Quantities' to cure gout. Cheyne went even further than Pringle and Linden by prescribing a multi-step process of alcohol and mineral water consumption to cure the first 'fits' of Gout. Arguing 'Dilution is the only remedy', Cheyne suggested that sufferers should first consume 'Fine, clear, old small Beer, with a little old Mountain, or Madera Wine; Water boil'd with a few Spicy Seeds, mix'd with these Wines; Water Gruel with some Wine'. He continued to note, 'During the whole Fit, Liquors may be more freely and safely indulg'd, than Solid foods', including 'light bitters infused in wine' and a final 'course of *Bath* or *German Spaw* Waters' washed down with 'generous Wines drunk temperately' (Cheyne 1720, 15, 23–24, 28).

Pro-temperance British physicians not only instigated our modern notions of alcohol and physical health, but also ushered in ideas of mental illness, withdrawal, disease, and addiction surrounding alcohol consumption. Rallies against alcohol overconsumption were nothing new, as clergymen had spent the past two centuries decrying alcoholism. Yet the 'over' in consumption is key here, for even most clergymen had to accept alcohol as a part of British society: as historian Roy Porter explained, how could the Church condemn alcohol entirely 'given the mystery of the eucharist, and when so many Bible passages commended it' (Porter 1985, 387)? Thus, while clergymen and reformation societies had long extolled the virtues of alcohol consumption in moderation, certain physicians' assertion of outright temperance broke new ground. No longer was it good enough to enjoy a pint of ale with friends or a nip of whiskey to ward off the cold. Nay, even the most innocent tipple might prove the stumbling block which led to depression, disease, poverty, and death.

Various temperance advocates—e.g. Bernard Mandeville, George Cheyne, Thomas Wilson, Richard Mead, and John Lettsom—wrote tracts demonstrating the evils of alcohol throughout the eighteenth century.

Yet Thomas Trotter's *An Essay, Medical, Philosophical, and Chemical, on Drunkenness and Its Effects on the Human Body* (1804, originally published as Trotter's University of Edinburgh dissertation in 1788) proved critical in both compiling and extending the study of alcoholism (Porter 1985, 390–393; Nicholls 2009, 65–67; Hirsh 1949, 230). Trotter's scholarship was especially important in its advancement of alcoholism as a disease: in a sentence which would fit in a twenty-first-century psychology textbook, Trotter asserted, 'the habit of drunkenness is a disease of the mind'. After providing a concise definition of drunkenness—'a disease produced by a remote cause, and giving birth to actions and movements in the living body, that disorder the functions of health'—Trotter detailed the symptoms, effects, and physical ailments relating to what we today would term 'alcoholism'. Compiling a list that would make anyone think twice about a tipple, Trotter specified alcohol-related diseases ranging from apoplexy to gout to inflammation of the liver to emaciation to madness. Once again demonstrating the advancement of the study of alcohol according to modern medicine, moreover, Trotter concluded his volume with a chapter on 'the method of correcting the habit of intoxication, and of treating the drunken paroxysm' (Trotter 1804, 8, 136, 172).

The eighteenth-century physician prescribed a relatively advanced rehabilitation programme. From identification to convalescence, Trotter laid out a clear programme of temperance for his fellow Britons, who he especially worried about, as 'it cannot be doubted that the convivial disposition of the inhabitants of Great Britain and Ireland, has a strong tendency to extend the habit of ebriety'. He continued, 'there is no business of moment transacted in these islands without a libation to Bacchus. It prevails among the Peers of the realm down to the Parish committee' (Trotter 1804, 141). Trotter and those various physicians before him believed they had the cure, but that didn't mean anyone would listen.

Eighteenth-century Britons loved their drink. Cheyne had made the same complaint regarding mass alcohol consumption and class fifty-two years earlier, exclaiming

> Did only the Profligate, the Scoundrel, the Abandoned run into these Excesses, it were as vain to endeavor to reclaim them, as it were to stop a Tempest, or to calm a Storm: but now the Vice is become Epidemical, since it has got not only amongst Mechanics, and the lowest Kind of People,

> but amongst persons of the highest genius, and finest taste, and most accomplished Parts. (Cheyne 1736, 45–46)

Of course, Cheyne published his tract at the height of London gin craze; a time when Hogarth mocked the debauched, drunken mother in his colourful prints and London harboured 1500 distillers of hard alcohol (Clark 1988, 64). Just because physicians had 'discovered' addiction and laid out a clear path to reform did not mean that their ideas would infiltrate popular culture, especially since popular Western culture was so tied to the consumption of alcohol.

British physicians were also, problematically, battling to upend the dictums their forebears had so efficiently established regarding the medicinal qualities of alcohol. Like in their views of mineral water, physicians and laypeople alike had long considered alcohol a potentially healthy consumable if administered with care and moderation. In 1542, the English physician, Andrew Boorde, lauded wine because it 'doth quicken a man's wits, it doth comfort the heart, it doth scoure the liver; specially, if it be white wine, it doth rejoice all the powers of man, and doth nourish them; it doth ingender good blood, it doth nourish the brain and all the body' (Clark 1983, 112). Sixteenth- and seventeenth-century British doctors stocked their cupboards with alcohol, which they prescribed to patients according to various diseases, while poorer colonists who could not afford a doctor's visit consumed ale and cider to fight everything from the common cold to cancer. These beliefs thrived through the eighteenth century: Dr. Richard Blackmore recommended medicinal concoctions with white and red wine as the base of a cure for melancholy (i.e. depression) (Blackmore 1726, 170), and various physicians reminded their patients that periodic alcoholic intoxication (like mineral water intoxication) 'was beneficial because it purged the body of noxious humors' (Meacham 2009, 9–10; Porter 1985, 385–390). Yet all should be in moderation. As the British doctor Hugh Smythson explained in 1785, 'the inordinate use of a cordial [alcohol], originally intended to "*strengthen the heart of man*", but perverted in the abuse of it to a sure and deadly poison' (Smythson 1785, 97).

To add even more confusion to the mix, those same eighteenth-century temperance writers often contradicted themselves in their views towards alcohol. After baring his soul regarding his past alcohol addiction, George Cheyne assured readers that he had spent the past twenty years '*sober*, *moderate* and *plain* in my diet, and in my greatest health drank not above a quart, or three pints at most, of *wine* any day [...] for near one-half of the time from thirty to sixty I scarce drank any strong liquor at all [...] I drank very little above a pint of wine, or at most not a quart one day with another, since I was near thirty' (Boswell 1837, 27). So, which was it? Should Britons live a life of 'Temperance, Sobriety, and Virtue', as Cheyne argued in the opening pages of his *English Malady* (1733), or should they follow his own lead, and consume pints of wine daily (Cheyne 1733, n.p.; Shaw 1726, 477)?

The contradictions did not stop with Cheyne. Having provided enough cautions against drinking alcohol to make the most seasoned toper think twice, Trotter added an odd caveat on wine: 'as an article in the medicine the virtues of wine are sovereign in their kind: there are some diseases for which it is the best remedy'. Trotter was especially ardent in his belief that 'the stimulus of wine is favourable to advanced age'. The physician argued that wine, 'and all fermented liquors', quickened 'the circulation of the blood' and generated heat, and thus should be increasingly consumed between the ages of forty and sixty, with 'six glass *per diem*' for those sixty and over. Yet, after prescribing wine and 'all fermented liquors' to citizens over forty, he went back to railing against alcohol as a medicine, exclaiming, 'there can be no doubt that many persons have to date their first propensity to drinking to the too frequent use of spirituous tinctures as medicines, rashly prescribed for hysterical and hypochondriacal complaints' (Trotter 1804, 150–151, 167).

These contradictions made their way across the Atlantic, with the most notorious British American temperance advocate, Benjamin Rush, exclaiming in 1772, 'why all this noise about wine and strong drink? Have we not seen hundreds who have made it a constant practice to get drunk almost everyday for 30 or 40 years, who, notwithstanding, arrived to a great age, and enjoyed the same good health as those who have followed the strictest rules of temperance' (Levine 1978, 168)? In a final flourish, Benjamin Franklin provided readers of his popular *Poor Richard's Almanack* with more incongruous advice regarding alcohol. In 1736, Franklin foreshadowed Rush's 1772 reflection, quipping, 'there's more old Drunkards than old Doctors' (Franklin 1961). Yet, by 1750, the British American physician warned fellow Britons, 'Drunkenness, that worst of Evils, makes some Men Fools, some Beasts, some Devils' (Franklin 1987, 1270).

Eighteenth-century physicians seemed to drown in questions regarding the health of mineral water and alcohol, finding one answer at the same time that they contradicted another. Quacks doled out mineral water and alcohol as long as the money kept coming, laughing off more established physicians like Cheyne and Linden who damned their prescriptions as initiated 'without Distinction and without Choice' (Cheyne 1720, 74). Yet, at the same time that self-congratulatory physicians chastised their colleagues 'fitted to the vulgar Capacity' (Cheyne 1720, 74) they were walking contradictions, squabbling among themselves and leaping from opinion to opinion at random. Like their quack counterparts, moreover, physicians also relied upon monetary returns and social capital, as 'eighteenth-century medicine operated more like a trade than the lofty profession with which it has since sought to be identified' (Porter 1997, 286). Through all of this, physicians became sounding boards for larger arguments over societal development and health. Unfortunately, there was hardly as much agreement there, either.

4 Intoxicating Spaces

When eighteenth-century British physicians reflected upon, argued over, and analyzed mineral water and alcohol, they were referring to more than just bodily health—they were also debating the health of civil society. It was no coincidence that writers often compared society to the human body: 'different individuals were cells, different human associations were organs, and those responsible (for history, for society, for the state) commanded and ruled those organs, playing the role of doctors' (de Baecque 2001, 185). Societal health, like human health, was ever-fluctuating, ever pervious to an almost endless variety of vagaries. And, as alcohol and mineral water became two sides of the same intoxicating coin, so too did their booming consumption force physicians, public officials, philosophers, and businessmen to reflect upon how the two public spaces most related to mineral water and alcohol—spas and taverns—might shape the health of civil society.

It would be easy to treat spas and taverns as necessarily separate entities. One, after all, was directed at health, cleanliness, and respite, while the other was often the resort of drunkenness, debauchery, and disintegration. Yet this oversimplification misses a key point: spas and taverns, like mineral water and alcohol, were necessarily overlapping entities in the social psyche of the eighteenth-century Atlantic World; battlegrounds of bodily and societal health where a diverse company engaged with complicated, even dangerous, forms of overt consumption.

From London to Leeds, Barbados to Boston, taverns were the social foundation of British, and eventually American, society. London, which harboured around 600,000 souls by the early eighteenth century, boasted over ten thousand drinking establishments (Porter 1994, 171). The largest British American cities like New York City, meanwhile, supported around 220 taverns, or one tavern for every 115 people, by midcentury. Taverns dotted British country roads and served as central meeting places for smaller towns and villages. And these numbers only account for *licensed* taverns, as a thriving network of unlicensed 'disorderly' houses also tucked into the corners, alleys, and nooks of British cities. Ultimately, taverns emerged as the most numerous, popular, and accessible public spaces in the eighteenth-century Atlantic World (Scribner 2019, 14).

Though less numerous, spas also became key nodes of societal development where diverse sets of Britons gathered for intoxication and sociability. While Bath rose to prominence as the most popular spa centre in Great Britain by the mid-eighteenth century, London alone supported seventeen separate spas, while another 134 bubbled up throughout England by the end of the eighteenth century (Hembry 1990, n.p. (inside cover); Borsay 2000, 775–803; Borsay 1999). Colonists in British North America and the Caribbean also cultivated a handful of spas on the English model in the second half of the eighteenth century (Scribner 2016, 409–449; Bridenbaugh 1946, 151–181). With 'Health-promoting Waters, of every kind' as their central consumables, British spas were shrines to health; carefully cultivated arenas where customers might improve themselves in a safe, orderly environment (Linden 1768, ii).

Yet these two spaces were hardly distinct or oppositional. In fact, spas and taverns often grew out of each other. Historian Peter Borsay argued that many 'polite towns' proved 'remarkably adept at "finding" an adjacent spring which could be dressed up as a spa, to provide a fashionable accessory' (Borsay 2012, 160). Tavernkeepers did the same (Curl 2010, 32). In 1739, the owner of 'a noted house of good entertainment, known as the Green Man' discovered a chalybeate spring behind his tavern in Dulwich. Realizing his luck, the owner 'built a handsome room on one end of his bowling green for breakfasts, dancing, and entertainments; a part of the fashionable luxury of the present age which every village for ten miles round London has something of' (Sydney 1891, 49). Linden remarked that most of London's wells began as 'mere Tippling-houses and Assemblies of entertainment' (Linden 1752, 139).

But these efforts did not always work. Benjamin Rush discovered a spring in central Philadelphia in 1773, which he described as medicinal, if a bit foul: 'the water, when it first comes from the pump, has a slight faetid smell, is somewhat turbid, and after standing a few hours exposed to the air, deposits a yellow sediment. The smell of the water is increased by rest. It has a strong ferruginous [iron-impregnated] taste'. Thus far, the description of the water fits plenty of other mineral springs. The owner of the property was delighted, and opened the pungent spring to eager Philadelphians. Unfortunately, 'the water lost its virtue within a few months after investigation owing to the contents of a neighboring necessary (i.e. cesspit)'. Rush had unknowingly urged Philadelphians to drink from a spring which issued through human waste. They had drunk it dry, only to realize that 'the well communicated with the necessary which gave the smell and sediment' (Drinker 1937, 25).

Sidestepping Benjamin Rush's blunder, it would be easy to assume that spas were spaces of temperance: yet they also often spawned a diverse network of taverns and drinking establishments. As historian Phyllis Hembry explained, 'Although visitors [to Bath] came ostensibly to drink the waters, much alcoholic liquor was consumed and some of the many inns took in lodgers'. Hembry continued to describe Buxton as 'another spa where social life focused on the inns', and labelled the 'social life' of England's northern spas as 'inn-centred' (Hembry 1990, 156, 217–218). Ironically, spa-goers seemed disappointed if there was only water to drink. The owner of Pennsylvania's Yellow Springs spa was thus sure to advertise in 1771 that his spa boasted a 'fine dwelling house [...] used as a public house, and is so well accustomed, as to have from 100 to 300 people daily for the summer season' (*Pennsylvania Gazette*, March 14, 1771), while the owners of Kilburn Wells (just outside London) ushered spa goers to the Bell Tavern, where the 'politest companies' could enjoy equal doses of ale and water (Walford 1870, 246).

The Kilburn Wells notation of the 'politest companies' is key, for taverns and spas acted like prisms and mirrors, refracting peoples into distinct groups while also forcing leaders to reflect upon the health of British civil society. Like with alcohol and mineral water, thinkers could not necessarily agree on how they felt about taverns and spas. Leaders might celebrate certain taverns as centres of mirth and erudition at the same time they damned others as 'bawdy houses'. The same went for spas: just as physicians like Trotter argued that the 'waters of Bath are in considerable repute for their efficacy in recruiting the worn down constitution of inebriates' (Trotter 1804, 181), the English essayist, Daniel Defoe, described Bath as 'the resort of the sound, rather than the sick; the bathing is made more a sport and diversion, than a physical prescription for health; and the town is taken up in raffling, gaming, visiting, and in a word, all sorts of gallantry and levity' (Defoe 1962 [1727], 34). Taverns and spas, like alcohol and mineral water, were hotbeds of debate and contradiction. In these arguments, however, eighteenth-century Britons and Americans revealed much about their ideas of societal health.

Debates over public spaces like taverns and spas often hinged upon class, as officials generally considered 'upper-class' public spaces as encouraging societal health and order, and 'lower-class' taverns and spas/'watering places' as nurturing incivility and disorder (Scribner 2019, 1–19; Tomory 2014, 500–505). Elite taverns and coffeehouses (establishments which grew out of taverns and served coffee and alcohol) often enjoyed praise as 'penny universities' where Britons could engage with ideas, peoples, and consumables from around the world (Ellis 1956; Cowan 2005, 89). In a clear link between societal improvement and tavern going, the *Spectator* explicitly advertised itself as bringing 'Philosophy out of Closets and Libraries, Schools and Colleges, to dwell [...] in Coffee-Houses' (Addison March 12, 1711).

The same class-based ideals extended to upper-class spas. The daily operations of Bath and Tunbridge Wells were overseen by Richard 'Beau' Nash, who Oliver Goldsmith praised in 1762 for teaching 'a familiar intercourse among strangers at Bath and Tunbridge, which still subsists among them'. This civilizing process—'that ease and open access first acquired there'—extended beyond the spa, as 'our gentry brought back to the metropolis, and thus the whole kingdom by degrees became more refined by lessons originally derived from [Nash's spas]' (Goldsmith 1966 [1762], 288–289). Trotter echoed Goldsmith's effusions in 1788, explaining to potential customers 'that species of *etiquette* which one is forced to go through in fashionable circles [at Bath], and among trifling entertainments, may, on particular people, have a powerful influence in introducing new trains of thinking' (Trotter 1804, 181). If approached by the 'right' people (i.e. civilized elites) in the 'right' ways (through agreed-upon modes of sociability and civility), taverns and spas could be stimulating vehicles of social health.

But both could do just as much harm as good. Eighteenth-century London fostered a staggering variety of 'lower-class' alehouses, grog shops, taverns, and 'bawdy houses' which elite and ordinary Britons alike frequented. That aspiring Scottish gentleman, James Boswell, is well known for patronizing London's litany of seedy spaces: already drunk on the night of June 4, 1763, Boswell went 'roaring along' to 'Ashley's Punch-house and drank three threepenny bowls [of rum punch]'. From there, he stumbled to the Strand where he paid for a prostitute's services, but finding 'the miscreant refused me performance', he 'pushed her up against a wall' before verbally accosting her with a group of passersby's (Boswell 1950, 272–273). It need not be said, but his casual discussion of sexual violence hardly represented the actions of a civilized gentleman. Yet, like so many 'rakes' and 'libertines' throughout the British Atlantic World, men like Boswell made up the rules as they went, damning lower-class taverns as 'Gate[s] to Debauchery […] the Nurse of Riot and Fury' and their lower-class customers as '*indisposed* to Virtue […] His *Neighbor's* Contempt and Derision' at the same time that they often proved their most destructive patrons (*Boston Gazette*, August 29, 1763; Bryson 1998, 244).

The social anxieties continued into spas. Though Linden considered Tunbridge Wells unmatched in 'Conveniences' and 'Accommodation for the Reception of Company of the first Distinction', an over-charging landlord made Linden feel 'no Body could however use fairer Words, or more Civility; but then no Body accommodated worse, or brought in more exorbitant bills'. His landlord—a 'Cut-throat' of low social station—sullied Linden's otherwise civil experience (Linden 1752, 100–101). Worried that the Somersham Spa might fall into vulgarity, elite subscribers issued an order in 1767 which required a license for 'servants to sell wine, spirituous or malt liquors […] as also to dress any provisions, and entertain company, provided good hours be kept, and no rioting or debauchery of any sort be suffered' (Layard 1767, 23–24).

Plenty of other British mineral springs boasted nowhere near the accommodations of Tunbridge Wells or the Somersham Spa, and were thus viewed by elite Britons as watering-holes for the 'poorer sort' sort of people (labourers, servants, artisans) where little-to-no improvement or civility occurred (White 2012, 325). Take one spring in the supposed 'wilderness' of Virginia, for example. An Englishman who resided in America during the Revolution recalled, 'in the summer months it is very common to make a party on horseback to a limestone spring, near which there is usually some little hut with spirituous liquors'. Already considering 'the indolence and dissipation of the middling and lower classes of white inhabitants' so severe that they displayed 'a barbarity worthy of their savage neighbours [Native Americans]', the Englishman was aghast when he was 'accidentally drawn into one of these parties, where I soon experienced the strength of the liquor, which was concealed by the refreshing coolness of the water'. Matters only grew worse when 'a veteran Cyclops' and his gang arrived at the spring looking for a boxing-match. Drunk and debauched, the Englishman escaped into the woods before the cyclops' eye fell upon him (de Chastellux 1827, 292–293).

5 Conclusion: Through a Glass Darkly

Mineral water and alcohol, spas and taverns; it seems their 'health' was all in the eye of the beholder. Labelled as 'intoxicants' by eighteenth-century physicians, mineral water and alcohol might do as much harm as good if not consumed correctly. Ordered and classified according to strength, certain mineral and alcoholic 'liquors' cured certain ailments. All, however, must be taken in moderation, which required the careful guidance of professional medicine practitioners. Of course, many of those same practitioners offering their supervision were little more than quack doctors out to make a quick pound off of hypochondriacs, thereby negating the whole process before it even began. Then again, even supposedly 'professional' physicians could not decide if mineral waters were even good for their patients. These same debates often merged with arguments over alcohol. Physicians railed against alcohol as the 'bane of the nation' (Wilson 1736) in multi-volume tracts, yet included in those same tracts various suggestions on the efficacy of alcohol for curing illness. Mineral spas and taverns, finally, necessarily entered the larger conversation over the supposed health civil society: might they be civilizing schools or dens of debauchery? Who should attend them and why? Who shouldn't? To make matters even more complicated and contradictory, this eighteenth-century scientific and social debate often ran counter-current to the very advice that physicians and officials had been pushing on the public for the past century. All was certain and nothing was certain.

Yet, progress—no matter how fleeting and inadvertent—is often made in contradiction and disagreement. In their seemingly rudderless debates, eighteenth-century Britons throughout the Empire both complicated and advanced their understanding of science, health, and society. They weren't necessarily looking for consensus, and that is not necessarily a bad thing. We still describe doctors as 'practicing' medicine, after all, and modern science still vacillates over topics of health, diet, and commerce regarding water (Oatsvall 2019, 1–31). Mineral water and alcohol—as well as their attendant public spaces—provided eighteenth-century physicians with inverse, reciprocal, and competitive intoxicants and institutions through which to deliberate the future of human and societal improvement. In doing so, they revealed just how contradictory 'modern' humans had become. We are still uncovering those various contradictions, pitfalls—and progressions—in our supposedly 'enlightened' present. Hopefully we won't stop any time soon.

Acknowlegements The author would especially like to thank Sophie Chiari and Samuel Cuisinier-Delorme for organizing the conference upon which this edited volume is based, and for their help throughout the entire process of publication. Special thanks also goes out to the conference's participants, as well as the Department of History at the University of Central Arkansas, for travel funding.

Works Cited

Primary Sources

Addison, Joseph. 1711. *Spectator* (10): March 12.

Baynard, Edward. 1715. *Psychrolousia, or, the History of Cold Bathing: Both Ancient and Modern*, Part Two. London: William Innys.

Beddoes, Thomas. 1793. *Observations on the Nature and Cure of Calculus, Sea Scurvy, Consumption, Catarrh, and Fever.* London: J. Murray.

Bergman, Torbern. 1784 [1779]. *Physical and Chemical Essays*, vol. 1, trans. Edmund Cullen. London: J. Murray.

Blackmore, Richard. 1726. *A Treatise of the Spleen and Vapours: Orr, Hypocondriacal and Hysterical Affections, with Three Discourses on the Nature and Cure of the Cholick, Melancholy, and Palsies*, 2nd ed. London: J. Pemberton.

Boswell, James. 1837. *Boswell's Life of Johnson*, vol. 3, ed. George Birkbeck Hill. Oxford: Clarendon Press.

Boswell, James. 1950. *Boswell's London Journal, 1762–1763.* New York: McGraw-Hill Book Company.

Cheyne, George. 1720. *Essay on the Gout, with an Account of the Nature and Qualities of Bath Water.* London: G. Strahan.

Cheyne, George. 1733. *The English Malady: Or, a Treatise of Nervous Diseases of All Kinds.* London: Strahan.

Cheyne, George. 1736. *Two Discourses, Shewing the Fatal Consequences of the Habitual Drinking of Distilled Spirituous Liquors.* London: J. Roberts.

de Chastellux, Marquis. 1827. *Travels in North America, in the Years 1780, 1781, and 1782*. New York: White, Gallaher, & White.

Defoe, Daniel. 1962. *A Tour Through the Whole Island of Great Britain*, vol. 2, ed. G.D.H. Cole and D.C. Browning. London: Everyman.

Franklin, Benjamin. 1961. *The Papers of Benjamin Franklin*, vol. 2, *January 1, 1735, Through December 31, 1744*, ed. Leonard W. Labaree. New Haven: Yale University Press.

Franklin, Benjamin. 1987. *Writings*. New York: The Library of America.

Goldsmith, Oliver. 1966. The Life of Richard Nash. In *The Collected Works of Oliver Goldsmith*, vol. 3, ed. A. Friedman. Oxford: Clarendon Press.

Hales, Stephen. 1739. *Philosophical Experiments: Containing Useful, and Necessary Instructions for Such as Undertake Long Voyages at Sea*... London: W. Innys and R. Manby.

Johnson, Samuel. 1785. *A Dictionary of the English Language*. London: J.F. and C. Rivington.

Layard, Daniel Peter. 1767. *An Account of the Somersham Water, in the County of Huntingdon*. London: Daniel Peter Layard.

Lewis, William. 1784. *An Experimental History of the Materia Medica, or of the Natural and Artificial Substances Made Use of in Medicine*. London: J. Johnson.

Linden, Diederick Wessel. 1752. *A Treatise on the Origin, Nature and Virtues of Chalybeat Waters, and Natural Hot Baths*. London: T. Osborne.

Linden, Diederick Wessel. 1768. *A Medicinal and Experimental History and Analysis of Hanlys-Spa*. London: John Everingham.

Monro, Donald. 1770. *A Treatise on Mineral Waters*, vol. 1. London: D. Wilson and G. Nicol.

Priestly, Joseph. 1772. *Directions for Impregnating Water with Fixed Air; In Order to Communicate to It the Peculiar Spirit and Virtues of Pyrmont Water, and Other Mineral Waters of a Similar Nature*. London: J. Johnson.

Pringle, John. 1764 [1752]. *Observations on the Diseases of the Army*, 4th ed. London: A. Millar.

Prior, Matthew. 1835. *The Poetical Works of Matthew Prior*, vol. 2. London: William Pickering.

Ruddy, John. 1757. *A Methodical Synopsis of Mineral Waters*. London: William Johnston.

Shaw, Peter. 1726. *A New Practice of Physic*, vol. 2. London: J. Osborn and T. Longman.

Short, Thomas. 1734. *The Natural Experimental and Medicinal History of the Mineral Waters*... London: F. Gyles.

Smythson, Hugh. 1785. *The Compleat Family Physician; Or, Universal Medical Repository*. London: Harrison and Co.

Steele, Richard. 1829. *The Guardian and the Tatler, Complete in One Volume.* London: Jones and Co.

Sutherland, Alex. 1764. *An Attempt to Ascertain and Extend the Virtues of Bath and Bristol Waters by Experiments and Cases*, 2nd ed. London: W. Frederick and S. Leake.

Trotter, Thomas. 1804. *An Essay, Medical, Philosophical, and Chemical, on Drunkenness and Its Effects on the Human Body.* London: T.N. Longman and O. Rees, originally submitted as a dissertation in 1788.

Wilson, Thomas. 1736. *Distilled Spirituous Liquors the Bane of the Nation.* London: J. Roberts.

Secondary Sources

Borsay, Anne. 1999. *Medicine and Charity in Georgian Bath: A Social History of the General Infirmary, c. 1739–1830.* Burlington, VT: Ashgate.

Borsay, Peter. 2000. Health and Leisure Resorts 1700–1840. In *The Cambridge Urban History of Britain Vol. II, 1540–1840*, ed. Peter Clark, 775–803. Cambridge: Cambridge University Press.

Borsay, Peter. 2012. Town or Country? British Spas and the Urban-Rural Interface. *Journal of Tourism History* 4 (2) (August): 155–169.

Bridenbaugh, Carl. 1946. Baths and Watering Places of Colonial America. *William and Mary Quarterly* 3 (April): 151–181.

Brodie, Allan. 2014. Scarborough in the 1730s—Spa, Sea, Sex. In *Mineral Springs Resorts in Global Perspective: Spa Histories*, ed. John K. Walton, 15–44. London, Routledge.

Bryson, Anna. 1998. *From Courtesy to Civility: Changing Codes of Conduct in Early Modern England.* Oxford: Clarendon Press.

Clark, Peter. 1983. *The English Alehouse: A Social History 1200–1830.* New York: Longman Inc.

Clark, Peter. 1988. The 'Mother Gin' Controversy in the Early Eighteenth Century. *Transactions of the Royal Historical Society* 38 (December): 63–84.

Coley, Noel G. 1982. Physicians and the Chemical Analysis of Mineral Waters in Eighteenth-Century England. *Medical History* 26 (2) (April): 123–144.

Coley, Noel G. 1990. Physicians, Chemists, and the Analysis of Mineral Waters: 'The Most Difficult Part of Chemistry'. In *The Medical History of Waters and Spas*, ed. Roy Porter, 67–81. London: Wellcome Institute for the History of Medicine.

Cowan, Brian. 2005. *Social Life of Coffee: The Emergence of the British Coffeehouse.* New Haven: Yale University Press.

Curl, James Stevens. 2010. *Spas, Wells, & Pleasure-Gardens of London.* London: Historical Publications.

de Baecque, Antoine. 2001. Representations of Body. In *Encyclopedia of the Enlightenment*, vol. 1, ed. Michel Delon, 185. London, Routledge.
Drinker, Cecil K. 1937. *Not So Long Ago; A Chronicle of Medicine and Doctors in Colonial Philadelphia*, 1937. New York: Oxford University Press.
Ellis, Aytoun. 1956. *The Penny Universities: A History of the Coffee-Houses*. London: Secker and Warburg.
Hardy, Anne. 1984. Water and the Search for Public Health in London in the Eighteenth and Nineteenth Centuries. *Medical History* 28 (3) (July): 250–282.
Harley, David. 1990. Honour and Property: The Structure of Professional Disputes in Eighteenth-Century English Medicine. In *The Medical Enlightenment of the Eighteenth Century*, eds. Andrew Cunningham and Roger French, 138–164. Cambridge, Cambridge University Press.
Hembry, Phyllis. 1990. *The English Spa, 1560–1815: A Social History*. London: Athlone Press.
Hirsh, Joseph. 1949. Enlightened Eighteenth-Century Views of the Alcohol Problem. *Journal of the History of Medicine and Allied Sciences* 4 (2) (Spring): 230–236.
Humphrey, Nicholas. 2001. Introduction: Altered States. *Social Research* 68 (3) (Fall): 585–587.
Jennings, Paul. 2016. *A History of Drink and the English, 1500–2000*. London: Routledge.
Levine, Harry G. 1978. The Discovery of Addiction: Changing Conceptions of Habitual Drunkenness in America. *Journal of the Study of Alcohol* 39 (1) (January): 43–57.
McIntyre, Sylvia. 1973. The Mineral Water Trade in the Eighteenth Century. *Journal of Transport History*, New Series 2 (February): 1–19.
Meacham, Sarah H. 2009. *Every Home a Distillery: Alcohol, Gender, and Technology in the Colonial Chesapeake*. Baltimore: Johns Hopkins University Press.
Nicholls, James. 2009. *The Politics of Alcohol: A History of the Drink Question in England*. Manchester: University of Manchester Press.
Oatsvall, Neil. 2019. Bottling Nature's Elixir: The Mountain Valley Spring Water Company, Environment, Health, and Capitalism. *The Arkansas Historical Quarterly* 78 (1) (Spring): 1–31.
Porter, Roy. 1985. The Drinking Man's Disease: The 'Pre-history' of Alcoholism in Georgian Britain. *British Journal of Addiction* 80 (4) (1985): 385–396.
Porter, Roy, ed. 1990. *The Medical History of Waters and Spas*. London: Wellcome Institute for the History of Medicine.
Porter, Roy, ed. 1994. *London: A Social History*. Cambridge, MA: Harvard University Press.

Porter, Roy, ed. 1997. *The Greatest Benefit to Mankind: A Medical History of Humanity*. New York: W. W. Norton.

Rorabaugh, W.J. 1991. Alcohol in America. *OAH Magazine of History* 6 (2) (Fall): 17–19.

Salinger, Sharon V. 2002. *Taverns and Drinking in Early America*. Baltimore: Johns Hopkins University Press.

Scribner, Vaughn. 2016. "The Happy Effects of These Waters": Colonial American Mineral Spas and the British Civilizing Mission. *Early American Studies* 14 (3) (Summer): 409–449.

Scribner, Vaughn. 2019. *Inn Civility: Urban Taverns and Early American Civil Society*. New York: New York University Press.

Sydney, William Connor. 1891. *England and the English in the Eighteenth Century: Chapters in the Social History of the Times*, vol. 2. London: Ward & Downey.

Thomson, Thomas. 1812. *History of the Royal Society, From Its Institution to the End of the Eighteenth Century*. London: Robert Baldwin.

Tomory, Leslie. 2014. The Question of Water Quality in London's New River in the Eighteenth Century. *Social History of Medicine* 27 (3) (July): 488–507.

Walford, Edward. 1870. *Old and New London: A Narrative of Its History, Its People, and Its Places*, vol. 5. London: Cassell, Petter & Galpin.

White, Jerry. 2012. *London in the Eighteenth Century: A Great and Monstrous Thing*. London: Vintage Books.

Withington, Phil. 2014. Introduction: Cultures of Intoxication. *Past and Present* 222 (Suppl. 9) (April): 9–33.

Website

Superior Bathhouse Brewery. https://www.superiorbathhouse.com (accessed October 26, 2020).

PART IV

Coda. New Ecocritical Perspectives

CHAPTER 14

All Is Deep: All Is Shallow—Literary Springs, Wells and Depths, from Shakespeare to Ecocriticism

Richard Kerridge

What are the literary and artistic traditions that run alongside, and draw upon, the belief in the healing power of deep spring water? And, more generally, what are the meanings of watery depths, in tradition and now in our time of ecological crisis? As a Coda to the collection of essays, this chapter will examine these meanings and tropes, and their historical shifts, using examples from English literature.

There is a long tradition of literary springs and wells endowed with symbolic and metaphorical meaning. Water rising from deep underground represents renewed contact with long-lost origins. Old vitality and wisdom rise suddenly into a present that has lost touch with them. Deep reserves of love, compassion or understanding can flow again, now that a blockage has gone, or a hidden place has been found. Usually the effect is healing and strengthening, but sometimes the old energies,

R. Kerridge (✉)
School of Creative Industries, Bath Spa University, Bath, UK
e-mail: r.kerridge@bathspa.ac.uk

S. Chiari and S. Cuisinier-Delorme (eds.), *Spa Culture and Literature in England, 1500–1800*, Early Modern Literature in History,
https://doi.org/10.1007/978-3-030-66568-5_14

long suppressed, are dangerous. So it is with pastoral more generally. One version brings delight, good humour and renewed natural health to the fictional character and—the hope is—the real audience. Another releases passions with chaotic or destructive potential. The origins that rise up into the present may be personal, as in memories of childhood. They may also be cultural, as in renewed contact with a primal mythic or poetic tradition. Writers sometimes use springs and wells figuratively, and sometimes present actual encounters, real or fictional, that combine the experience of the place, in a dramatic moment, with the symbolic or metaphorical meaning. This is the trope I will introduce first. How should ecocritics—critics concerned with the cultural representation of ecological processes—react to this tradition? What are its environmentalist uses? How are writers deploying it now?

1 Enchanted Springs in Petrarchan Sonnets

One of the earliest sonnets in English features two enchanted springs with contrasting properties. It is a poem that complicates the simple distinction I make above between health-giving and violently passionate effects upon the person who drinks the water. 'Complaint of the Lover Disdained', by Henry Howard, Earl of Surrey (1517–1547), was first printed in *Tottel's Miscellany* (1557), and has sometimes appeared since then under the title 'In Cyprus Springs'. This sonnet, in the Petrarchan tormented lover genre, describes first 'a well so hotte' that 'who tastes the same/Were he of stone as thawed yse should melt' (Howard 1557, 13). Venus gave this well its powers, and the heat is the intensity of amorous desire. The sonnet's dramatic speaker is a Petrarchan lover consumed by this hot desire, as if he has drunk the spring's water. He calls it 'moist poyson', but this is only because the woman he desires rejects his advances and is cold towards him. If she were receptive, his heat would be joyful. It is the conflict with her feeling that makes the hot passion a curse that robs him of freedom. Two enchantments have counter-acted each other, since to the speaker it is as if his beloved has drunk from the other well, a source of icy water 'Whose chilling venome of repugnant kind / The fervent heat doth quenche of Cupides wounde' (Howard 1557, 13). The effect of one spring opposes that of the other; together, the two have produced the Petrarchan dramatic situation of thwarted, eloquent love, exquisite and agonised. One elemental force, heat, represents passionate desire. The other, ice, represents the ability to resist unwanted approaches from others and painful longings of one's own. In the poem, the heat and the iciness are properties sometimes to be welcomed and sometimes feared. The speaker seems to regret the triumph of the 'crepyng fire' over the coldness of his limbs. There are circumstances in which coldness is to be valued: the same fire pains his heart that once 'harborde freedom'. In the historical context of this genre, the woman's iciness may be seen either as coyness or chastity and modesty, but present-day readers may value it as the confidence that enables her to refuse. Taken in either context, the poem expresses ambivalence about the power of amorous desire, and relativises the hotness and coldness that might otherwise seem to be simple antagonists.

Shakespeare's Sonnet 153 and Sonnet 154, the last in his sequence and among the most conventional, feature the same motif. Each tells the story of how a maid in the service of Diana, goddess of chastity, stole from beside the sleeping Cupid a brand burning with the fire of love. She plunged the brand into a cool well or fountain, which became instantly a hot spring with healing properties (Shakespeare 1997, 1975–1976). The speaker declares that this well is now famous for its power to cure 'strange maladies' (some scholars interpret this phrase as a reference to sexually transmitted diseases, and identify the bath mentioned in both sonnets with the hot wells in Bath). Nevertheless, the well's water is no remedy for the speaker's love-sickness, and he then surmises that Cupid must have relit the doused brand by exposing it to the lovely eyes of the woman the speaker adores. Her beauty and chastity combined have the power to ignite a loving flame that the enchanted cold water cannot quench. That is his compliment to her, and his way of protesting, perhaps as a renewed entreaty, that though his love is hopeless he has no wish to be cured of it.

2 Biblical Springs and Allegorical Landscapes

In the Bible, springs frequently represent God's provision of nourishment, material and spiritual, to those of faith who find themselves in arid and infertile places, literally and metaphorically. When the children of Israel come to the desert of Zin and protest bitterly to Moses about the lack of food and water (*King James Bible*, *Numbers*, 20, 2–12), God tells Moses that if he gathers the people and, in front of them, speaks to a rock, 'thou shalt bring forth to them water out of the rock'. Moses smites the rock twice: 'and the water came out abundantly'. Later, when they reach Beer, the gift of spring water appears again, this time in response to a song:

'Spring up, O well; sing ye unto it' (*Numbers*, 21, 16–18). In the Book of Isaiah, the prophet tells the children of Israel that after the coming of the Lord, 'with joy shall ye draw water out of the wells of salvation' (*Isaiah*, 12, 3–4). Similarly, in the Book of Joel, God's message is that 'the mountains shall drop down new wine and the hills shall flow with milk, and all the rivers of Judah shall flow with waters, and a fountain shall come forth of the house of the Lord, and shall water the valley of Shittim' (*Joel*, 3, 18). In Christian allegorical landscapes, springs and wells are generally sources of renewal of hope, vision and spiritual strength and purity. The clarity of the newly emerged spring water stands in contrast to confusion and impeded vision. One of the most famous of these landscapes is the country crossed by Christian in Bunyan's Puritan allegory *The Pilgrim's Progress* (1678). In this landscape, springs and wells are a feature of the Delectable Mountains, a place on the way to the Celestial City, and a source of hope, as the first point from which the gates of the City are visible. Places in *The Pilgrim's Progress* have been matched with real sites in Bunyan's home landscape near Bedford (the Delectable Mountains are said to be inspired by the Chiltern Hills). In dialectical relationships like this, between a real place and the traditions of mythical or symbolic meaning that are attached to its landscape-type, the encounter with the real renews and gives flesh to the tradition, while the tradition gives cultural meaning to the real. In turn, that meaning entwines with the personal meaning the place may have for an individual. This continuing exchange adds to the complexities of meaning already present when, for example, a Roman tradition of sacredness has been superimposed on a previous Celtic tradition, as with Sulis Minerva at Bath.

3 Restorative Springs and the Romantic Sublime

Romanticism took up the trope of wells and springs as a source of revitalising power, adapting the classical and biblical traditions. In William Wordsworth's poetry, natural springs and fountains represent the re-emergence in someone's life of feelings of joyful responsiveness to the infinity and complexity of the world. The joy rises up from childhood and youth, as seventy-two-year-old Matthew declares in 'The Fountain', composed in 1798 and published in *Lyrical Ballads* (1800):

> Down to the vale this water steers,
> How merrily it goes!

'Twill murmur on a thousand years,
And flow as now it flows.

And here, on this delightful day,
I cannot chuse but think
How oft, a vigorous Man, I lay
Beside this Fountain's brink.

My eyes are dim with childish tears,
My heart is idly stirred,
For the same sound is in my ears,
Which in those days I heard. (Wordsworth 2004, 67)

Sensations that seem unchanged from childhood bring the past, and Matthew's original, formative vitality, into the present, and at the same time situate his life in relation to the far distant future, practically infinite, into which the water seems to be flowing.

A defining feature of the Romantic natural sublime was that vast landscapes such as mountains, forests or seas, reaching to the horizon and beyond, represented infinite distances of time as well as space. Here are huge prospects, presenting a surface that contains immense local intricacy. Positioned at a distance, the observer knows about this intricacy but cannot see it; the difference of scale is too great. Usually, this observer—often the poet in the persona of dramatic speaker—is gazing from a point of elevation, such as the mountains of Wordsworth's Lake District. Alternatively, they may be at the foot of the mountain, gazing upwards. Figuratively, as well as literally, this protagonist is a small figure set heroically against the immensity of the prospect. Caspar David Friedrich's paintings place this figure in the foreground, representing a triumph that is defiant but frail against the vastness of time and space. Or sometimes, that heroic position is occupied by small upright edifice, such as an arch or a crucifix, weathered or decaying.

These great landscapes represent long-term, far-reaching processes that only have shape from a distance. Close-up, they are too large to see. The protagonist and the reader—or the person who looks at the painting—are alike in that they see the landscapes as if from outside. Yet these landscapes represent processes that we do not stand outside. We are in the midst of them. They produce us continuously. The separateness of that standing figure is a provisional triumph, a necessary dramatic illusion. To cross into the landscape, descending into it from the point of vantage, would be to lose sight of the vast processes. Soon, the complexity of the immediate surroundings would enmesh us, making us unable to see far ahead. Therefore, in the classic pattern of the sublime, the protagonist has to fall back from the brink, retreating from an encounter that has been almost overwhelming to the senses.

This drama of approach and retreat mimics the trajectory of another Romantic desire. One of the great themes of the continuing Romantic tradition is the wish for escape from the alienated self-questioning self-consciousness that modernity is perceived to have brought. What might a return to a natural way of life mean? How far should it go? There is a range of answers. At the far end stands the idea of living by unselfconscious instinct, without concern for the future or doubt about identity, as animals are supposed to live. This is the wholly unalienated condition: the impossible vision that attracts self-conscious Romantic desire. At the 1998 ASLE-UKI conference, philosopher Kate Soper used the striking phrase 'envy of immanence' for this tradition of Romantic yearning. It is a long tradition, very much still alive, and in literature it characteristically produces moments of climactic, arrested poise on the part of a protagonist who has advanced to a brink and can go no further, since to do so would be to cross into a place from which no messages could reach the reader. The desire is for wholeness, health and healing, yet a real, thorough, committed return to an instinctual, unselfconscious natural life is unattainable and would be morally problematical. It is also unimaginable and un-narratable, since the transition into this animal life would require the renunciation of language, a medium that entails self-consciousness and time-consciousness.

Such a return, or sublimation, would therefore be incompatible with the activity of composing or reading poetry. The poems can only achieve visionary, momentary glimpses. Romantic poetry in the genre of the natural sublime is therefore concerned primarily with the heightened emotional intensity that occurs in the moment of yearning contemplation, and with the dramatic build-up, aftermath and consequence. Poetic intensity functions, here, as a diversion of that impossible desire. It offers a consolatory, secondary and fleetingly transcendent resolution, and a way of giving the desire its due expression while preserving a route back to critical distance. This is why, in John Keats's 'Ode to a Nightingale' (1819), the taste of water from an ancient sacred spring is a sensation yearned for, and represented by means of expansive metaphor, rather than something directly experienced or described:

O, for a draught of vintage! that hath been
 Cool'd a long age in the deep-delved earth,
Tasting of Flora and the country green,
 Dance, and Provençal song, and sunburnt mirth!
O for a beaker full of the warm South,
 Full of the true, the blushful Hippocrene,
 With beaded bubbles winking at the brim,
  And purple-stained mouth;
 That I might drink, and leave the world unseen,
 And with thee fade away into the forest dim. (Keats 2007, 193)

With its intense beauty, the nightingale's song provides the sublimity elsewhere found in vast landscapes. The Hippocrene was a Greek spring on Mount Helicon, formed by the hoof-print of Pegasus and infused with the spirit of the Muses. Its water empowers the drinker to compose true poetry. In the dramatic scene set up by the poem, Keats longs for this inspiration, and in expressing the longing he receives the gift of the Muses. The ode is the result: both plea and reward. What prompts him, in the drama, to this achievement is the song of the nightingale, a creature that represents the animal instinctual life that lies out of reach. The nightingale's song is the poet's muse, yet what seems wrong to him about the bird and the song is their confinement in space and time. 'Thou wast not born for death, immortal Bird!' he says. Yet, there is a sense in which the bird, for Keats, is not in the grip of mortality, as humans are. The vision we project onto nonhuman animals is that they do not foresee and lament their own deaths; their unconsciousness of self and time protects them from this transformative knowledge. Keats identifies here a form of immortality belonging not to the individual bird, which will die very soon, but to the species-continuity that keeps the bird's characteristics unchanged across centuries. Because of this continuity, which stands in contrast to human cultural history, the nightingale's present song is the same as the one heard in classical and biblical times. Like the immersion of narratable selfhood into immediate moment, this dissolution of the individual into the continuity of the species is part of the relinquishment that a deep return to nature would involve. Unchanged song is one image for this. A spring enchanted long ago and still flowing is another.

To 'leave the world unseen' and 'fade away into the forest dim' with the nightingale would be to cross over and join the bird in that state of nature. A person who did so fully would begin to live only in the present moment, which, if it were really true, would mean there was no going back. The Keats character longs to be troubled no longer by 'the weariness, the fever and the fret' that human beings endure, and for a few lines he tries to imagine that he has crossed over, drawn by the song and enchanted by the spring. What would it feel like? Immediately, he is trying to do the impossible, paradoxical thing: send back descriptions from this state to the reader, dispatches from the other side.

Darkness is his immediate sensation. He cannot see the flowers that surround him with 'soft incense'. In one kind of Keatsian 'negative capability', the loss of one sense gives an almost transcendent intensity to the others. He is able to catch sensations normally off the human scale, such as the last faint scent of the violets whose season is all but over, and the first faint perfume of the musk rose whose time is about to begin. His nonhuman point of view seems to start with the nightingale and then become a succession of different perspectives, taking him down among the leaves that cover the fading violets, and into the open rose among murmuring flies. The nightingale could not enter these places, and, though each moment brings great intensity, the poet's power of ranging movement also signals the impossibility of what he desires, and the unwillingness of his imagination to be constrained by any particular point of view in time and space. Even as he achieves these almost overwhelming intimacies, it is clear that the work is being done by his imagination, however muse-inspired. He remembers the seasons of the different flowers; that is how he puts names to their scents. At the heart of the moment, he casts outside it, and thus is already withdrawing. He has attempted to scale down rather than up, but like the protagonist on the high vantage-point, he is unable to go further and has to retrace his steps. Minutes later, the nightingale's song is no longer so close. It fades:

> Past the near meadows, over the still stream,
> Up the hill-side; and now 'tis buried deep
> In the next valley-glades. (Keats 2007, 194)

Whether the bird has flown or the speaker walked on is not clear, but the description of the route suggests the latter. Removed now from the intensity of the experience, the Keats character cannot say whether it really happened or occurred in dream. In admitting this, he makes another absolute separation of the two worlds.

That emphasis on separation—on the isolation, exquisiteness and precariousness of the moment, compared to the continuity of ordinary life—gives this version of Romantic sublime, or pastoral enchantment, a tone that is near to tragedy. The Keats character identifies his longing to join the nightingale with a dangerous wistfulness for death. In contrast, the version in Wordsworth's 'The Fountain' is much gentler. Matthew is relaxed beside the spring, and able to visit it easily. The dramatic, reflective moment conjured by the poem's narrative is profound, but not so exalted as to hold out the prospect of a form of experience incompatible with the continuation of ordinary life and selfhood. Instead, the spring, with its unchanged sound, gives Matthew a sense of contact with his early childhood and the future beyond his lifespan, and so enables him to situate his life in longer processes of time. The shift of scale, from that of a single life to longer perspectives, is there, but does not demand an impossible choice.

Wordsworth's more famous poem 'Lines Written a Few Miles above Tintern Abbey On Revisiting the Banks of the Wye During a Tour, July 13, 1798' presents similar circumstances, except that here the protagonist is the poet in persona rather than a character such as Matthew. Flowing water again prompts memories and represents them symbolically, while remaining present as real, particular water. Looking down from a natural height onto the river, the speaker reflects on the water's sources:

> again I hear
> These waters, rolling from their mountain-springs
> With a sweet inland murmur. (Wordsworth 2004, 61)

For this Wordsworth character, the continuing flow of the waters recalls not only his childhood but moments since, when 'in lonely rooms, and mid the din / Of towns and cities', he has remembered the natural landscapes he knows:

> I have owed to them,
> In hours of weariness sensations sweet,
> Felt in the blood and felt along the heart,
> And passing even into my purer mind
> With tranquil restoration. (Wordsworth 2004, 62)

The movement of water—its passage underground, emergence in springs and confluence in rivers—resembles to him the way his blood flows, sustaining his physical body. It also resembles the surfacing and flow of restorative thoughts and feelings (we can also see these connections in Keats's use of the adjective 'blushful' for the Hippocrene: blood and long-lost emotion come to the surface). These resemblances serve to place the Wordsworth character's physical and emotional life, conscious and unconscious, back into the larger and longer natural and temporal processes of which he has lost sight and in which he has lost confidence, alienated from nature by his adult and urban experiences. The river and its sources emerging from underground become metaphorical without ceasing to be present as physical realities. That reconciliation between the literal and metaphorical assists the other reconciliations the poem makes.

4 J. H. Prynne: Taking Knowledge 'Back to the Springs'

Passages from Wordsworth, including this one, are a returning reference-point in the work of the modernist poet J. H. Prynne, whose poetry, especially that of the late 1960s, shows us some of the recent life of the trope of springs and wells. My account of the 'Tintern Abbey' lines above owes much to his Cambridge lectures and his 2010 essay 'Mental Ears and Poetic Work', in which he reads these lines and others for their interplay between soft and hard endings of words. Prynne's 1968 poem 'Die A Millionaire (pronounced 'diamonds in the air')' begins with: 'The first essential is to take knowledge / Back to the springs' (Prynne 2015, 13). What springs are these? Prynne's work at this time brought together several complementary visions of the possibility of finding revitalisation through renewed contact with distant origins seen as reserves of value and energy. These origins are hidden, but they are springs that still flow and have never stopped flowing. One such origin can be approached by means of the history of certain words. Prynne's intricate and revealing account of poetic composition and reading in 'Mental Ears and Poetic Work' proceeds at one point, for example, by means of the uncovering of a buried history in the word 'blessed', as used in 'Tintern Abbey':

> 'blessed' locates the endowment of benefit in the past tense of 'bless'. This in turn traces a formal link with 'blood' and 'bleed', as deriving from ME *blessen*, OE *bletsian*, *bloedsian*, all linked through the sense-development of 'to make sacred or holy by ritual shedding of blood. (Prynne, 2010, 136)

It is not so much that older meanings should return to displace current ones, as that when we consider the old and the new together, and the historical line between them, the activity generates critical, dialectical processes. Punning in general has this potential. An example in 'Die a Millionaire' is the word 'purchase', used emphatically four times so that it becomes a returning note that the poem finds repeatedly. In the poem's argument, the organisation of desire in consumer capitalism is imagined as a grid pattern, compared to the grids on maps and graphs, and to the national 'grid' that stores and releases electricity. The example that takes us from spring to river to grid is hydroelectric power, the form of power-storage cited by Heidegger in his challenge to the industrial concept of 'standing reserve'. *Grid*, as an organisational structure, thus appears in oppositional contrast to *flow*, including the flow of linguistic history that the poem seeks to release:

Otherwise it's
purchase, of a natural course, the alteration
or storage of current like dams in the
river: what starts as irrigation ends up
selling the megawattage across the grid. (Prynne 2015, 14)

The British imperialist acquisition of the Suez Canal was technically a purchase. Prynne moves from this instance ('merely/a blatant example') to a double sense of that word. Purchase is the taking of water into commercial possession, and also the way in which the dam uses the water's resistance and weight to gain purchase on the water and thus maintain control. This double sense—purchase as buying and purchase as gripping—persists through the poem, until we find the spring water now fully contained and available for purchase: 'the water of life/is all in bottles & ready for invoice' (Prynne 2015, 15). Faced with such commodification, what alternative flow from a point of origin can we find?

A poem published a year later, 'The Wound, Day and Night' (1968), proposes a geological answer. After a reference to argon dating, a method of aging rocks by analysing the products of radioactive decay, the poem refers immediately to 'song as echo of the world' (Prynne 2015, 64). Like a stream from a spring, this song 'runs sweetly by' (Prynne 2015, 64). It seems likely that 'echo of the world' refers, among other things, to the continuing thermal radiation from the Big Bang 13.8 billion years ago, known as Cosmic Microwave Background. American radio astronomers discovered the phenomenon in 1964. If we identify this CMB reverberation, detectable only by means of highly specialised technology, with the poetic lyricism to which Prynne aspires, or with Wordsworthian lyric intimations of long continuity, we will abruptly bring together two durations or scales so extremely contrasting as to be barely commensurable. What happens when they touch? It is an early example of a gesture that recurs in Prynne's work throughout his career. Something unmanageably large from one point of view is far too small from another. A tiny moment expands until its horizons are out of sight, while the whole life to date of the earth contracts to a flash, a twinkling or single musical note. *Down Where Changed* (1979) has 'Nearly too much/is, well, nowhere near enough' (Prynne 2015, 307). Note the word 'well' here. *The Oval Window* (1983) has 'Less won't do,/more isn't on either' (Prynne 2015, 317). Sometimes the device seems intransigent, signalling hopeless or sardonic incompatibility, but sometimes the act of combining the two scales in one phrase or poetic line holds out a rare possibility of overlap, in which each scale encompasses and gives recognition to the other. A non-poetical example of this overlap comes in the format of the critical commentaries Prynne has recently published on three short lyric poems by Shakespeare, William Wordsworth and George Herbert. Prynne reads these poems word by word and line by line, giving each word and phrase an extensive analysis that takes in its history and surveys the range of meanings and implications. Sometimes he gives a single word several pages. The method is an extreme version of 'close reading', so close that one can get lost in the localities, which become worlds of infinite implication (as in the encounter with sublime landscape described above). A deep reading like this could in principle continue indefinitely, but, at the end of the book, a folded page opens to show the whole poem. If that page is kept open, it sits alongside every other. Deep, slow reading and the unbroken lyrical experience of the whole poem contain each other. The eye moves between the two.

Alex Latter, in his study of the journal *The English Intelligencer*, set up by Prynne and others in the mid-1960s, identifies 'The Wound, Day and Night' as also a poetic response to another scientific discovery, one that coincided more or less exactly with the work's composition. Research on the Continental Drift indicated with increasing certainty 'that Europe and the Americas had once formed a single landmass'. Two lines in the poem seem to refer explicitly to this view: 'I am born back there, the plaintive chanting / under the Atlantic and the unison of forms' (Prynne 2015,

64). The discovery, Latter observes, confirmed 'Prynne's sense of trans-Atlantic brotherhood' (Latter 2017, 66) with Charles Olson, Edward Dorn and the Black Mountain poets. For Prynne, the geological discovery provided a physical historical correlative, of immense temporal and spatial proportions, to a shared transatlantic effort to reinvigorate Modernism and find renewed contact with that movement's springs. Latter argues that the break-up of the journal in 1968 marked a shift in Prynne's aspirations: a movement towards a more exacting perception of ways in which lyricism might be justified—a perception connected to the rare overlap described above. An earlier poem from 1968, 'If There is a Stationmaster at Stamford S.D. Hardly So', had used the phrase 'deep wells / of the spirit' (Prynne 2015, 45) so as to set the reader a dilemma. How can we choose between the idealistic meaning, in the tradition I have partly described, and an industrial-military meaning of 'wells' and 'spirit' suggested by references earlier in the poem to 'essential oils' and Vietnam? Each challenges the other, and the first meaning flickers between lyrical confidence and irony. By 1983, in *The Oval Window*, a line from the biblical song in Numbers appears surrounded by jargon from the financial markets, itself highly metaphorical and full of puns waiting to be activated:

> Spring up, O well; sing unto it: but
> the answer is a pool of values in prime
> hock to a pump and its trade-offs. (Prynne 2015, 321)

The 'values' here are stock market values in continual fluctuation, and the pump gives us the oil-based economy. As well as the biblical tone in these lines, I hear a resigned and laconic 'Oh well'.

'If There is a Stationmaster at Stamford S.D. Hardly So' ends with a vision of fluid release and melting that can be taken ambiguously. The statement that 'the icecap will/never melt/again' is followed by an enigmatic 'why/ should it' (Prynne 2015, 46). Do we read this as a reassuring 'why should it?', meaning that there is no reason to fear that the icecap will melt? Or do we attach more force to the line-break? If we do, perhaps there are two questions making a challenge: 'Why? *Should* it?' This must be why there is no question mark. The poem asks us to position the mark, or position more than one, and how we make, or ponder, this decision now will surely differ from what might have happened in 1968, for now there is much evidence that the real icecaps are indeed melting, a circumstance that shifts the balance in ideas of melt and flow from promise to threat. So, what uses can writers concerned with ecological dangers make of the tradition I have outlined, and what are the meanings that ecocritics – literary and cultural critics who prioritise environmental values – might attribute to springs, wells and depths?

5 Ecocriticism and the Meaning of Watery Depths

Ecocriticism asks readers to take an ecological view, which means that urgent, prioritising attention must be given to the interdependency of the different life-forms and other components in each local ecosystem, and in the global system or biosphere. In the broad ecocritical community there are differences of focus and priority. Topics include nature writing and the place of nature in popular and literary culture, environmental justice, ecofeminism, ecocriticism as a postcolonial and decolonising project, and, recently, 'new materialism' and associated fields such as biosemiotics. Sometimes these different ecocritical movements are seen as successive waves, and it is true that some emerged earlier than others, and that at any given moment some will be more influential and widely followed than others, but there isn't simply a wavelike pattern of succession. All of these approaches remain current. They still interact with each other.

When we come to the question of what springs, wells and underground or underwater depths might now mean, suggest and symbolise in literature, in the context of ecological crisis, what comes to the fore is the need to recognise the pervasiveness of interdependency, and therefore to move between different scales of perception. All the approaches I have mentioned share this need. The ecocritic Timothy Clark has identified 'scale derangements' as an important reason why ecological threats generally, and global warming in particular, defy representation, require new literary genres and forms, and challenge what Clark calls 'the foundational assumption of liberal thought'—the idea that 'a human being is an essentially private, atomistic and apolitical individual' (Clark 2015, 103).

A change, at least of emphasis, is required. Several recent movements in cultural theory converge on the perception that instead of thinking in terms of entities with hard boundaries, we should shift our attention to relationships of interdependency and mutual shaping. These relationships are a continuing flow. In the Heideggerean phrase, they are 'always already' taking place. Instead of the relatively hard-boundaried entities to which we are accustomed—individuals, species, societies, ecosystems, culture, nature—we see co-evolution, energy flow, symbiosis, hybridity, assemblages, actor-networks, culturenature and post-humanism. All of these terms refer to the continuous mutual constitution of entities, and their collective constitution of the world. Timothy Morton calls this perception 'the ecological thought' and refers to 'the mesh' and to 'hyperobjects'. Karen Barad, the theoretical physicist and cultural theorist, proposes the term 'intra-action' as a replacement for 'inter-action' (Alaimo and Hekman 2008, 133), since the latter term assumes two entities already relatively fixed in form. Ecocritic Hannes Bergthaller summarises the project of new materialism as:

> a redescription of the world that dissolves the singular figure of the human subject, distinguished by unique properties (soul, reason, mind, free will or intentionality), into the dense web of material relations in which all things are enmeshed. (Bergthaller 2014; Iovino and Oppermann 2015, 37)

Stacy Alaimo uses the term 'trans-corporeality' to refer to 'the material interchanges across human bodies, animal bodies, and the wider material world' (Alaimo 2016, 112). Combined with cultural, scientific, political and economic networks, these continuous interchanges constitute 'a swirling landscape of uncertainty' from which the individual self 'cannot be disentangled'. Alaimo is a leading theorist and critic in 'the blue humanities', the field of ecocriticism concerned with oceans and marine life, taken both as specific study and exemplar. 'Hydrofeminist' Astrida Neimanis extends this approach to water in general, with a strong emphasis on fluid elements of the human body, and on aquatic evolutionary origins. An important term in Neimanis's thought is 'gestationality', which she uses to shift the emphasis in descriptions of selfhood from identities already formed to those in the process of becoming (Chen et al. 2013; Neimanis 2017).

These approaches ask for depth of perception in several directions: physical depth, depth of time and origin, depth of complexity. Another term signalling this is 'Chthulucene', proposed by Donna J. Haraway as an alternative or desired successor to 'Anthropocene', the name in wide use currently for the period in which collective human activity has become a major forcing agent in global ecological systems such as climate and geological deposition. Haraway finds the term problematical because of its attribution of responsibility to a general personified humanity, rather than to those with economic and political power. 'Capitalocene' and 'Plantationocene' are substitutes Haraway offers, but she also argues that the period to which these three names apply should be kept as short or thin as possible (Haraway 2016, 100). Our collective endeavour should be to move as soon as possible into an epoch in which the biosphere is widely perceived as the product of multi-species partnerships or kinships. Haraway says that 'we need a name for the dynamic ongoing symchthonic forces and powers of which people are a part, within which ongoingness is at stake' (Haraway 2016, 101). Such a name will look back into origins and forward into consequences; it does not simply enclose one period. 'Chthulucene' comes from 'chthonic', meaning 'of the underworld' or 'of the deep earth'. The word's Greek origins connect it with underworld gods, and it is sometimes used for forces or spirits emerging from deep underground and from deep in the past. For Haraway, the term 'Chthulucene' 'names earthwide tentacular powers and forces'. It points us towards entangled 'myriad temporalities and spatialities and myriad intra-active entities-in-assemblages – including the more-than-human, other-than-human, inhuman and human-as-humus' (Haraway 2016, 101).

In the context of these ideas, the potential significance of springs and wells is that they carry things from the depths to the surface, and thus reveal parts of the system normally invisible, far removed and mysterious. Traditionally, the sacred springs that gods had enchanted were portals between worlds. They might carry traces of the gods' world, the underworld, the paradise lost or the mysterious deep past. Now, in the ecocritical frame I describe above, such springs may be portals between different parts of our one biosphere, bringing us evidence that the invisible depths are none the less parts of the system. I will conclude by looking briefly at two recent literary texts that seek to explore this sense of connection, and might therefore be called Chthulucene writing.

Jean Sprackland's non-fiction work *Strands* (2012) describes a series of objects that she encountered while taking recreational walks on Ainsdale Sands, a beach near Liverpool. There is a mixture here of domestic, familiar space and potential sublimity. A beach like this is a popular place of holiday relaxation. It is also the threshold of an immense and mysterious alien world that we must understand as part of our own. Each of Sprackland's chapters is about a different item that the tide or the people have left on this beach. Some are underworld creatures, such as an apparently fur-covered burrowing worm called a sea-mouse. An uncanny trace from the far distant past appears in the form of Neolithic footprints, animal and human, exposed by the retreating tide that takes with it a layer of mud-surface. Other objects are familiar, but their appearance here makes them strange and opens up distances. In one chapter, Sprackland attempts an inventory of the items of plastic litter she finds on a single walk. This is part of it:

> Petrol can–1
> Drinks carton–2
> Sanitary towel wrapper–13
> Sweet wrapper–39
> Chocolate bar wrapper–49
> Toy dinosaur–1
> Rope–2
> Crisp packet–4
> Bart Simpson stencil–1
> Ice-lolly wrapper–7
> (Sprackland 2012, 111)

Timothy Clark sees derangements of scale as one of the most challenging features of the ecological crisis. His list includes the disruption of our sense of distance, spatial and temporal. What is far away, and what is close? He also points to a loss of clarity about what is important and what is trivial. These derangements are present on Sprackland's beach. Some of the objects she finds have a touching innocence. They are small; they belong to the inconsequential tasks of an ordinary day. Many are childish. How could they do harm? Yet they are filling the world. The disparity reveals a gap between the small-scale world of daily tasks that we barely consider, and the large-scale world of cumulative ecological consequences. A scale that is too small flips instantly into one that is too large, and then back again. The toy dinosaur gives us this flip in a single object. We are with Sprackland on a short walk close to her home; then we are carried, abruptly, out to the Great Pacific Garbage Patch, said to be twice the size of Texas. The same effect happens with time. Plastic, it seems, is astonishingly new:

> Can we even imagine a world without plastic? What was life like before it so thoroughly colonised our homes, offices, vehicles, streets, shops, gardens and parks? Its success story has been so phenomenal that it's hard to say

> what we would be without it. But our grandparents would know. We've only been mass-producing plastic since the 1930s: there was a time within living memory when plastic was a rare sight, and a novelty. (Sprackland 2012, 106–107)

A lifetime, so short when compared to geological or evolutionary epochs, expands suddenly to contain such a transformation. The world as it was when that lifetime began seems impossibly close yet impossibly distant. Similarly, the footprints that have lain hidden, keeping their shape, for 5,000 years will be destroyed when the tide returns a few hours after their exposure. Nearly too much turns at once into nowhere near enough. Sprackland's book reaches out across great distances of space and time, but contains these distances in the space of the story of a short walk, an interlude in the ordinary business of her life. The separateness of these perspectives is a cause of our environmental inaction.

Another separation of worlds, extreme, tragic and irrevocable, marks J. M. Ledgard's novel *Submergence* (2011). Two lovers, James and Danielle, disappear from each other into invisible folds of the earth. James is a British intelligence agent posing as an expert on water supply in Kenya. Jihadi militia men snatch him, transport him away in a shark-fishing boat and keep him prisoner in a series of secret camps in the 'badlands' of Somalia. At one point they force him to wade into the sea, pretending that they will execute him there. Danielle is a marine biologist studying deep-sea microbial life. Her work takes her down into deep ocean trenches. The book cuts repeatedly between these two locations, with their different forms of terrifying depth. After holding out hope of a conventional plot-denouement, in which some form of rescue or resolution will re-unite the two lovers and unite their different deep enclaves in some larger picture of the world, the novel allows this hope to fade slowly. James's story becomes a matter of stasis, of endless waiting. Danielle's becomes a descent into uninhabitable places; she can penetrate their darkness and strangeness, but has no knowledge of James's whereabouts or the true nature of his work. Implicit, throughout, is a sense of the narrator's desire to bring the two characters, places and different forms of knowledge together by finding a vantage-point from which they can be seen as parts of a single system. Tantalisingly, there are moments that seem to reveal such a wholeness, but they are trivial, and their effect is merely uncanny: on the wall of one of the rooms in which James is interrogated there is a poster of Thierry Henry playing for Arsenal (Ledgard 2011, 50). Or the connections are confined to personal memory, and coincidences in the two characters' histories. James's family ancestors were whalers, and at one point in his captivity he recalls the story of one of these forebears who survived being swallowed by a whale and lying in its stomach a day and a night (Ledgard 2011, 30). Perhaps at the moment when James remembers this story, Danielle, enclosed in her small submersible deep in the ocean, imagines a whale:

> The ocean was hungry. It was a mouth and a grave.
>
> A beaked whale has a heart attack in the Ligurian sea and dies. It sinks and its head is mashed on the sides of an underground canyon. Immediately its cheeks are flushed with bacteria. There are worms, spider crabs, and all manner of creatures feeding on a single vertebra. [...] That life can't be destroyed, it feeds on death – or less than death – it reconfigures and goes further in, into hotter water. (Ledgard 2011, 178–179)

Wholeness recedes as a possibility. The novel becomes, in structure, more like a poem, holding two worlds apart, as images, with space between them, each conditioning the way we receive the other. Near the book's end, a passage occurs that is not obviously from the viewpoint of either character. It is the external narrator's comment, or it could come from either or, just possibly, both:

> You will be in Hades, the staying place of the spirits of the dead. You will be drowned in oblivion, the river Lethe, swallowing water to erase all memory. It will not be the nourishing womb you began your life in. It will be a submergence. You will take your place in the boiling-hot fissures, among the teeming hordes of nameless microorganisms that mimic no forms, because they are the foundation of all forms. (Ledgard 2011, 180)

Dissolution into the deep digestive processes of the biosphere seems to be the only reunion likely to happen, and the only view that a vantage-point, authorial or scientific, currently offers. This is the warning that comes from the depths in this novel.

A paradox, in the ecocritical schools of thought that I have been discussing, is that the need to acknowledge and take account of myriad forms of interdependency leads both to a sense of the sublime and to a much more deeply knowable world. Would such a world necessarily be one without the mystery of inaccessible places? I try to capture this paradox in my title: the world is becoming both deeper and shallower.

In 2017, a photograph circulated on the Internet of a tin of spam—a popular processed pork product that often features in British jokes—lying at a depth of 4,947 metres in the Mariana trench in the Pacific, described as the deepest place in the world. Dropped by a ship, the spam rests on grey dust that also looks familiar, as if the place is not really the deep sea-floor but the floor of a neglected attic or garage. This picture, a fine example of the ecological uncanny, gives us, again, Clark's derangements of scale. Is it far or close, trivial or important, familiar or strange? We need both sides of each opposition. Neither can cancel the other.

Works Cited

Primary Sources

Howard, Henry, Earl of Surrey. 2011. Complaint of the Lover Disdained (1557). In *Tottel's Miscellany: Songs and Sonnets of Henry Howard, Earl of Surrey, Sir Thomas Wyatt and Others*, ed. Tom MacFaul and Amanda Holton. London: Penguin Classics.

Keats, John. 2007. Ode to a Nightingale (1819). In *John Keats: Selected Poems*, ed. John Barnard. London: Penguin Classics.

Ledgard, J.M. 2011. *Submergence*. London: Jonathan Cape.

Prynne, J.H. 2015. *Poems*. Hexham: Bloodaxe Books.

Shakespeare, William. 1997. Sonnet 153 and Sonnet 154. In *The Norton Shakespeare*, ed. Stephen Greenblatt, Walter Cohen, Jean Howard, and Katharine Eisaman Maus. New York: W. W. Norton.

Sprackland, Jean. 2012. *Strands: A Year of Discoveries on the Beach*. London: Jonathan Cape.

Wordsworth, William. 2004. *Selected Poems*. London: Penguin Books.

Secondary Sources

Alaimo, Stacy. 2016. *Exposed: Environmental Politics and Pleasures in Posthuman Times*. Minneapolis: University of Minnesota Press.

Barad, Karen. 2008. Posthuman Performativity: Towards an Understanding of How Matter Comes to Matter. In *Material Feminisms*, ed. Stacy Alaimo and Susan Hekman. Bloomington: Indiana University Press.

Bergthaller, Hannes. 2014. Limits of Agency: Notes on the Material Turn from a Systems-Theoretical Perspective. In *Material Ecocriticism*, ed. Serenella Iovino and Serpil Oppermann. Bloomington: Indiana University Press.

Chen, Cecilia, Janine MacLeod, and Astrida Neimanis, eds. 2013. *Thinking with Water*. Montreal: McGill-Queen's University Press.

Clark, Timothy. 2015. *Ecocriticism on the Edge: The Anthropocene as a Threshold Concept*. London: Bloomsbury Academic.
Haraway, Donna J. 2016. *Staying with the Trouble: Making Kin in the Chthulucene*. Durham: Duke University Press.
Iovino, Serenella, and Serpil Oppermann. 2015. *Material Ecocriticism*. Bloomington: Indiana University Press.
Latter, Alex. 2017. *Late Modernism and the English Intelligencer*. London: Bloomsbury.
Neimanis, Astrida. 2017. *Bodies of Water*. London: Bloomsbury Academic.
Prynne, J. H. 2010. Mental Ears and Poetic Work. *Chicago Review* 55 (1) (Winter): 126 157.

Index

S. Chiari and S. Cuisinier-Delorme (eds.), *Spa Culture and Literature in England, 1500–1800*, Early Modern Literature in History,
https://doi.org/10.1007/978-3-030-66568-5

T

The manufacturer's authorised representative in the EU is Springer Nature Customer Service Centre GmbH, Europaplatz 3, 69115 Heidelberg, Germany. If you have any concerns regarding our products, please contact ProductSafety@springernature.com

Printed and bound by CPI Group (UK) Ltd, Croydon, CR0 4YY

30/09/2026

02225700-0007